AF477201

Intellectual Property Rights in Pharmaceutical Industry: Theory and Practice

(Appended with Validation, Audits, National Phase Entry and Prosecutions)

Second Edition

Intellectual Property Rights in Pharmaceutical Industry: Theory and Practice

(Appended with Validation, Audits, National Phase Entry and Prosecutions)

Second Edition

Dr. Bayya Subba Rao

M. Pharm, FAGE (MAN), P.G. Diploma
in Patent Laws (NALSAR), IAO, Ph.D

Professor (Formerly – Patent Analyst at
IPR & Regulatory Centre, Pharmexcil, Hyderabad).

Dr. P.V. Appaji

M. Pharm, Ph.D

Director General, Pharmexcil, Hyderabad.

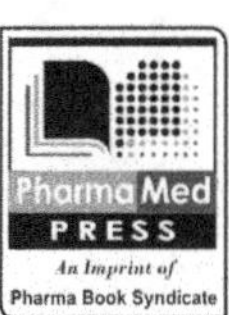

PharmaMed Press

An imprint of Pharma Book Syndicate

A Unit of BSP Books Pvt. Ltd.
4-4-309/316, Giriraj Lane,
Sultan Bazar, Hyderabad - 500 095.

Intellectual Property Rights in Pharmaceutical Industry: Theory and Practice
by Dr. Bayya Subba Rao and Dr. P.V. Appaji

© 2018, 2015, *by Publisher,* All rights reserved.

Second Edition 2018
First Edition 2015

Published by

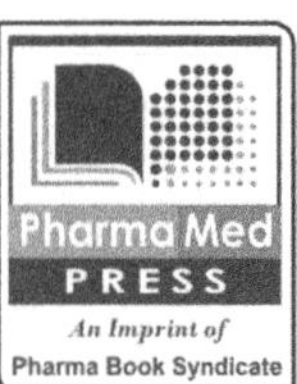

PharmaMed Press
An imprint of Pharma Book Syndicate

A unit of BSP Books Pvt. Ltd.
4-4-309/316, Giriraj Lane, Sultan Bazar, Hyderabad - 500 095.
Phone: 040-23445688, 23445600; Fax: 91+40-23445611
e-mail: info@pharmamedpress.com
www.pharmamedpress.com/pharmamedpress.net

ISBN: 978-93-87593-38-1 (Hardback)

Message

I am happy to know that Dr. Bayya Subba Rao and Dr. P.V. Appaji have authored a book on "Intellectual Property Rights in Pharmaceutical Industry: Theory and Practice, Second Edition" which is mainly aimed at academic and pharmaceutical industry for the benefit of students, teachers, researchers, scientists, regulators and policy makers.

I wish the authors and their proposed book all success.

Dr. Gopakumar G. Nair
Gopakumar Nair Associates

Preface to Second Edition

Intellectual property rights and their protection have gained importance in the last one and a half decade after India signing the World Trade Organisation agreement and obliging to fulfill the Trade Related Aspects of Intellectual Property Rights agreement.

During the transition period, Indian government has taken necessary steps in vesting new intellectual property legislations and upgrading already existing legislations. Simultaneously, Indian government has built up necessary infrastructure in modernizing intellectual property offices, availability of applications and grants of various intellectual properties to public by providing free access to databases online. Introduction of product patent system and national treatment of internationals to fulfill reciprocity has imparted more challenges in the field of pharmaceuticals.

Having realized the importance of intellectual property protections, several Indian universities have introduced topics relating to intellectual property rights in the academic curriculum especially in the field of pharmaceuticals.

We personally realized the importance of intellectual property rights and their protection. However, exclusive books on intellectual property rights emphasizing on pharmaceuticals is rarely observed.

The need of a book on intellectual property rights relating to pharmaceuticals is realized and the information provided was tuned exclusively for pharmaceuticals. The book provides the basic understanding of the concepts with more emphasis on Indian patent system so that, pharmaceutical fraternity that includes students, scientists, teachers, regulators and policy makers in better understanding the intellectual property protection system and its need.

Several times legislation is framed or amended after court's judgment of a case. Several times a better understanding of the legislation is possible with reading the details of a case. An attempt is made by providing as examples as annexure.

The book titled Intellectual Property Rights in Pharmaceutical Industry: Theory and Practice, Second Edition is expected to impart the fundamentals especially at the   B. Pharm, Pharm D, M. Pharm, and Ph. D levels along with other science educational programs in all the Universities of India and working science professionals, industry in understanding the concepts, finally leading to an orientation of research development that ensure intellectual property protection.

The book is an outcome of interpretation of the 'Bare Act' especially The Patents Act, 1970 concentrating relating to pharmaceuticals with inclusion of related judgments made at US, Indian courts, etc.

Propagation of knowledge resources is expected to be the growth of the pharmacy profession and we hope fruitful information is gained after reading the book. We look forward from the student, teacher, industry, regulatory and scientist community providing their valuable comments and suggestions.

Dr. Bayya Subba Rao

Dr. P.V. Appaji

Acknowledgements

We take the opportunity in thanking the almighty, parents, teachers and family members. Our special thanks to Committee of Administration, Pharmexcil and Government of India for all the opportunities and strengths.

Dr. Bayya Subba Rao
Dr. P.V. Appaji

CONTENTS

Message ....(v)

Preface to Second Edition .... (vii)

Acknowledgements...(ix)

CHAPTER 1

Introduction and History of Intellectual Property Rights 1

1.1 Introduction 1

1.2 History of Intellectual Property Rights.................................... 1

1.3 Classification of Intellectual Property Rights............................ 3

CHAPTER 2

International Agreements, Treaties and Conventions............ 6

A. Intellectual Property Protection **8**

2.1 Paris Convention (1883)... 8

2.2 Berne Convention (1886) 9

2.3 Madrid Agreement (1891) 9

2.4 Trademarks Law Treaty (1994).. 9

2.5 WIPO Copyrights Treaty-WCT (1996)...................................... 10

2.6 Patent Law Treaty (2000) 10

2.7 Singapore Treaty (2006) 11

B. Global Protection System **11**

2.8 Hague Agreement (1925) 11

2.9 Lisbon Agreement (1958)... 12

2.10 Patent Co-operation Treaty (1970)....................................... 12

2.11 Budapest Treaty (1977) 13

2.12 Madrid Agreement and Protocol (1989).................................... 14

C. Classifications... **15**

2.13 Nice Agreement (1957)... 15

2.14 Locarno Agreement (1968) 15

2.15 Strasbourg Agreement (1971) 15

2.16 Vienna Agreement (1973) 16

CHAPTER 3

Introduction to Different Components of Intellectual Property Rights 17

    3.1 Industrial Property Rights 17

        3.1.1 Patents 17

        3.1.2 Trademarks 17

        3.1.3 Trade Secrets 18

        3.1.4 Geographical Indications 19

        3.1.5 Designs 19

        3.1.6 Integrated Circuits 20

        3.1.7 Plant Varieties 20

    3.2 Copyrights 21

CHAPTER 4

Introduction to Traditional Knowledge and Biological Diversity 22

    4.1 Traditional Knowledge 22

    4.2 Biological Diversity 23

CHAPTER 5

Introduction to WTO Agreement 24

    5.1 Origin, Objective and Role of GATT 24

    5.2 Origin, Objective and Role of WTO 24

CHAPTER 6

Trade Related Aspects of Intellectual Property Rights Agreement 26

CHAPTER 7

The Patents Act, 1970 31

    7.1 Inventions not Patentable 31

    7.2 Patentable Subject Matter 32

        7.2.1 Novelty 33

        7.2.2 Non-Obviousness 33

7.2.3 Use-Full 33

7.2.4 Enable 33

7.3 Contents of a Patent 34

7.3.1 Title 34

7.3.2 Abstract 34

7.3.3 Field of Invention 34

7.3.4 Prior Art 34

7.3.5 Summary of the Invention 35

7.3.6 Figures/Drawings/Chemical Structures/Tables 35

7.3.7 Detailed Description of the Invention/Embodiments 36

7.3.8 Claims 36

7.4 Types of Patent Applications 39

7.4.1 Provisional Application 39

7.4.2 Complete Application 40

7.4.3 Patent of Addition 40

7.4.4 Divisional Application 41

7.4.5 Convention Application 41

7.4.6 PCT Application 41

7.5 Rights of Inventor/Patentee 41

7.6 Term, Grant of Patent 42

7.7 Infringement 43

7.7.1 Direct Infringement 43

7.7.2 Doctrine of Equivalence 44

7.7.3 Prosecution History Estoppel 44

7.8 Time Line of Indian Patent Office Procedure 45

7.9 Compulsory Licensing 47

7.10 Oppositions 48

7.11 Powers of Controller of Patents 48

7.12 Patent Agents 50

7.13 International Arrangement 50

7.14 Penalties 51

CHAPTER 8

Surrender, Revocation, Lapse, Restoration of Patent and Register of Patent.................53

8.1 Surrender of Patent 53

8.2 Revocation.. 53

8.3 Lapse and Restoration 54

8.4 Register of Patents... 54

CHAPTER 9

Expenditure for Application, Follow Patent Office Procedure, Grant of a Patent..........55

CHAPTER 10

Application Procedure and Time Line for Grant of Patent through PCT 56

CHAPTER 11

Non-Patented and Patented Literature Search 58

11.1 International Patent Classification........................... 59

11.2 Date of Expiry of a Patent 59

11.3 Title 59

11.4 Abstract 59

11.5 Claims... 59

11.6 Text of the Patent... 60

11.7 Name of Patentee... 60

CHAPTER 12

Comparison of the Principal The Patents Act, 1970 with The Three Amendments (1999, 2002, 2005)..........61

12.1 The Patents Act, 1970 (The Principal Act)............... 61

12.2 Patents (First Amendment) Act, 1999 Dt. 26-3-1999 w.e.f 1-1-1995 62

12.3 Patents (Second Amendment) Act, 2002 Dt. 20-5-2003
w.e.f 20-5-2003 62

    12.3.1 Patentable Inventions.................................... 62

    12.3.2 Not Inventions 62

    12.3.3 Term of Patent 62

    12.3.4 Application Requirements 62

    12.3.5 Compulsory Licence.................................. 63

    12.3.6 Right to Import and Parallel Imports 63

    12.3.7 Bolar Provision.. 63

    12.3.8 Burden of Proof 63

    12.3.9 Provision for Traditional Knowledge and
           Biological Diversity... 63

12.4 The Patents (Amendment) Ordinance, 2004 63

CHAPTER 13

Differences in The Patents Act, 1970 with other Countries

**Differences in The Patents Act, 1970
with other Countries** **65**

CHAPTER 14

Administrative Structure of WTO, Membership and Dispute Settlement as per TRIPS Agreement

**Administrative Structure of WTO, Membership and
Dispute Settlement as per TRIPS Agreement** **66**

14.1 Administrative Structure of WTO 66

14.2 Membership... 68

14.3 Dispute Settlement.. 68

14.4 Issues 69

    14.4.1 Anti-Dumping... 69

           14.4.1.1 Issue of India with South Africa................. 70

           14.4.1.2 Issue of Chinese Taipei (customs territory
                    of Taiwan, Penghu, Kinmen and Matsu)
                    with India 70

    14.4.2 Hindrance of Import of Pharmaceutical Products.......... 71

           14.4.2.1 Issue of India with Argentina 71

    14.4.3 Transit issue of Pharmaceutical Products 71

           14.4.3.1 Issue of India with European
                    Union and the Netherlands 71

14.4.4 Implementation of Patent/Intellectual
Property System.. 72

14.4.4.1 Issue of United States and
European Communities with India 72

14.4.4.2 Issue of European Community with
Canada and India as Third Party 73

14.4.4.3 Issue of United States with Brazil and
India as a Third Party 73

14.5 Representation of Indian Government to
EU Over the Transit/Border Issue 74

CHAPTER 15

Technology Transfer **75**

CHAPTER 16

**Hatch-Waxman Act of United States-A Relation to
Drug Discovery, Regulatory and Market Approval** **77**

16.1 Origins of US Drug Law 78

16.2 Drafting the Hatch Waxman Act 78

16.3 Overview of Drug Discovery, Regulatory and
Market Approval Process 78

16.3.1 Investigational New Drug (IND) Application 78

16.3.2 New Drug Application (NDA) 79

16.3.3 Hatch Waxman Act and Abbreviated NDA 79

16.3.4 Impact of Hatch Waxman Act on
Patent System: The Bolar Amendment.......................... 80

16.3.5 Role of Filing Patent Information.................................. 80

16.3.6 Patent Term Extension.. 80

16.3.7 Certification and Notification Requirement of the Act . 81

16.3.8 Market Exclusivity Provision by Hatch Waxman Act... 82

16.3.9 Market Exclusivity Provision not under the
Provision of Hatch Waxman Act.................................. 82

16.3.10 Provisions for Antibiotics.. 83

16.4 Case Studies 83

    16.4.1 Barr Laboratories vs. Eli Lilly 83

    16.4.2 Glaxo Smith Kline vs. Apotex 83

    16.4.3 Teva vs. Pfizer 84

    16.4.4 Mova vs. Upjohn 84

    16.4.5 Inwood Laboratories Inc vs. Young 84

    16.4.6 Purepac, Teva vs. FDA 84

CHAPTER 17

Intellectual Property Validation

Intellectual Property Validation 86

CHAPTER 18

Intellectual Property Audits

Intellectual Property Audits 92

CHAPTER 19

National Phase Entry for IP Protection

National Phase Entry for IP Protection 94

CHAPTER 20

Intellectual Property Litigation Prosecution

Intellectual Property Litigation Prosecution 97

CHAPTER 21

FAQs in Pharmaceuticals on Patents - Regulatory - Marketing

FAQs in Pharmaceuticals on Patents -
Regulatory - Marketing 99

Annexure 1 Anatomy of a US Patent 127

Annexure 2 Trademarks Registered 131

Annexure 3 Geographical Indications Registered and Guidelines 137

Annexure 4 Designs Registered 151

Annexure 5 Plant Variety Registered 157

Annexure 6 Patent Application Forms 1, 2, 3, 5, 28 (SME) 171

Annexure 7 Doctrine of Equivalence Case Study 179

Annexure 8 Judgement Relating First Indian Compulsory Licensing 193

Annexure 9   Rejection of Compulsory License Application Case Study... 257

Annexure 10 Pregrant Opposition Case Study 273

Annexure 11 Postgrant Opposition Case Study.. 289

Annexure 12 Notice of Working of Patent 319

Annexure 13 Revoking of Patent by Gazette Notification 323

Annexure 14 Fee for Patent Application, Office Procedure and
Maintenance….. 327

Annexure 15 IPO as Receiving Office … 367

Annexure 16 PCT Application 373

Annexure 17 IPO as International Search Authority 389

Annexure 18 ISA Report Case Study 393

Annexure 19 IPO as International Preliminary Examination Authority..... 403

Annexure 20 IPEA Report Case Study... 407

Annexure 21 Japanese Guideline on Technology Transfer 417

Annexure 22 Statistics and Relavant Publications 445

    (i)   An Overview of Patent System

    (ii)   An Overview of Trade Marks in Pharmaceuticals

    (iii) Influence of Intellectual Property Matters in Pharmaceutical Manufacturing and Exports

    (iv) An Analysis of Para IV Certifications of USFDA

    (v)   An Overview of Innovation Policy and Innovation Index

    (vi) Challenges Ahead for New Government in Pharmaceuticals in Intellectual Property Matters

    (vii) Strategies and Lead Resources for Generic Drug Development

Annexure 23 List of Global Countries and their Membership with
International Conventions/Treaties/Agreements.................... 483

Annexure 24 List of Indian Organisations Active in
Patenting Pharmaceutical Technologies (Indicative)............. 495

Annexure 25 CGPDTM Organisation Structure.. 501

Introduction and History of Intellectual Property Rights

1.1 INTRODUCTION

Creations of brain are called as intellect. Since these creations have commercial value, are called as property. As these creations are belonging to an individual, they are the rights of the individual and hence the word coined as intellectual property rights. Intellectual property rights are governed by intellectual property law. Intellectual property rights are believed to increase the economy of the country and it is the duty of every country to have necessary laws to safe guard the intellectual property of the citizens. Government of every country grants exclusive rights for the creations and it is the duty of the holder of the rights to monitor the act of infringement of his rights. Forth coming chapters are expected to impart basics and practice of IPR matters.

1.2 HISTORY OF INTELLECTUAL PROPERTY RIGHTS

Intellectual property rights are granted since ancient times in India. During the Harappa civilization, special marks were identified on the pottery indicating as trademarks. With respect to global scenario, in 1300s at Alp Mountains, the people who identified the mines for the first time used to dictate terms on the surrounding available resources like water, wood. In Germany, in 1409, a special privilege was given in construction of model mill to store grains. In order to encourage creators, exclusive rights were granted for stained glass in England. An exclusive right was not granted by English for playing cards as they already existed in the public domain. In United States, exclusive rights were granted for hopper boy. French have taken a step ahead in registration and examination of the intellectual property rights before grant of exclusive rights.

Initially, inventions were kept secret so that it is well protected. As technology developed, as a matter of national prestige the inventions were exhibited. In 1867, Germany received the first genuine recognition as an industrial nation in an exhibition held at Paris. During Vienna exhibition, in 1873, it was the American who refused to participate in the exhibition to safeguard the intellectual property creations from German nations. This led to origin of an international understanding as Paris Convention for protection of intellectual property rights. The convention provided a right of claiming priority among the countries who are the members of the convention.

In Indian context, in 1856, the Act VI on protection of inventions based on the British Patent Law of 1852 was established. During this period certain privileges were granted to inventors of new manufacturers for a period of 14 year. In 1859, the act was modified as Act XV in which making, selling, using of inventions in India and authorizing others to do so for 14 years from the date of filing the specification. In 1872, the act was re-named as the The Patents and Design Protection Act, in 1883 as The Protection of Inventions Act, in 1888 consolidated as The Inventions and Designs Act and in 1911 as The Indian Patents and Designs Act.

In 1893, to carry out the administrative tasks relating to intellectual property at the international level, an international organization called United International Bureaux for the Protection of Intellectual Property (BIRPI) was established in Berne, Switzerland.

After the World War II, economy in many European and Asian countries was shattered. After the United Nations Organisation (UNO) was born, three bodies were born in 1947 i.e., World Bank, International Monetary Fund (IMF) and International Trade Organization (ITO). It was the US senate that blocked the ITO. The objective of these organisations was to revive the economy especially in developing countries. General Agreement on Tariffs and Trade came into existence to revive the economy of the countries by increasing international trade that is predictable by reducing the tariffs. On January 1, 1948, twenty three contracting states including India ratified GATT. The objective of GATT agreement is to bring international stable and predictable trade, as a mediator in settling disputes among the countries, hold frequent negotiations, and encourage reductions in tariffs to expand World trade. India signed the GATT agreement to import oil, industrial raw materials, machines, new technology that is domestically needed in exchange with export of indigenous products.

In 1960, with increasing in awareness of intellectual property rights, in order to bring closer to United Nations, BIRPI was shifted from Berne to Geneva. In 1967, to modernize and for better administration of the unions with respect to protection of the intellectual property and artistic works, while fully respecting the independence of the each of the union, the name of the international organisation United International Bureaux for the Protection of Intellectual Property (BIRPI) was changed to World Intellectual Property Organisation (WIPO).

The objective of World Intellectual Property Organisation is to promote international cooperation with respect to creation, dissemination, use and protection of works of the human mind for economic, social, cultural progress of all mankind. The organisation enhances a worldwide balance of the creation by protecting moral, material interests of the creators and providing access to the socio-economic and cultural benefits to others. The organisation promotes intellectual property and brings out cooperation among countries of the union by setting norms, standards, executing legal, technical assistance, registration activities for intellectual property protection to member countries.

1.3   CLASSIFICATION OF INTELLECTUAL PROPERTY RIGHTS

Intellectual property rights are basically classified in to industrial property rights and copy rights, Figure 1.1. Intellectual properties that are having commercial importance and use to an industry are called as industrial property rights. While, copy rights are rights relating to artistic and literary works.

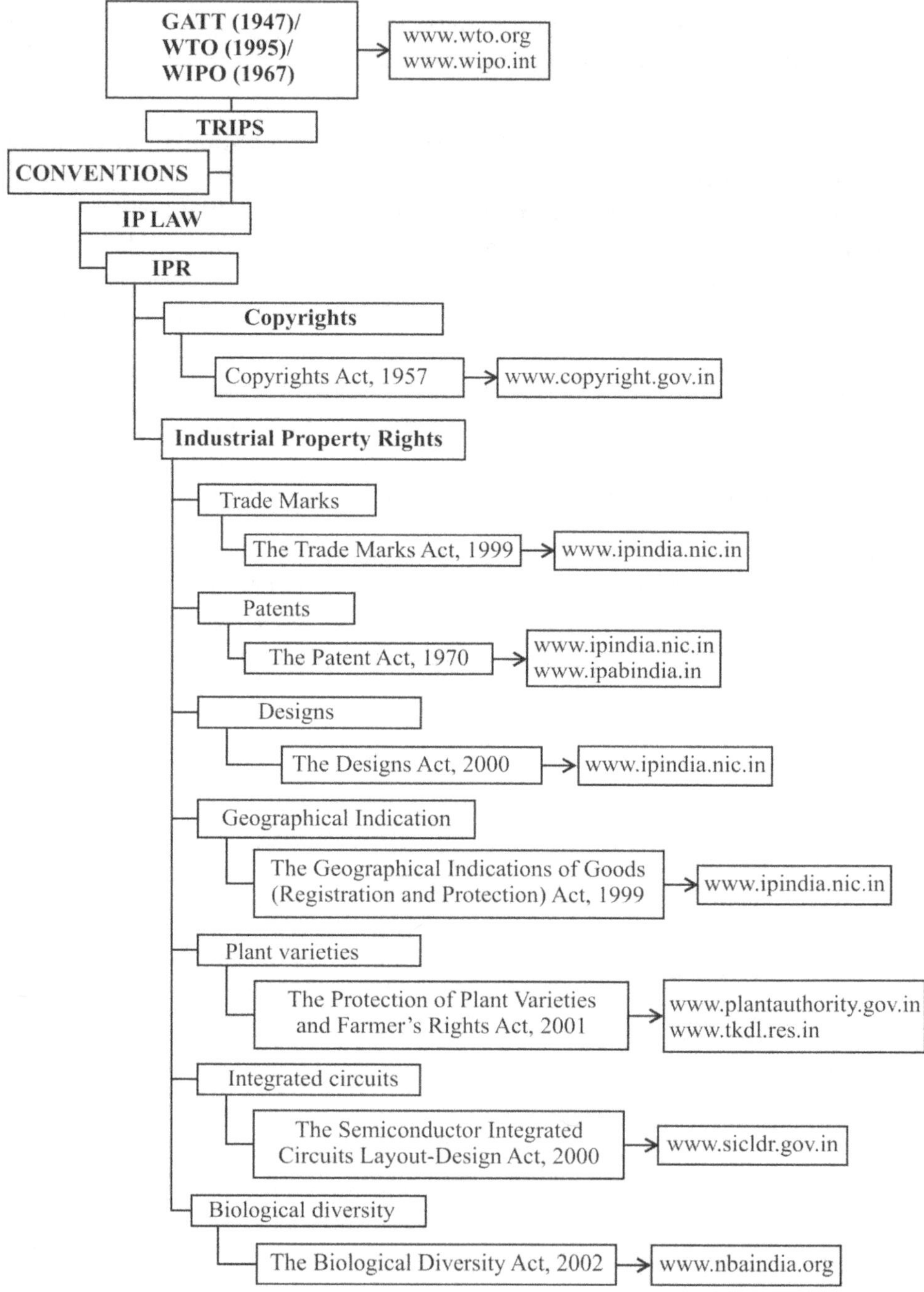

Figure 1.1 Classification of Intellectual Property Rights.

QUESTIONS

1. Define intellectual property rights and brief about its origins?
2. What is the history of intellectual property rights?
3. Classify intellectual property rights?
4. What are the Acts that are governing intellectual property rights in India?

CHAPTER 2

International Agreements, Treaties and Conventions

Since 1300 several understandings were made among countries to encourage, safeguard intellectual property of nationals in foreign countries. Such provisions were fruitful in harmonization of application procedures, examination procedures, granting procedures among countries. However, the international convention, agreement or treaties were able to bring out minimum guidelines for the implementation, protection of intellectual property rights of its citizens leaving upto the discretion of the individual country in maintaining the stringency of the legislations to the local needs. Table 2.1 illustrates the treaties, in chronological order for understanding the harmonizations made in different components of intellectual property rights. The conventions, agreements or treaties are categorized with respect to Intellectual Protection, Global Protection System, and Classification and they are either regional or international. Several regional treaties are now international treaties. Several treaties are in status of in force or not yet in force. Limiting to pharmaceuticals and more concerned to, the relevant treaties concerned are discussed.

Table 2.1 List of Treaties/Conventions/Agreements

IP Protection		
Year	**Name of Treaty**	**Purpose**
1883	Paris Convention	Protection of Industrial Property
1886	Berne Convention	Protection of the rights of authors in their literary and artistic works
1891	Madrid Agreement (Indication of Source)	Repression of false or deceptive indications of source of goods
1961	Rome Convention	Protection of performers, producers of phonograms and broadcasting organisations
1971	Phonograms Convention	Protection of producers of phonograms against unauthorized duplication of their phonograms
1974	Brussels Convention	Distribution of programme-carrying signals transmitted by satellite

Table 2.1 Contd...

IP Protection		
Year	**Name of Treaty**	**Purpose**
1981	Nairobi Treaty	Protection of the Olympic symbol
1994	Trademarks Law Treaty	Standardize and streamline national and regional trademark registration procedures
1996	WIPO Copyrights Treaty (WCT)	Protection of works and the rights of their authors in the digital environment
1996	WIPO Performances and Phonograms Treaty (WPPT)	Protection of rights of performers, producers of phonograms particular in digital environment
2000	Patent Law Treaty	To harmonize and streamline formal national and regional application, patent procedures
2006	Singapore Treaty	Creation of a modern and dynamic international framework for the harmonization of administrative trademark registration procedures
2007	Washington Treaty	Intellectual property in respect of integrated circuits
2012	Beijing Treaty	Intellectual property rights of performers in audiovisual performances
2013	Marrakesh VIP Treaty	Facilitate access to published works by visually impaired persons and persons with print disabilities

Global Protection System		
Year	**Name of Treaty**	**Purpose**
1925	Hague Agreement	Concerning the international registration of industrial designs
1958	Lisbon Agreement	Protection of appellations of origin and their international registration
1970	Patent Cooperation Treaty	Patent protection for an invention simultaneously in each of a large number of countries by filing an "international" patent application
1977	Budapest Treaty	International recognition of the deposit of microorganisms for the purpose of patent protection
1989	Madrid Agreement (Marks)	Protect a mark in a large number of countries by obtaining an international registration
1989	Madrid Protocol	Relating to the Madrid agreement concerning the international registration of marks

Classifications		
Year	**Name of Treaty**	**Purpose**
1957	Nice Agreement	The international classification of goods and services for the purposes of the registration of marks
1968	Lacarno Agreement	Establishing an international classification for industrial designs
1971	Strasbourg Agreement	The international patent classification
1973	Vienna Agreement	International classification of the figurative elements of marks

A. Intellectual Property Protection

2.1   Paris Convention (1883)

Initially inventions were kept secret so that it is well protected. As technology developed periodically, as a matter of national prestige the inventions were exhibited. At Paris exhibition, in 1867, Germany received the first genuine recognition as an industrial nation. In 1873, during the Vienna exhibition, it was the Americans who refused to participate. The reason was that the Americans need intellectual property protection of their creations from German nations so that ideas are well protected. This led to the initiation of international conventions, international understandings, first of its kind with Paris Convention.

Paris Convention applies to industrial property relating patents, trademarks, industrial designs, utility models (a kind of "small-scale patent" provided for by the laws of some countries), service marks, trade names, geographical indications (indications of sources and appellations of origin) and repression of unfair competition.

A provision of 'national treatment' is provided wherein countries which are members of convention treat foreign nationals as country's own nationals. A term 'right of priority' was introduced pertaining to patents, utility models, marks and industrial designs. Where a first application filed in a contracting state, he shall have the equal rights of priority of date of filing in all the contracting states. Within 12 months (for patents, utility models) or within 6 months (for industrial designs, marks) he can make a decision to file the application in contracting states. The subsequent filings in the contracting states shall be considered as the same date of filing of the first application. A provision of 'compulsory licence' shall be granted in conditions of abuse of exclusive rights, not worked for at least three years from date of grant or four years from date of filing patent application.

With relating to trademark, Paris convention indicates filing and registration among the contacting states as independent to domestic law. This indicates flexibility in the contracting states depending on the local condition of the trademarks; an exclusive right may be granted or refused. However, a registered trademark is compulsory in contracting states. Each contracting state should refuse use and registration of marks relating to state emblems, official signs, and hallmarks of contracting states. A provision of collective marks is made for a grant.

Effective protection relating to industrial designs, trade names, indications of source, unfair competition as exclusivity is indicated.

2.2   BERNE CONVENTION (1886)

In pharmaceuticals, several books, scientific works as literature are authored. Berne convention deals with protection of works and rights of authors and provides minimum guidelines for protection among contracting states with special provision to developing countries. The convention insists on national treatment, automatic, indicating that if protected in one country, must be considered in all contracting states. The contract state has the independence in the grant or refuse of exclusivity for the work.

As per the convention, a work should be expressed and shall be protected for a minimum of 50 years after the death of the author. In other cases such as anonymous, pseudonymous works only for 50 years of exclusivity shall be considered. In case of audiovisual, the minimum term of protection is 50 years. In case of photographic works, the minimum term of protection is 25 years. In several cases the exclusivity term is from the date of availability of the work to the public.

If a contracting state provides a longer term of protection than minimum prescribed by the convention and the protection ceases in the country of origin, protection may be denied once protection ceases in country of origin.

The convention indicates the contracting states in providing provision of right to translation, make adaptations, arrangement of work, perform in public, recite literary works in public, communicate to the public, broadcast subject to the provisions provided by the contracting state. The convention provides moral rights in claiming or objection authorship.

2.3   MADRID AGREEMENT (1891)

The agreement mainly deals with false and deceptive indication of source (country of origin). Where a contracting state wrongly indicates source of origin directly or indirectly, the goods must be seized or such importation must be prohibited. The agreement provides in detail the manner in which seizure may be requested, goods prohibited for use, sale, display/ publicity.

2.4   TRADEMARKS LAW TREATY (1994)

The objective of the treaty is to harmonize applications, registrations of trademarks among the contracting states. The treaty is mainly to harmonize procedures in the trademark offices in the contracting states.

The treaty indicates three phases such as application for registration, changes after registration and on renewal. The treaty seeks to collect and have information relating name of applicant, address of application, address of representative, the goods and services a registration is sort along with indication of number of class as per the harmonized Nice classification. A single request by the applicant may be made for any changes in the registration made with respect to all contracting states or all the trademarks belonging to one applicant.

The treaty has provided with uniform initial duration of registration and periodic renewal after every 10 years.

2.5   WIPO Copyrights Treaty-WCT (1996)

World intellectual property organisation copyrights treaty is a special agreement under the Berne convention and deals with protection of works and the rights of their authors in the digital environment. All the contracting states must comply with Paris Act, 1971 and Berne Convention, 1886. The treaty provides a provision of protection as copyright for computer programs in whatever mode or form being expressed, compilations of data or other materials (databases) which constitute intellectual creations.

The treaty grants rights of distribution, rental, and communications to public, subject to provisions provided. The treaty provides a 'three step' test to determine limitations and exceptions and the limitations may be extended to local needs, provided the local law fulfills Berne convention. The treaty provides a minimum period of at least 50 years as term of protection for any kind of work. The treaty indicates the contracting states with legal, infringement remedies ensuring the boundaries of rights of the holder.

2.6   Patent Law Treaty (2000)

The objective of the treaty is to harmonize the official national and regional application, patent procedures that are user friendly with exceptions in filing date requirements. The treaty provides the flexibility for the contracting states with respect to the requirements to be furnished for the benefit of the applicant for exclusive rights. The treaty harmonizes the requirements in obtaining the filing date in order to minimize the risks by fulfilling three formal requirements. The elements that should be furnished indicate that the applicant is seeking for a patent for an invention along with applicants address, contact details and description of the invention. Elements with respect to international application through PCT such as PCT request form, application with respect to national application should be received by the contracting state to minimize procedural gaps between national, regional and international patent systems.

The treaty established standard model of international forms that should be accepted by contracting states. The treaty facilitated the applicants with respect to reduction in costs, providing procedural time limits implementation of electronic filing with co-existence of both paper and electronic communications.

2.7   SINGAPORE TREATY (2006)

The objective of the treaty is to harmonize administrative trademark registration provisions and to facilitate a modern, dynamic international frame work fulfilling Trade mark Law Treaty, 1994 with wider scope of application along with developed communication technologies. The Singapore treaty is applicable to all types of marks. Time limits for registrations are specified and the classification may be followed on the ground of Nice classification. Unlike Trademark Law Treaty, the Singapore treaty applies to all the marks that can be registered and additionally includes acceptance of non-traditional marks such as non-traditional visible marks, holograms, three dimensional marks, color, position and movement marks, and non-visible marks such as sound, olfactory, taste and feel marks. The applications shall be accompanied with non-graphic, photographic reproductions.

The treaty provides the flexibility in choosing the form, furnishing the form either in paper or electronic form subject to the provisions indicated. The treaty accepts the provision of Trade mark Law treaty without authentication, certification or attestation of signature on paper communication. However, the contracting states are free in making elements for authentication of electronic communications.

The treaty provides a provision of relief measure of extension of time limit, continued processing, reinstatement of rights under un-intentional conditions. A provision for recording of trademarks along with establishing the elements to be fulfilled has been made. The treaty does not hinder registration of new type of marks, and provides flexibility in implementation of electronic filings and automations.

B. GLOBAL PROTECTION SYSTEM

2.8   HAGUE AGREEMENT (1925)

The agreement deals with international agreement concerning the international registration of industrial designs. The agreement streamlines administration and registration of designs among the contracting states. The agreement is governed by Act, 1960 and Act, 1999. The application may be obtained from a natural person or a legal representative. The agreement provides the provision of filing single application at the International Bureau (IB) of World Intellectual Property Organisation (WIPO).

An international application as per the agreement may be governed by Act, 1960, the Act, 1999 or both depending on the contracting party with which the applicant has connection. An international application may be filed directly at the international bureau or at the native country intellectual property office.

An international application may contain up to 100 designs, provided they belong to same class as per international classification for industrial designs (Locarno classification). The agreement provides a provision of submitting the application in English, French or Spanish. The international application must contain one or several reproductions of industrial designs and must designate at least one contracting state.

The agreement provides a provision of publication of designs in Industrial Designs Bulletin issued weekly online for public access. Depending on the contracting state, the applicant may defer up to 30 months from publishing from the priority date or from the date of international registration.

If the contracting party does not indicate the refusal of the application within the prescribed limit, the international registration has effect as grant of protection by the contracting with respect to the law of the contracting party.

As per the agreement, the term of protection is 5 years, renewed for one five years under the Act, 1960, or two such periods under the Act, 1999. However, a contracting party may extend the term of protection subject to the provisions of the local law.

2.9   LISBON AGREEMENT (1958)

The agreement deals with protection of appellations of origin, that is, geographical denomination of country, region or locality designating the origin of the product for its unique characteristics of quality either with respect to geographic environment either due to natural or human factor. The agreement provides a provision of registration of such products by the international bureau of WIPO upon request by the contracting party. The agreement indicates that the international bureau to maintain a register, publish Lisbon's system official bulletin and periodically update the status to the contracting parties.

The agreement provides a provision of up to one year from the date of receiving the notice that a contracting party not ensure in grant of exclusivity as registration in its territory. In such cases of refusal of grant by the contracting party, necessary grounds of refusal has to be furnished.

2.10   PATENT CO-OPERATION TREATY (1970)

The objective of the treaty is to provide patent protection for an invention simultaneously in each of the large number of countries by filing one single international patent application. Such application can be filed by anyone who is a national or resident to a PCT contracting state. As per the treaty, an application may be filed at native intellectual property office or directly submitted at the international bureau of the WIPO.

If an applicant is a national or resident to the contracting state party of European Patent Convention, the Harare protocol, the Bangui agreement, or the Eurasia Patent Convention, the international application may be filed also at European Patent Office (EPO), the African Regional Intellectual Property Organisation (ARIPO), the African Intellectual Property Organisation (OAPI) or the Eurasian Patent Office respectively.

The agreement indicates that filing an application through PCT with indication of contracting states, shall be deemed as a national patent application in all the designated states. The agreement provides a provision of international search by any one of the chosen International Searching Authority (ISA) as per the PCT. The authority provides with a written, preliminary, non-binding written opinion of the invention whether meets patentability criteria. Based on the written opinion, the applicant has the independence to continue the grant procedure or to withdraw the application, or amend the claims to fulfill patentability criteria. If the international application is not withdrawn, it is published by the international bureau together with the international search report. At this stage, the written opinion is not published.

Before the expiration of 19 months from the priority date, the applicant has another option requesting Supplementary International Search Authority (SISA) to conduct another search more in precise in particular languages to reduce the likelihood of relevant subject matter coming into limelight prior entry into the national phase that would likely hinder the grant. The treaty provides a time period of 30 months from the date of priority date to enter the national phase during which all the necessary procedures with respect to language translation, paying the necessary fee, acquiring patent agent may be made.

After making necessary changes, amendments in the application after the search report and written opinion of the international search authority, the applicant may request International Preliminary Examination Authority under the PCT for a report that is non-binding to further ensure the patentability of the subject matter and to decide to proceed further for grant of a patent. If no international preliminary examination authority report is requested, the international bureau establishes an international preliminary report on patentability based on the ISA opinion and communicates with the designated states.

The agreement sets single application procedure, single examination procedure, setting time frame to meet the protocols, minimizing translations and expenditure and attain a granted patent in several countries.

2.11 BUDAPEST TREATY (1977)

The treaty mainly deals with international recognition of the deposit of microorganisms for the purposes of patent procedure. It is mandatory that an invention should be disclosed and described in a specification. Invention of microorganisms and their disclosure and description is not possible. In a broader meaning, the biological material has to be available for the public. Instead of depositing the biological material at every country, the treaty provides a provision by depositing at any 'international depository authority'. The treaty indicates that the depository authority is a scientific institute collecting culture and capable of storing microorganisms. The treaty benefits the applicant in reduced cost by single deposition. In India, Microbial Culture Collection Centre (MCC), Pune is recognized as the International Depository Authority (IDA) for the deposit of the microorganisms for the purpose of patent procedure.

2.12 Madrid Agreement and Protocol (1989)

The agreement deals with international registration of marks. The agreement is governed by two treaties i.e., the Madrid agreement and the Madrid protocol. The system provides protection of the mark in large number of countries by one international application filing. The agreement indicates that the international application for a mark shall be considered for only such mark is registered in the country of origin. An international application must be presented at the international bureau of WIPO through the office of origin and the application must indicate one or more contracting states where the applicant seeks for protection. An international application may be filed in English, French or Spanish irrespective of treaties governing the international application.

The international application is accepted subject to payment of basic fee, a supplementary fee for each class of goods and/or services beyond the first three classes and a complementary fee for each contracting party designated. As per the protocol provisions, individual fee to the contracting state shall be paid instead of complementary fee and the amount is specified by the contracting state and shall not be higher than the amount payable for the registration of the mark.

Soon after receiving the application by the international bureau, the application is examined with respect to the requirement of the agreement, protocol and for common requirements. Once it fulfills, the application is examined for classification with respect to good and/or services. If no irregularities, the international bureau records the mark in the international register, publishes the international registration in the WIPO gazette of international marks and notifies to contracting parties. Individual contracting party provides individual information regarding the mark whether can be accepted or refused with respect to its legislation and local needs. An indication of refusal by the contracting party shall be furnished by valid grounds within twelve months (extended up to 18 months in case of protocol) from the date of notification. The refusal is communicated to the applicant or his representative as indicated in the register and published in the gazette by the international bureau. The applicant may decide at a later stage for appealing or reviewing with the competent authority without involvement with the international bureau. The final decision of refusal shall be communicated with the international bureau for recording and publishing.

The effect of international registration is from the date of international registration. The term of international registration is for 10 years and renewed for further 10 years on payment of prescribed fee.

The advantages with the agreement are one single international filing with protection in several countries, minimized cost, any one language filing,

C. CLASSIFICATIONS

2.13 NICE AGREEMENT (1957)

Nice agreement also called as Nice classification. The agreement establishes a system of classification of goods and services. The agreement indicates a uniform designation of number of class for a category of goods and services so that contracting states indicates the numbers wherever necessary and bring out uniformity in accepting applications, examination and registering of trademarks.

The classification consists of 34 goods and 11 services. The latter consists of 11,000 items.

2.14 LOCARNO AGREEMENT (1968)

Locarno agreement also called as Locarno classification. The agreement deals with establishing of classification for industrial designs. The agreement indicates a uniform designation of number of class and subclasses for a category of goods to which design belong or to be incorporated so that contracting states indicates the numbers wherever necessary and bring out uniformity in accepting applications, examination and registering of designs.

The classification consists of 32 classes and 219 subclasses. The latter comprises approximately 7000 items.

2.15 STRASBOURG AGREEMENT (1971)

The agreement deals with establishing of classification of patents as International Patent Classification (IPC). The agreement indicates a uniform designation of number for the field/technology of the invention for which patent application is filed. The classification brings out uniformity in receiving, examination, searching and granting of patents among the contracting states.

As per the International Patent Classification, technology is divided into 8 sections with approximately 70, 000 subdivisions. Each subdivision is denoted by a symbol consisting of Arabic numerals and letters of Latin alphabet.

The classification made easier the process of examination, providing search reports, submission of examiner reports of an application for an early grant of a patent within the stipulated time.

2.16 VIENNA AGREEMENT (1973)

Vienna agreement is also called as Vienna classification. The agreement deals with establishing of classification of the figurative elements of marks. The agreement indicates a uniform designation of numbers based on figurative elements to which mark belong or to be incorporated so that contracting states indicate the numbers wherever necessary and bring out uniformity in accepting applications, examination and registering of marks.

The classification consists of 29 categories, 145 divisions and some 1,700 sections in which the figurative elements of marks are classified.

QUESTIONS

1. What is the objective of origin of various treaties/ conventions/ agreements relating to intellectual property rights?

2. What are the different international treaties relating to pharmaceuticals and that are governing intellectual property rights?

CHAPTER 3

Introduction to Different Components of Intellectual Property Rights

3.1 INDUSTRIAL PROPERTY RIGHTS

Intellectual property rights that are of industrial application leading to increase in business are considered as industrial property rights.

3.1.1 Patents

The word patent was coined from a Latin term 'patent-em' meaning open. A patent is a document (Annexure 1) issued by government to the inventor granting him exclusive rights to make, sell, use or import upon disclosure of the invention for a definite period of time.

The criteria for an invention to be a patentable subject matter, the invention must be novel, non-obvious, useful and enable. It is necessary that the invention should fulfill all the criteria and not any one. In India, The Patents Act, 1970 governs the protection of inventions as intellectual property. Indian intellectual property offices located at Kolkata, Delhi, Mumbai and Chennai receive applications and grants patents for inventions. Department of Industrial Policy and Promotion, Department of Commerce under the Ministry of Commerce & Industry, Government of India bring out policy, implements the intellectual property of Patents in India.

The term of a patent is for 20 years from the date of filing.

Using, International Patent Classification -A61K, several patents relating pharmaceuticals granted for a process, product, and formulation can be observed.

3.1.2 Trademarks

A trademark is an indication of a product originated from an individual or a company signifying the quality of the product and distinguishes from its competitor. A trademark is an alphabet, numerical, alphanumerical, device or a combination of these (Annexure 2). Several trademarks in terms of colour, three dimensional signs, audible signs (sound marks), olfactory marks (smell marks), invisible signs (touch) are in use. Thus a trademark indicates the quality of the product originated from a company. The criteria for a trademark to be registered is that it should be unique, distinctive, does not deceive public, does not confuse public, does not use emblems or names covered under "Prevention of Improper Use" Act, 1950, an exclusive right. The Trademark Act, 1999 governs the registration of intellectual property. Trademark registry located at Mumbai, Kolkata, Delhi, Chennai, Ahmedabad receives applications and registers the marks. Department of Industrial Policy and Promotion, Department of Commerce under the Ministry of Commerce & Industry, Government of India bring out policy, implements the intellectual property of trademarks in India.

Services are also recognized internationally for their role in the economic growth of a country. Service marks are registered at the registry relating to transportation, banking etc.

Collective marks as registered marks are issued to several companies having same product with individual trademarks. Such collective marks indicate the product is fulfilling the quality guidelines set by the organisation issuing the collective mark.

In pharmaceuticals, several trade names are used and are registered as trademarks indicating the product is from a specific company.

The term of a trademark is for 10 years and renewed from time to time.

World Health Organisation has listed all the active substance used as drugs that are available in the market with their International Non-proprietary Names (INN) commonly called as generic names of drugs. Trade names should neither be derived from INNs nor contain common stems used in INNs.

Class 5, class 9 and class 10 include goods relating to pharmaceuticals, scientific and medical devices respectively. With respect to services class 42, 44, and 45 deals with scientific-technological services, medical-veterinary-hygiene, beauty care for human and animal. For a trade or service mark, the corresponding class number has to be indicated in the application form.

Examples of trade names as trademarks are Gelusil, Wokadine, Sinarest, Ferox, Ala-100, Cholestat, and Disprin. Trade name as trademark for services is Apollo Hospitals.

3.1.3 Trade Secrets

All the intangible assets of an organisation are trade secrets. Trade secrets are also called as 'know how'. A trade secret in pharmaceutical industry may be a business method, method of manufacture etc. A trade secret is a secret forever until and unless the secret is revealed. In India, there is no legislation with respect to protection of trade secrets. Several countries in the world have legislations as data exclusivity where in crucial data is protected for a certain period of time. In pharmaceuticals, data relating to pharmacodynamics, pharmacokinetics of New Chemical Entities (NCE) submitted to regulatory authority is being protected as data exclusivity so that generic companies are facilitated in using the data after a certain period of time only in filing generic drug applications. If a provision of data exclusivity is provided in India, entry of generic drugs into the market might still be delayed.

Examples of trade secret, know how or data exclusivity are such as protection of pharmacodynamic and pharmacokinetics data of the new chemical entities by the innovators.

3.1.4 Geographical Indications

Geographical indication of goods indicates that the good is produced in a particular geographical region and its quality characteristics are due to the unique climatic, geographic conditions. Hence such goods are indicated by the geographical location of origin (Annexure 3). In several countries, geographical indications are also called as Appellations of Origin. Unlike trademarks belonging to an individual, geographical indication of goods belongs to a group of individuals who are skilled in the art of producing the good in that location. Hence, it is necessary that all the people skilled in the art form a union and register the good for geographical indication. The criteria for registration of a good as geographical indication are that the good should not deceive, not confuse public, contrary to a law, does not hurt the religious class.

In India, The Geographical Indications of Goods (Registration and Protection) Act, 1999 governs registration of goods as geographical indicators. Geographical Indication registry located at Chennai receives applications and registers. Department of Industrial Policy and Promotion, Department of Commerce under the Ministry of Commerce & Industry, Government of India bring out policy, implements the intellectual property of geographical indications in India.

The term of a geographical indication is for 10 years and renewed from time to time.

Examples of geographical indications are Mysore sandal soap, Tirupati laddu, Basmati rice etc.

3.1.5 Designs

An aesthetic appearance of an article is considered as a design. An article which is already existing earlier but its new aesthetic appearance brings out industrial application, leading to increase in business, economic growth of the country. The criterion for a design to be registered as an exclusive right is that it should be unique, original, not in public domain, distinctive.

In India, The Designs Act, 2000 governs registration of goods for their designs. Indian intellectual property offices located at Kolkata, Delhi, Mumbai and Chennai receive applications and register goods for their design. Department of Industrial Policy and Promotion, Department of Commerce under the Ministry of Commerce & Industry, Government of India bring out policy, implements the intellectual property of designs in India. In pharmaceuticals, several tablet designs, packing designs are protected as registration exclusivity (Annexure 4).

The term of design is for 10 years and may be extended for further 5 years.

Under the class 24, medical device designs are registered. Examples of designs registered in pharmaceuticals include tablet shapes, blister packs, and medical devices such as intraocular lens, implantation device etc.

3.1.6 Integrated Circuits

Design layout of circuits of hardware is playing a critical role in bringing out especially electronic goods into more compact, aesthetic appearance. Such circuits are found to possess very high industrial application leading to increase in business, economic growth of the country.

In India, The Semiconductor Integrated Circuits Layout Design Act, 2000 governs registration of designs of circuit layouts. Semiconductor integrated circuit layout design registry located at New Delhi receives applications and register the design of the layout of the circuits. The criteria for registration of semiconductor integrated circuit layout design are, the design layout should be original, not commercially exploited, and distinctive. Department of Electronics and Information Technology, Ministry of Communications and Information Technology, Government of India implements the intellectual property of semiconductor integrated circuit layout design in India.

The term of semiconductor integrated circuit layout design in India is for 10 years.

3.1.7 Plant Varieties

Plants that are cultivated leading to new variety by cultivators are protected as exclusive right since they have industrial application and commercial value. Several extant varieties, farmers' varieties are protected as exclusive rights (Annexure 5). The criteria for a plant variety for registering as an exclusive right are that the variety should be novel, distinctive, uniform, stable, capable of identifying such variety, does not mislead characteristics, does not confuse characteristics, different from botanical/registered species, does not deceive/confuse public, does not hurt religious sentiments, does not contain a name or emblem covered under "the Emblems and Name (Protection of Improper Use) Act, 1950", does not contain solely or partly of geographical name.

In India, The Protection of Plant Varieties and Farmers' Rights Act, 2001 governs registration of plant varieties as exclusive right. Department of Agriculture and Co-operation, Ministry of Agriculture, Government of India implements the intellectual property of protection of plant varieties in India. The registration authority is located at New Delhi.

The term of exclusivity of plant variety is 18 years for trees and vines, 15 years for extant varieties, 15 years for other cases.

At the authority, cultivation of a crop of sunflower with number KSFH-7032 was registered for distinguishing character as short seed length.

3.2   COPYRIGHTS

Intellectual properties belonging to artistic and literary work are protected as exclusive property since such works are having commercial value, leading to economic growth of the country. The criteria of an artistic or literary work to possess exclusive right as copyright are that the work should be original, published where the author (citizen of India) is dead at the time of publication, unpublished work, should not infringe a work already copyright protected. An exclusive intellectual property as copyright is granted for literary, dramatic, musical, artistic works, cinematographic films, sound recording, work of architecture, computer programme. Several privilege rights are granted as performers rights, neighbouring rights, broadcasting rights where rights are shared among the creators of the intellectual property.

In India, The Copyright Act, 1957 governs registration of a work as a copyright. Department of Higher Education, Ministry of Human Resources Development (HRD), Government of India implements the intellectual property of protection of literary and artistic work as copyrights. Applications are received at New Delhi office, relocated from HRD office to intellectual property office.

The term of a copyright is life time of author plus 60 years for anonymous and pseudonymous works (literary, dramatic, musical or artistic work other than photography) provided the identity of the author is disclosed before the expiry of the said period else only 60 years; 60 years for posthumous work; 60 years for photographs; 60 years for cinematograph films; 60 years for sound recording; 60 years for government works; 60 years for works of public undertaking; 60 years for works of international organisations.

Several pharmaceutical text books, figures, questionnaires are copyright protected either directly by the author or through a publisher.

QUESTIONS

1. Define and classify intellectual property rights and write in detail about various components of intellectual property rights?
2. What are the different ministries for various intellectual property rights are implemented in India?
3. What is the exclusivity term of various intellectual property rights in India?

CHAPTER 4

Introduction to Traditional Knowledge and Biological Diversity

4.1 TRADITIONAL KNOWLEDGE

Several methods of cultivation, methods of manufacture, methods of treatment of disease, several naturally available resources either plant, animal or mineral origin are being used for cure of disease. Such knowledge is passed from generation to generations. Such information is only known to a region.

After the issue of a foreign company filing for patent for strain of rice and giving the name of Basmati, after the issue of foreign department filing for a patent for a neem oil composition and after the issue of foreign university filing turmeric for wound healing property, Indian scientists through Government of India brought legal injunctions at the foreign country courts not to grant patents for India's widely used and well known traditional knowledge. The foreign patent offices and courts have dismissed the applications for patents relating to rice naming as Basmati, neem oil composition and turmeric as there was an international understanding among countries as International agreements and conventions.

Since then, Indian government assigned Council of Scientific and Industrial Research, Ministry of Science and Technology, Government of India and Department of AYUSH, Ministry of Health and Family Welfare, Government of India in collecting, compiling all the traditional knowledge being practiced in various parts of India and has brought a database available to public so that such knowledge is never claimed for exclusive intellectual property right by an individual of national or international origin.

In the Indian traditional knowledge digital library, several herbs being used since ages are indicated.

4.2   BIOLOGICAL DIVERSITY

Indian government has brought a new legislation as The Biological Diversity Act, 2002 governed by Ministry of Environment and Forests, Government of India. Under the provisions of the Act, a National Bio-Diversity Authority was constituted for the first time and the role of the authority is for deposition of sample, grant of permission to use, conduct research, apply for an intellectual property rights for the resources used from natural origin. It is mandatory for several of the intellectual property grants, approval by the National Biological Diversity Authority to be submitted at the intellectual property office or the registry.

QUESTIONS

1. What is traditional knowledge and why it gained its importance?

2. What is the objective and role of Biological Diversity?

3. What are the governing bodies, Acts that implement traditional knowledge, biological diversity in India?

CHAPTER 5

Introduction to WTO Agreement

5.1 ORIGIN, OBJECTIVE AND ROLE OF GATT

After the World War II, economy in many European and Asian countries was shattered. After the United Nations Organisations was born, three bodies were born in 1947, i.e., World Bank, International Monitory Fund (IMF) and International Trade Organization (ITO). It was the US senate, which blocked the ITO. The objective of these organisations was to revive the economy especially in developing countries. An international agreement called as General Agreement on Tariff and Trade (GATT) came into existence. The objective of GATT is to encourage international trade. On January 1, 1948, 23 contracting states including India ratified GATT. The role of GATT is to bring out trade liberalization through multilateral trade negotiations. GATT provides a stable and predictable international trade system. It acts as a mediator in settling the disputes between countries regarding trade. Additionally, GATT holds frequent negotiations, encourages reductions in tariffs so that expansion in world trade becomes possible. The objective of India signing the GATT agreement is to export indigenous products and in turn purchase oil, industrial raw materials, machines, new technology and other things that are domestically needed. During 1950s and 1960s, continuous reductions of tariffs led to high rate of world trade growth. Thus in the GATT era, trade liberalization helped in trade growth consistently instead production growth.

5.2 ORIGIN, OBJECTIVE AND ROLE OF WTO

Reduction in tariffs led to trade growth internationally, however competition prevailed and economic recessions among countries came into existence. Economic recessions led to high rate of unemployment, factory closures. To overcome, bi-lateral agreements came in practice. Advances in science, individual needs, world trade became more complex. Trade services were identified as a promising world economy, but rules were not covered under GATT. This led new discussion among countries and Uruguay round of negotiations were the last and largest round of discussions of GATT. The discussion led way for further international trade liberalization not only inclusion of trade but also the inclusion of trade in services, Trade Related Aspects of Intellectual Property Rights (TRIPS), approval of farm trade by services, market access, anti-dumping rules with the proposal of creation of new institution in place of GATT as World Trade Organisation (WTO).

The role of WTO is aspects relating to agriculture, textiles, clothing, banking, telecommunications, government purchases, industrial standards and products safety, food sanitation regulations and intellectual property. The objective of WTO is foundation of multilateral trade system by treating foreigners and locals equally, bringing free through negotiations, predicting through binding and transparency, promoting fair competition, encouraging development and economic reforms.

WTO has brought benefits like peace, solving disputes among countries, free trade that in turn reduce cost of living, choice of products, quality, economic growth and good government, thus improving welfare of people of the member countries.

When a comparison is made between GATT and WTO, GATT's commitments are being provisional, while WTO is being complete and permanent. GATT dealt with trade of merchandise goods whereas WTO is currently dealing additionally with trade services, trade-related aspects of intellectual property rights. In case of dispute settlements, WTO is faster, automatic and less susceptible to blockage when compared with GATT.

Hence, GATT established in 1947 ended with 1994 discussion converting itself by name with enhanced role and functions as WTO. On April 15, 1994 at Marrakesh, Morocco the ministries of 125 governments signed the agreement and from January 1, 1995 World Trade Organisation came into existence in place of GATT.

Upon signing the agreement all the countries became WTO members. Under the annex 1C of WTO agreement, an agreement relating to Trade Related Aspects of Intellectual Property Rights has to be fulfilled by the members.

QUESTIONS

1. What is the objective and role of GATT?

2. What is the objective and role of WTO?

3. When GATT and WTO originated?

Trade Related Aspects of Intellectual Property Rights Agreement

After GATT converted to WTO, the members who accepted the agreement are mandatory to comply with Trade Related Aspects of Intellectual Property Rights agreement. The objective of TRIPS agreement is to reduce distortions and impediments to international trade, taking into account the need to promote effective and adequate protection of intellectual property rights. The agreement ensures that measures and procedures to enforce intellectual property rights do not themselves become barriers to legitimate trade.

The TRIPS agreement insists on applying basic principles of GATT 1994 and relevant international intellectual property agreement and conventions, providing adequate standards and principles concerning the availability, scope and use of trade related aspects of intellectual property, effective and appropriate enforcement of intellectual property rights considering the differences in national legal systems, effective procedures for multilateral prevention and settlement of disputes between governments and transitional arrangement aiming at the fullest participation in the results of the negotiations. The agreement set forth guidelines relating to recognition of international trade in counterfeit goods, intellectual property as private rights, underlying public policy objectives of national systems for protection of intellectual property rights, providing flexibility for least developed member countries in respect of implementation of laws and regulations, reduce international tensions relating to disputes on intellectual property rights with strengthening relations between World Trade Organisation and World Intellectual Property Organisation.

TRIPS agreement comprises of seven parts with seventy three articles as guidelines to the member countries for implementation of legislations, enforcement and implementation of intellectual property rights within the member countries. The guidelines are considered to be the minimum guidelines and it is up to the countries discretion and local needs the stringency of the legislations prevails.

Part I of the guidelines discusses about the general provisions and basic principles indicating that the members are free in implementation of the agreement keeping in view of the local legal systems. Nationals of one country are also considered nationals of other country under the provision of Paris Convention (1967), the Berne Convention (1971), the Rome Convention and the Treaty on Intellectual Property in Respect of Integrated Circuits and are members of World Trade Organisation.

The agreement insists WIPO role relating to the acquisition or maintenance of intellectual property. Article 7 of TRIPS agreement reveals the objectives of promotion and enforcement of intellectual property rights as a means of promotion of technological innovation and to the transfer and dissemination of technology. Article 8 of the agreement insists on formulating new laws and amending already existing laws to current needs to protect public health and nutrition, promote socio-economic and technological development.

Part II of the TRIPS agreement has eight sections dealing with different components of intellectual property rights. With respect to copyrights, the agreement insists on fulfilling Berne Convention, computer programs and compilation of data within the purview, limiting rental rights with respect to cinematographic works preventing widespread copying with safeguarding exclusive rights. The agreement insists a minimum period 50 years as exclusive copyright to be implemented by the member countries. Performers, producers of phonograms and broadcasting organisations have a provision of exclusivity preventing un-authorized direct or indirect reproduction, re-broadcasting. Performers and producers of phonograms were provided with a provision of minimum 50 years of exclusivity while broadcasting exclusivity for a minimum of 20 years from the end of the calendar year.

Section 2 of part II of the agreement emphasizes on protectable subject matter relating to trademarks. Members may require, as a condition of registration, that signs be visually perceptible. The section emphasizes consideration and implementation of Paris Convention. An application shall not be refused solely on the ground that intended use has not taken place before the expiry of a period of three years from the date of application. The agreement insists on publishing of the mark before or after registration so as to receive petitions as opposition and cancel the registration if necessary.

Article 16 discusses about the rights provided to the trademark holder. The holder has the right to prevent a third party in applying for similar kind of signs for identical goods of trade or services thus preventing confusion to the public. Article 6 bis of the Paris Convention shall be taken into consideration, *mutatis mutandis*, to services. Hence, the trademark in checked whether well known in the relevant sector of the public and if the marks are found not similar a trademark is registered. The section provides a minimum period of seven years as exclusivity of sign as trademark and renewable indefinitely. A registration of a trademark may be cancelled after an uninterrupted period of at least three years of non-use. Compulsory licensing of trademark shall not be permitted as per the guidelines.

Section 3 of part II discusses about geographical indications indicating the fulfillment of Paris Convention. Registration of trademarks of goods misleading the public of the true place of origin shall not be encouraged. Article 24 of agreement emphasizes on international negotiations for increasing the protection of individual geographical indications. A member shall not diminish the protection of geographical indication that existed in that member immediately prior to the date of entry into force of the WTO agreement for at least 10 years prior 15[th]April 1994 or in good faith preceding that date.

Section 4 of part II discusses about Industrial designs and indicates that a design should be new or original for registration and speaks about owner rights. The minimum duration of exclusivity is 10 years.

Section 5 of part II discusses about Patents emphasizing on subject matter that is patentable. Subject matter that is excluded from patentability is highlighted. Members shall provide for the protection of plant varieties either by patents or by an effective *sui generis* system or by any combination thereof. Article 28 of the section emphasizes the rights conferred as exclusive rights on products, processes. The owner of the patent has the right to license as contracts. It is mandatory that the patent must disclose the invention along with the best mode in clear so that person skilled in the art can carry out.

Article 31 of the section 5 emphasizes on compulsory licensing indicating that a third party should approach the patent holder for licensing. The section also indicates the other conditions in which a compulsory license may be granted. Royalty for such licensing and termination of licensing are discussed. The term of protection of a patent under article 33 is 20 years from the date of filing. Article 34 emphasizes on burden of proof especially relating to process patents. The judicial authority shall have the authority to order the defendant to prove that the process to obtain an identical product is different from the patent process.

Section 6 of part II discusses about layout designs (topographies) of integrated circuits. The section indicates fulfillment of treaty on intellectual property in respect of integrated circuits and exclusive rights of the owner. The term of protection is for 10 years and may be extended another 5 years.

Section 7 of part II discusses protection of undisclosed information, commonly known as trade secrets or data exclusivity. The agreement insists on providing a provision to protect undisclosed information submitted as data to governments or government agencies. The section indicates data submitted by innovators relating to pharmacodynamics, pharmacokinetics of drug shall be protected against unfair commercial use. Members are necessary to protect such data against disclosure, except where necessary to protect the public or unless steps are taken to ensure that the data are protected against unfair commercial use. In the context of India, Indian government does not fulfill the criteria of protection as trade secrets keeping in view of the local needs. If a legislation relating to trade secrets is made in India, entry of generics into Indian market may further be hindered.

Section 8 of part II discusses on control of anti-competitive practices in contractual license. Article 40 of the section emphasizes on abuse of intellectual property rights to increase trade by licensing practices. A provision of consultation of one member with the other concerning alleged violation is made.

Part III, IV, V, VI and VII of TRIPS agreement discusses about enforcement, acquisition and maintenance of intellectual property rights and related *inter-partes* procedures, dispute prevention and settlement, transitional arrangements and institutional arrangements respectively. Emphasis on effective enforcement of action of act of infringement, with all preventive measures and the final decision by the judicial authorities are to be implemented by the members. A provision of injunction as a power to the judicial authority is provided relating to infringement act at the customs. The judicial has the authority to declare the damages as payment to be made to the rights holders during an act of infringement. Measures can be made by the members giving powers to the judicial authority to prevent act of infringements transnationally. In such case, the applicant might have to submit information necessary or lodge application for identification of the goods to the concerned authority. The rights holder has the provision of inspecting the goods detained by the customs. The agreement provides guideline for both civil and criminal proceedings where ever necessary. A transparency provision relating dispute prevention and settlement among members through the council of TRIPS is made. A transitional arrangement of 5 years to fulfill the agreement by the members, however some flexibility of additional 5 years to finally implement product patent system is made. A provision of exclusive marketing rights shall be granted for a period of five years after obtaining marketing approval in that member or until a product patent is granted or rejected, whichever period is shorter, provided that, subsequent to the entry into force of the WTO agreement, a patent application has been filed and a patent granted that product in another member and marketing approval obtained in such other member. The guideline provides a provision of institutional arrangement to TRIPS as a council in order to communicate, administer, monitor, receive and settle disputes of the members with simultaneous consultations with World Intellectual Property Organization.

India after becoming the member of World Trade Organisation, a ten year transition period was given during which infrastructure, legislations necessary were established. The Patents Act, 1970 was amended thrice in the years 1999, 2002 and 2005 to oblige TRIPS obligations.

Questions

1. What is TRIPS agreement?
2. When TRIPS agreement originated in India?
3. Write in detail about TRIPS agreement relating to pharmaceuticals?
4. Did India fulfill TRIPS agreement, explain in detail?

CHAPTER 7

The Patents Act, 1970

Prior 1950, Ayurvedic system of medicine prevailed in India. Herbs were cultivated and necessary demand was not fulfilled. Meanwhile, Allopathic system promised early cure of a disease and synthetic methods were adopted in India to meet the demands. Majority of the products were imported and drug prices were high and not reachable by common man. Indian government appointed justice Rajagopala Ayyangar committee in 1957 and it suggested for revision of patent law with process patent system so that drug prices come down. This led to enactment of The Patents Act 1970.

The Patents Act, 1970 has twenty three chapters with a total of 163 sections including repealed. The Act was amended for five times and post WTO three amendments are considered to be the most significant to the current scenario and usually considered as three amendments made to the Act.

7.1   INVENTIONS NOT PATENTABLE

Chapter II, Section 3, of the Act discusses about Inventions not patentable. Inventions that are frivolous, contrary to well established natural laws, mere commercial exploitation, contrary to public order or morality, serious prejudice to human, animal or plant life or health or to the environment, mere discovery of scientific principle, abstract theory, mere discovery of a new form of a known substance, mere new use, mere admixture, mere arrangement or re-arrangement, method of agriculture or horticulture, process of medicinal, surgical, curative, prophylactic or treatment of human beings or animals, plants or animals in whole or any part thereof other than microorganisms but including seeds, varieties of species, biological processes for production or propagation of plants and animals, mathematical or business method or a computer programme, literary, dramatic, musical, artistic work, mere scheme or rule or method of performing mental act or method of playing game, presentation of information, topography of integrated circuits, traditional knowledge, inventions relating to atomic energy are not patentable. Section 5 under the chapter was omitted indicating both process and product patent applications are accepted for a grant subject to fulfilling patentability criteria.

In relation to pharmaceuticals section 3d, 3e and 3f have a significant role. Section 3d emphasizes invention that are relating to mere discovery of a new form of a known form as not patentable. This indicates that drug substances in the form of new salts, esters, ethers, polymorphs, metabolites, pure form, particle size, isomers, mixtures of isomers, complexes, combinations and other derivatives of known substance shall be considered to be the same substance, unless they differ significantly in properties with regard to efficacy. In addition to this, a new use of a known substance shall not be considered as an invention.

Section 3e, emphasizes that a substance obtained by a mere admixture resulting only in the aggregation of the properties of the components thereof or a process for producing such substance.

Section 3f, emphasizes that the mere arrangement or re-arrangement or duplication of known devices each functioning independently of one another in a known way.

Several applications received at the patent office relating to section 3d, 3e or 3f were either granted or rejected for a patent based on case by case implying that such innovations should have clinically significant efficacy for a grant else rejected from a patent grant.

Section 3j, indicates that living things other than microorganisms are not patentable. This implies one side that microorganisms are livings things, on the other side that even though microorganisms are livings things, are patentable. Diamond *vs.* Chakraborthy is a revolutionary case in United States for the first time in the World, a living thing was granted with a patent. Chakraborthy is an Indian origin US settled microbiologist. He developed a strain of bacteria that is not naturally occurring in nature and can fragment crude oil. An application was filed for a patent and the judge Diamond of the US Courts argued as not a patentable subject matter as the microorganism is a living thing. Chakraborthy was successful and a patent was granted for the microorganism even though it is living thing since the microorganism did not exist naturally in nature and came into existence through human interference. Since then, a provision is made for patenting microorganisms that are developed through human interference.

7.2   Patentable Subject Matter

It is mandatory that subject matter involved in the invention should fulfill the criteria of patentability. A subject matter only when fulfill, novelty, non-obviousness, usefulness and is enabled is considered as a patentable subject matter. If any one of the four criteria is not fulfilled, an application may be rejected from grant of a patent.

7.2.1 Novelty

A subject matter is considered as novel when it has newness. Such inventive step should be assessed by the person skilled in the art. In several cases it is necessary to demonstrate the novelty of the invention with the existing inventions in the field. It is quite often to ensure novelty with obviousness.

7.2.2 Non-Obviousness

Obvious means easily seen. A subject matter that is already known to the public, persons skilled in the art indicates the technology under discussion is obvious. A subject matter to fulfill the patentability criteria it should qualify non-obviousness. To ensure the subject matter is non-obvious we have to look into all the knowledge resources for possible obviousness. Once the subject matter fails obviousness, it indicates that the subject matter is non-obvious and fulfills one of the patentability criteria.

A person skilled in the art ensure the subject matter is non-obvious either by checking prior art in available literature. Subject matter of discussion in thoroughly reviewed from research paper publications in journals, magazines, thesis books etc., as non-patented literature or in patented literature both at national and international levels. In several cases the person skilled in the art have to thoroughly assess his level of knowledge in the field of discussion, identify the problems encountered in the field of invention, solutions already available, the solution to the current invention provides and the amount of inventive activity taking place in the field. In several cases, the subject of discussion may not be available in literature but well-practiced by the public. Hence it is necessary to thoroughly review the prior art and ensure that the subject matter is not seen as obviousness and qualifying as non-obviousness.

7.2.3 Use-Full

Utility is also called as use-full. Use-full especially indicates industrial applicability indicating commercial use. An invention mere of commercial exploitation does not qualify patentability criteria. Hence, a subject matter if does not have any industrial applicability may not be considered for the grant of a patent.

7.2.4 Enable

A subject matter that has qualified for novelty, non-obviousness and useful, if not enabled, a patent is not granted. This means that enabling the invention indicates that the invention is disclosed. It is necessary in the complete specification the entire invention made is disclosed. Among the experiments conducted, the best method or best mode or best embodiment of the invention has to be emphasized by the inventor.

7.3   Contents of a Patent

A patent granted contains a title, patent number, bibliographic data, date of filing, abstract, field of invention, prior art, summary of the invention, figures/drawing/chemical structures/tables, detailed description of the invention, best mode, claims.

7.3.1 Title

A title should indicate what kind of technology is developed as an invention. A title should be short and should help in quick assessment of what the invention is about. Several times, a title does not match to the invention that the person skilled in that art is seeking for. An invention patented in several countries might not have the same title and may be changed to the local needs or as instructed by the examiner of the application. It is quite often observed that a common terminology is used as title, making critical for prior art search.

7.3.2 Abstract

An abstract of a patent gives a quick understanding in knowing about the invention made. After the title, it is the abstract of the patent that is made available in public domain especially in several databases. Chemical Abstract Services of American Chemical Society provide list of abstracts that are published in journals. An abstract must discuss the basis of taking up the work and that led to the invention. It should be precise, in short and must provide the conclusion drawn from the invention in brief.

7.3.3 Field of Invention

Before further reading of the complete invention discussed in the patent document, this section helps in knowing the exact technology developed in the current invention. A particular field of technology is further involved with different technologies and this provision helps the persons skilled in the art to further read the invention mentioned in the patent. For instance, in pharmaceuticals an indication of solid dosage form in the title indicates a broad scope to a person skilled in the art. Field of invention narrows down and indicates the exact technology to which the current invention is about.

7.3.4 Prior Art

Prior Art is also called as background of the invention. The lead for an invention is based upon the technology available in the field of interest. A thorough review of the technology helps to understand the extent of the development made in the field and the setbacks existing. Based upon this, new ideas are developed and new experiments are made and the results are fruitful, indicates that the current invention made has some advantages with respect to the past work. A patent examiner when reads the prior art or back ground of the invention, he will have the preliminary idea of the current invention indicating how it fulfill the patentability criteria. Hence, background of the invention has a critical role in judging whether the current invention fulfilled patentability criteria for a grant of a patent. Several patents are granted based on less number of steps involved in the invention, commercially viable process, clinically significant in efficacy. It is a common practice in quoting the published literature, their setback and how the current invention overcomes the problems with past work.

7.3.5 Summary of the Invention

In this part, a brief discussion relating to the invention is made. The chief points commonly called as embodiments are discussed in brief. A summary may end up with a few hundred words to several pages in a patent document. Several times, the broad scope of the invention can be understood which is not indicated in the detailed description of the invention or claims included in the patent document.

7.3.6 Figures/Drawings/Chemical Structures/Tables

In this section, any drawings, figures, chemical structures, tables relating to the invention are included. Several times, these are included at the right place where ever necessary along with text present in the document. In several patent offices, the patent document available for retrieval from online databases is either in complete format or in fragmented format. For instance, patent retrieval from the US patent office in html format is different from Tagged Image File Format (TIFF). Several figures, drawings are not possible to be included as html format, but possible in TIFF. In such conditions, the figures, drawing are present as separate documents in the database. Likewise, chemical structures are not feasible in html format and available in TIFF format. Markush was the first to implement several chemical structures using one general chemical structure and since then, all the patent offices in the world suggest for Markush chemical structure representations (Figure 7.1). Tables are usually the data that was established during the process of invention. Indian patent office provides complete text present in the patent document in html format and especially figures such as drug release profiles as a separate document.

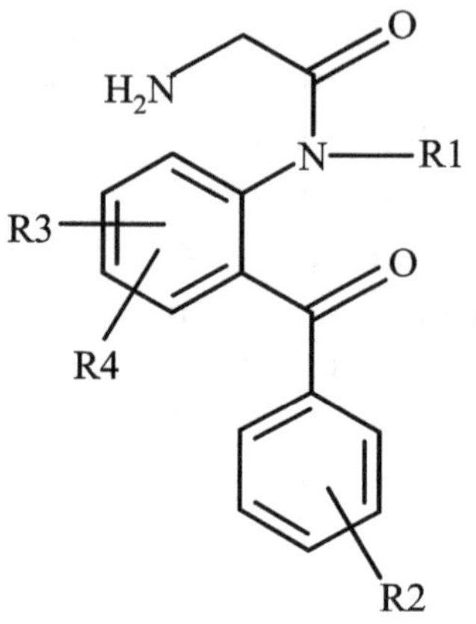

Figure 7.1 Markush Chemical Structure.

7.3.7 Detailed Description of the Invention/Embodiments

In this section, the inventor describes completely about the invention. Several times, the section is also referred to as embodiments. Several aspects that are not available in the summary section are being made available here. Reference numbers relating to biological materials submitted as per international treaties, approval by national biodiversity authority are included. Here, several methods followed, parameters monitored describing the sequence of methodology used to achieve the invention are described. Where ever necessary suitable figures/drawings/chemical structures/tables might be included. The scope of the invention is completely described with the limited experiments conducted by the inventor and may be understood. Suitable examples are quoted with respect to the experiments made. Several times, a patent document does not contain all the experimental data generated and the broad scope of the invention is specified, which a person skilled in the art easily understand.

Among the experiments conducted under the purview of the inventor, it is necessary that inventor emphasize and mentions the experiment in which the outcome of the invention is the best to his knowledge. In several cases, patents were revoked, invalidated and gained commercial importance to a third party, for the inventor being guilty in mentioning the best mode/best embodiment of his invention.

7.3.8 Claims

A patent document ends with the claims. A claim contains a preamble, transitional phrase and body. Claims determine the territory, boundary of the invention. It is the claims that describe the inventor's exclusivity. Drafting a claim is crucial and such claims should not be too narrow or too broad. In several cases, an improper claim drafting led to creation of new inventions leading to new patent grants. A person skilled in the art can develop a new invention based on the claims made.   In pharmaceuticals, claims help us whether the inventor has exclusivity for a process or product. A claim should describe the complexity of science and able to distinguish from prior art.   A complete specification contains one or more claims.   A claim starts with an independent followed by it's dependent.   A specification may contain multiple independent with corresponding dependent claims.   The word comprising instead of consisting is commonly used in claim drafting indicating that the parameters or ingredients or sequence of steps are flexible and not rigid in conducting the experiment giving broad scope of protection of the invention to the inventor.

For instance, US Patent 4,996,197 mentions an independent claim "an ophthalmic composition comprising Rhamsan gum and at least one ophthalmic pharmacologically active substance" indicating the patent is claiming a process for a pharmaceutical formulation made using Rhamsan gum.   The formulation can be formulated for any active pharmaceutical ingredient either in single or in combinations for said ophthalmic route of administration.

Indian patent IN 201928 mentions an independent claim "A compound of formula (I), a pharmaceutically acceptable ester, ether or N-alkyl derivative thereof, or a pharmaceutically acceptable salt thereof" indicating a product claim.

In Indian patent IN 209877, the text of the patent document "Further, active ingredients or substances, where applicable, may be present either in the form of one substantially optically pure enantiomer or as a mixture of enantiomers or polymorphs thereof. The active ingredient or substance can be poorly soluble, soluble or highly soluble. The active ingredients or substances are comprising of the following therapeutic classes but not limited to general anesthetics, angiotensin converting enzyme inhibitors, angiotensin receptor antagonist, antacids, anti-rheumatoid, anti-asthmatics, anti-allergics, antiarrhythmic, antibiotics, anti-convulsants, anti-depressants, anti-diarrhoeals, anti-emetics, anti-histamines, anti-infective, anti-bacterials, antiviral, antifungal, anti-protozoals, anti-inflammatory agents, anti-nauseants, anti-hyperlipidemic drugs, anti-parkinson, anti-helmintics, antipsychotics, antipyretics, anti-spasmodic, antithrombotic drugs, anticoagulants, anti-platelets, anti-tumor drugs, anti-uricaemic drugs, anxiolytic agents, appetite stimulants, appetite suppressants, bronchodialators, anti-hypertensives(diuretics, beta-blockers, ACE inhibitors, calcium channel blockers, vasodialators), chelating agents, cholecystokinin antagonists, cognition activators, cough suppressants, erythropoietic drugs, fertility agents, antidiarrhoeals, laxatives, antiulcer agents, growth regulators, immunomodulating agents, neuroleptics, neuromuscular agents, potassium channel blocker, potassium channel opener, prostaglandins, respiratory stimulants, selective aldosterone receptor blocker, sedatives & hypnotics, synthetic hormones, tachykinin nk 1 antagonist, vaso-constrictors and vertigo agents and vitamins.

Examples of active ingredients or substances comprise of, but not limited to AAE581, AAG561, abacavit sulfate, abciximab, ABT-510, ABT-751, acarbose, acetaminophen, acyclovir, aesloratadine, AG-1749, aldosterone antagonist, alendronate sodium, almotriptan, alprazolam, aminocaproic acid, amlodipine besylate, AMP397, amphetamine, anagrelide hydrochloride, anastrazole, aprepitant, aripiprazole, atorvastatin calcium, atrasentan, AZD0328, AZD0865, AZD0902, AZD2171, AZD3409, AZD4282, AZD4750, AZD5106, AZD7140, azelnidipine, azithromycin, balsalazide disodium, bazedoxifene, betaxolol hydrochloride, bicalntamide, BILN-2061, biperiden HC1, bisoprolol fumarate, bromfenac sodium, buformin, candesartan cilexetil, captopril, carboplatin, carvedilol, CCI-779, cefadroxil, ceftriaxone sodium, celecoxib, CEP 7055, cerivastatin, cetrizine HC1, CHC12103, chlorthalidone, CHS 13340, ciglitazone, cilastazole, ciprofloxacin, clindamycin, clofapine, clonazepam, clopidogrel bisulfate, clorazepate dipotassium, chlorpropamide, clozapine, CP-122,721, CP-526,555, CP-529, 414, CRF-1 antagonists, CS-003, CS-011, CS-023, CS-502, CS-505, CS-706, CS-747, CS-866, cyclophosphamide, cyclosporine, deloratadine, desloratadine, dexmethylphenidate HC1, dextroamphetamine sulfate, diclofenac sodium, dicyclomine hydrochloride, digoxin, diltiazem, divalproex sodium, docetaxel, dofetilide, domperidone, doxazosin mesylate, doxercalciferol, doxorubicin HC1, dronedarone, dulaxetine, emiglitate, enalapril maleate, enbrel, endesartan, englitazone, enoxaparin sodium, enzothiadiazine, eplernone, eplivanserin, epoetin alpha, eprosartan, eptifibatide, erythromycin, escitalopram, esomeprazole magnesium, esters of ampicillin, estradiol, estropipate, ethacrynate sodium, etoricoxib, exemestane, famotidine, fexofenadine HCl, fidalestat, fluoxetine, fluoxetine HCl, fluticazone propionate, fluvastatin sodium, fluvoxamine maleate, fondaparinux sodium, frovatriptan, FTY720, fudosteine, fulvestrant, gabapentin, galantamine HCl, galopentin, ganirelix acetate, gemitatrine HCl, glatiramer acetate, glibenclamide (glyburide), glibornuride, gliclazide, glimepiride, glipizide, gliquidone, glisoxepid, gosereline acetate implant, granisetron, guanabenz acetate, guanylate cyclase inhibitors, haloperidol, hydralazine, hydrochlorothiazide, hydromorphone HCl, hydroxyurea, ICL670, idraparinux, imatinib mesylate, indapamide, infliximab, ipratropium bromide, irbesartan, isosorbide 5-mononitrate, isosorbide dinitrate, isotretinoin, itrozole tablets, J695, ketorolac trimethamine, KUC 7483, lactobionate, 1AF237, lafutidine, lamotrigine, landiolol, latanoprost, leflunomide, letrozole, levetiracetam, levofloxaine, levonorgestrel, levothyroxine sodium, linezolid, levothyronine sodium, lisinopril, loperamide, loratidine, lorazepam, losartan, lovastatin, ludrocortisone acetate, mabthera, MCC-135, meloxicam, mephalam, metformin hydrochloride, methylphenidate HCl, MH-15E, miglitol, minoxidil, misoprostol, mometasone furoate-monohydrate, montelokast sodium, moxifloxacin HCl, MS 209, MS 275, naratriptan hydrochloride, nateglinide, nebirapine, nebivolol, neorecormon, niacin, nicorandil, nifedipine, nitricoxide, nitroprusside, NK-104, NKS 104, NM 283, norethindrone acetate, norgestrel,

NS 2330, octreotide acetate, olanzepine, olmesartan, omeprazole, ondensetron HCl, orlistat, osanetant, oseltamivir phosphate, oxaliplatin, oxcarbazepine, oxistat, oxprenolol, oxybutynin chloride, paloxetine HCl, pantoprazole sodium, paroxetine, paroxetine HCl, pazufloxacin, pemoline, pentoxyphylline, perindopril, phenbutamide, picotamide, pimecrolimus, pioglitazone, potassium chloride, pralnacasan, pravastatin sodium, propranolol, prucolapride, PTK787, quetiapine, quetiapine fumarate, quinapril, R1068, R1204, R-142440, R1439, R1440, R1453, R1487, R1518, R1549, R1559, R411, R450, R673, R701, R744, rabeprazole sodium, raloxifene HCl, ramipril, ranitidine hydrochloride, renzapride, RHIL-11, ribavarin, rimonabant, risedronate sodium, risperidone, rituximab, rivastigmine tartrate, rofecoxib, roloxifene HCl, ropinirol, rosiglitazone maleate, rosuvastatin, SAB378, salmeteyol xinafoate, saredutant, serm 6471, sertraline HCl, sildenafil citrate, simvastatin, sirolimus, sitafloxacin, sodium valproate, somatropin, sotalol, SR 123781, SSR 126517, SSR 180575, SSR 250411, SSR 591813, sulodexide, sumatriptan succinate, T-1249, TAK-013, TAK-370, TAK-559, TAK-637, tamsulosin HC1, TAP-144SR, TCH346, TCV - 116, telbivudine, telmisartan, temozolomide, terbinafine HC1, timolol, tipranavir, tirapazamine, tolazamide, tolbutamide, tolcyclamide, tolterodine tartrate, tolterodine tartrate, tomoxetine HC1, topiramate, topotecan HC1, tramadol, trandolapril, trastuzumab, troglitazone, UK-338,003, UK-369,003, valacyclovir HC1, valdecoxib, valsartan, valtorcitabine, vancomycin hydrochloride, venlafaxine, voriconazole, warfarin sodium, xaliproden, zafirlukast, zalcitabine, ziprasidone, ziprasidone mesylate, zofenopril calcium, Z01446, zoledronic acid, zolpidem tartarate, ZP 10, etc.

In a preferred embodiment of the present invention, the active ingredient or substance selected are venlafaxine HC1, sodium valproate, domperidone maleate, diltiazem HC1 and mixtures thereof.

In a most preferred aspect, in the invention venlafaxine is used in the form of venlafaxine hydrochloride indicating the invention is relating to a formulation design claimed for any category of the drug available in the market, but the invention was worked on specific drugs. Such patents are usually called as platform patent.

7.4 TYPES OF PATENT APPLICATIONS

Patent applications are of six types. They are provisional application, complete application, patent of addition/additional patent application, divisional application, convention application, PCT application. It is necessary to understand that necessary forms with required fee to be submitted.

7.4.1 Provisional Application

A provisional application is also called as provisional specification. An inventor during his experimentations, the invention is incomplete but the subject matter fulfills patentability criteria of novelty, non-obviousness and usefulness and under such circumstances, the inventor can apply for a patent based on the data available during that time calling as provisional application. A provisional specification need not have complete details of his invention but whatever information that fulfills the criteria has to be submitted. At this stage, the inventor need not have to submit figures, drawings, and claims. In brief, about the invention may be considered. The benefit of a provisional application is that the inventor has the right to claim priority of his invention. However, it is mandatory that the inventor has to submit his complete specification within 12 months from the date of filing provisional specification/application.

7.4.2 Complete Application

A complete application is also called as complete specification. An inventor can directly apply a complete specification without a provisional application provided he is sure of no such invention is made earlier or filed by others. In several cases, a thorough review of prior art may be necessary to ensure that the subject of invention is not in public domain made by others either in research journals, thesis books, patent application filings, patent grants, patent surrendered, patent revoked, patents invalid etc. A complete specification must fulfill all the contents of a patent. The advantage with direct filing of a complete specification is that the invention has better exclusive time which may be lost when a provisional application is submitted.

7.4.3 Patent of Addition

During the invention process, the inventor files an application for a patent based on the experiments conducted and information established. A patent might be granted for the invention. At a later stage, the inventor during his experiments has observed some improvements in his inventions and wishes to have exclusivity. Under such circumstances, the inventor may submit an additional patent application wherein the priority of the application is considered as per the main patent. This indicates that an additional patent or patent of addition have an exclusivity period of the left over time period of the main patent. In several cases, a main patent might be revoked under the grounds of not fulfilling patentable subject matter and the additional patent or the patent of addition application shall be considered as a fresh patent, claiming the exclusivity term leftover. A patent of addition shall not be granted before grant of the patent of the main invention. In developed countries, several patents are extended in their term due to improvements in the patented invention and being protected for the improvements. Such provision of ever green of patents is not permitted in India.

7.4.4 Divisional Application

A patent is granted for only one invention. Several times the inventor may file an application for a grant of patent and during the examination process, the examiner identifies the application consisting of more than one invention and in such situations, the examiner may suggest for a separate application as a divisional application indicating a separate patent application for another invention.

7.4.5 Convention Application

A convention application implies a Paris convention application. Patent application procedure, examination, granting procedures are considered at international and national phases (especially through PCT) and discussed at a later stage. An inventor may file application in a foreign patent office without a grant in the native country provided the native and foreign countries are members of Paris Convention. However, the inventor has to get prior permission from the controller of patent of the native country, for application in the foreign convention country. Several pharmaceutical companies have application filing strategies for effective exclusivity coverage saving money and time. The term of a patent granted through Paris Convention is 20 years from the priority date. In several cases, it is necessary to check whether the country of interest is a member of Paris convention.

7.4.6 PCT Application

An inventor in his native patent office may submit an application for grant of patent in the countries which are members of Patent Co-operation Treaty (PCT). After filing an application (Annexure 6) in the native country, the inventor can decide in deciding the countries he wishes to have a granted patent as PCT application within 12 months. An application through PCT helps the inventor in single application filing, minimum translations, single examination procedure, single international search report, minimized fee, saving time and getting patent protection in several countries. As per the TRIPS agreement, every country of the agreement has to provide provisions for receiving, examination of applications for grant in different countries through PCT.

7.5   RIGHTS OF INVENTOR/PATENTEE

The first inventor of an invention has the sole rights for submission of application for a patent. Necessary application form for grant of patent (form 1), provisional or complete specification (form 2), statement of undertaking (form 3), and declaration as to inventor ship (form 5) along with the prescribed fee has to be submitted. The first inventor can be an individual or an employee to an organisation where the employer becomes the applicant. In most of the cases, an application is filed by an authorized, qualified patent agent or patent attorney who is eligible for communicating with patent office and following the procedures until grant of a patent (See Annexure 6 for mentioned forms).

Once a patent is granted, the inventor becomes the patentee and has the exclusive right to make, sell, use or import the invention patented. The patentee has the right to prevent and monitor any third party is directly or indirectly making, selling, using or importing the invention for commercial benefits. The patentee has the right to claim damages from the date of grant of patent if a third party is violating the exclusive rights for commercial benefits. The patentee can voluntarily submit an application form with the description of the goods for which he possesses exclusivity to the regulatory authority especially to the customs authority for illegal entry of the goods into the country. The patentee has the rights to inspect any suspicious place of business of his product for which he possesses exclusive rights. Where two or more persons as co-owners have a granted patent and possess exclusive rights, each shall possess an equal undivided share in the patent. Where two or more persons are co-owners of a patent, unless written agreement among the co-owners, either of patentees does not have the rights to license it out to a third party. It is the duty of the patentee to identify the infringer.

7.6   Term, Grant of Patent

A term of a patent is 20 years from the date of filing. In several cases, multiple priorities are being made and it is necessary to identify the first filing.

In case of a patent of addition, the validity of the patent is the leftover term of the main patent. Where a main patent was revoked by the patentee or revoked by the controller of patents due to lack of patentability criteria, the patent of addition shall be having exclusivity with respect to first filing of filing of the invention considered and the patent of addition becomes independent patent.

In case of a divisional patent, the term of the patent is twenty years from the date of filing the main application from which multiple inventions were made as individual patent applications and were granted with individual patents.

In case of patent granted through PCT application, the term of the patent is for twenty years from the date of first international filing.

In case of patent granted through Paris convention, the term of the patent is for twenty years from the date of first filing either at national or international level whichever is earlier.

In several cases, multiple provisional specifications, multiple complete specifications being submitted, multiple amendments were made in complete specifications, claims and under such circumstances, the term of the patent has to be individually assessed. In case of provisional and complete specifications, the earliest date of disclosure is considered for priority date. In several cases, the subject matter is disclosed in both provisional and complete specification and the later date is considered upon genuine reasons.

In several cases, claims are not submitted at once but several times. Under such situations, the priority date of that claim shall be the date of the filing of the application accompanied by that specification. A situation may arise, the subject matter is claimed partly in one and partly in another, and the priority date of that claim shall be the date of the filing of the application accompanied by the specification of the later date.

Where a claim in a complete specification has two or more priority dates, the earliest among the dates is considered as priority date of the claim.

A provision of postdating is accepted when the inventor feels to cancel provisional application and wants to consider date of complete specification as the date of filing. On genuine reasons it might be considered and postdated to complete specification date.

In several cases, a term of a patent is extended to encourage the inventor on certain grounds. Especially veterinary, pediatric, orphan drug patents are extended with respect to patent term as the business is limited, subject to genuine reasons, especially in the United States.

An application when fulfilled all the criteria, shall be placed in order of grant and shall be granted. The controller directs the patent document available to the public. The date of patent shall be the filing date of application and is entered in the register.

7.7   INFRINGEMENT

When a third party without the notice of the patent holder violates and on commercial grounds make, sell, use or import the patented invention, the act is considered as infringement. It is the duty of the patentee to monitor and identify potential infringers of his patented subject matter. The patentee has the right to file a case on the infringer. Infringement can be classified into three types i.e., literal (direct) infringement, doctrine of equivalence, and prosecution history estoppel.

7.7.1 Direct Infringement

When a third party knowingly or un-knowingly make, use, sell or import a product that is under the purview of the claims made for an invention that was already patented, then the third party's act is considered as direct or literal infringement.

7.7.2 Doctrine of Equivalence

In several cases, the third party's act cannot be concluded as direct infringement. In such circumstances, a triple identity test is being conducted. The triple identity test, work on the principle of same function, same use, same result. If the third party's act justifies the triple identity test, it is concluded as an act of infringement. For instance, a bicycle was patented by innovator A and later innovator B came up with a tricycle and applied for a patent. Innovator A can file a case as an act of infringement. Upon review, a bicycle might be different from tricycle in a lay man's point of view, but for a person skilled in the art can judge that tricycle has same function, same way and same result like that of bicycle. Hence, on the grounds of doctrine of equivalence (Annexure 7), a patent may not be granted for the innovation made by B.

7.7.3 Prosecution History Estoppel

In several infringement cases, the judge might not be able to decide whether an act of infringement has taken place with respect to direct infringement or doctrine of equivalence. Especially in chemical, pharmaceutical industries, a few parameters might not have significance in consideration initially. Later on, such parameters might have a significant role and lead to crucial decisions to judge whether a patent to be granted or not to be granted on the grounds of infringement.

For instance, scientist 'A' has developed a method and claimed for pH range of 6-9. Later, another scientist 'B' has developed a method and claimed for pH 5. Scientist 'A' when filed a case against 'B' as an act of infringement on the grounds that pH 5 has no significant difference with pH 6, it is the person skilled in the art/judge to decide whether a patent to be granted to 'B'. In order to decide, the judge might review several other non-related infringement cases and their judgment. Interestingly, it was found that scientist 'A' has amended his claims during his prosecution for pH 6-9 based on an already granted patent prior to his application filing for the sake of getting a patent. This piece of history of prosecution has given an indication and a patent was granted to scientist 'B'. Such amendments made by scientist 'A' are called as 'prosecution history estoppel'. The case of Hilton Davis Chemical Co *vs*. Warner Jenkinson addresses the parallel grounds of doctrine of equivalence and prosecution history estoppels (Annexure 7).

Parallel import is a provision by which importing patent products from an authorized license holder being exempted from an act of infringement.

Several disputes were witnessed in the past relating to transit of pharmaceutical goods from India to destination country. The goods were considered as an act of infringement while halting at a different country before reaching the destination country. Such infringement issues arose either due to non-uniformity of patent grants, same product of different process patents, or a product patent. Such act of infringement can be resolved under genuine reasons else, the product may be destroyed by the customs or the regulatory authority.

Some of the crucial (pharmacodynamics, pharmacokinetics) data generated by the innovators of new drug is being submitted to the drug regulatory authority for approval and release into the market. Such data is safeguarded in several countries (unlike India) and prevent use by the generic industries where it is mandatory to submit the innovator's data as reference and generic company's bioequivalence data for comparison. Use of such data during the data, patent, market exclusivity period may be considered as an act of infringement. However, such data may be referred and submitted under the provision of Bolar amendment along with generic manufacturer's data for research purpose; regulatory approval purpose provided no commercial activity is made. A stock piling of the patented invention for commercial activity before a patent has expired in considered as an act of infringement.

Several generic drug manufacturers try to file drug approval applications, especially at USFDA for early entry of their product into the market before the patent term expire, challenging as an act of non-infringement, invalidating the patent for various reasons.

In circumstances, where an accidental entry of a vessel, aircraft into the Indian territory with patented products, it is not considered as an act of infringement.

7.8   TIME LINE OF INDIAN PATENT OFFICE PROCEDURE

The procedure involved in application submissions to grant ranges from simple to very complex conditions depending on various parameters. If very well planned, an application filed may be granted with a patent at the earliest possible stipulated time schedules mentioned in The Patents Act, 1970 and The Patent Rules, 2003. In several cases, it might take at least three years for an application to be granted with a patent.

Figure 7.2 Indicates the Indian patent office procedure for receiving and grant of a patent.

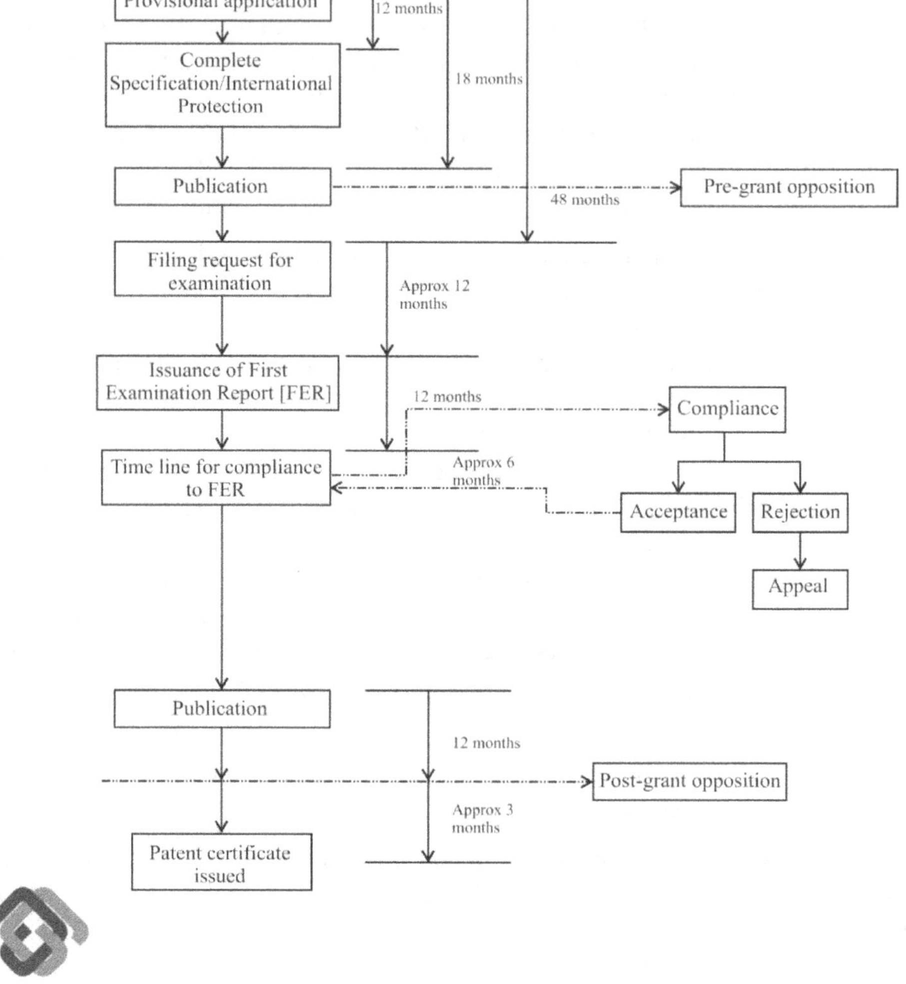

Figure 7.2 Indian Patent Procedure.

Soon after filing a provisional with necessary application form, the filing date is considered as the first reference date of filing. From the date of filing a provisional application, within 12 months a complete specification has to be submitted. The patent office within eighteen months publishes the application for a patent mentioning the details such as title, bibliographic data, and abstract of the invention on every Friday of every week in a journal. Such publication gives a provision of making the invention to be known to the public inviting for pre-grant oppositions. A party can file a pre-grant opposition at the patent office at any time before the grant of a patent. Meanwhile, the inventor or the applicant within 48 months from date of filing, can request for examination of his application. Within 6 months from the date of making a request by the inventor, the controller of patent assigns an examiner within stipulated time (1 month) for the examination of the application of the patent and the examiner submits his report to the controller of patents within stipulated time (1-3 months) and finally the patent office issues a first examination report (within the stipulated time of 12 months from the date of making the request). The inventor is provided with a provision of 12 months from the date of receiving the first examination report from the patent office to submit, amend, clarify, make changes in the specification etc. The patent office scrutinizes all the information furnished by the inventor with compliance of first examination report. If the information furnished with respect to first examination report complies, an intimation of grant communication from patent office may be made within 6 months. From the date of intimation made, within 3 months, the patent office publishes in the journal that an application for an invention has been granted with a patent. From the date of publication in the journal that a patent has been granted, a third party may submit a post grant opposition to revoke the patent grant. If no post grant opposition is observed, a patent certificate is issued within three months after twelve month expiry from the date of publication in the journal of the granted patent.

7.9   COMPULSORY LICENSING

When an invention was granted with a patent and if not worked for 3 years after grant of the patent, a third party may approach the inventor for a license to the patented invention to work and bring into industrial and commercial application. When the patentee is not willing, the third party might approach the Indian patent office, the controller of patents by submitting prescribed application form with necessary fee for grant of a compulsory license. The grounds on which the applicant is requesting for grant of a compulsory has to be justified, furnished with necessary documentary proof.

A compulsory license is also granted to a third party, when a patented invention is commercially exploited, commercially not at the reach of the public, where a country does not have the facility to manufacture drugs, and under national emergency conditions. Where a patented invention not able to fulfill the market demands, a compulsory license may be sought.

A compulsory license is for a limited term and may further be extended. However, devoid of the grounds on which the compulsory license was issued to the third party, proportional royalty with respect to the sale of the invention have to be paid to the patent holder. A compulsory license issued may not be to one individual and may be to several individual. The controller of patents has the rights to grant (Annexure 8) a compulsory license and may be revoked as and when needed. (See Annexure 9 for rejection of compulsory license application).

In India, the first compulsory license order was granted to NATCO for the Bayer's product 'Sorafenib' useful in the treatment of advanced stage of liver and kidney cancer. NATCO vs. Bayer case provides the complete prosecution history, decision, grounds on which the compulsory license was granted.

7.10   Oppositions

An opposition can be filed for an invention either as a pre-grant (Annexure 10) or post-grant opposition (Annexure 11). A patentee or third party upon valid grounds and legal provisions may oppose. An opposition is filed, usually at the patent office, as a pre-grant opposition any time before the grant of the patent. An opposition is filed at the courts (district courts) or at the Appellate Board (equivalent to high court) as a post-grant opposition with simultaneous notice to the controller. Several third parties such as social welfare organisations are playing a key role in filing oppositions. Several applications and patents granted were successfully opposed on the grounds of the invention lacking novelty, commercial exploitation, subject being obvious, lack of inventive step, subject matter being traditional knowledge, and based on the provisions of section 3. A post grant opposition must be filed within 12 months by an interested party from the date of publication in the journal indicating a patent was granted for an invention. The Patents Act, 1970 made clear indication of the eligibility criteria of an interested party to oppose for pre-grant or post-grant.

Intellectual Property Appellate Board (IPAB) was established by Central Government in the year 2007 for speedy disposal of cases present at the High Courts. Appeals can be made within three months at the Board against a decision/order/direction made by the registrar, controller etc. The controller of patents has a provision to hear the legal proceedings for an appeal. Indian IPAB located at Chennai, is constituted with chairman, vice chairman, technical members (patents, trademarks) and a deputy registrar. To become a technical member of the Board, the individual must have exercised at least five years the functions of controller or at least ten years as a registered patent agent. IPAB is currently limited to Patents, Trade marks and Geographical indications.

7.11   Powers of Controller of Patents

Soon after receiving the application at the patent office, and after publication in the journal, the inventor has to file an application to the controller of patents requesting for examination of the application. The controller within one month direct and appoint an examiner for the application. After receipt of the report from the examiner, the controller directs/issues (within 6 months from date of request made for examination) the First Examination Report (FER) to the applicant/inventor indicating to furnish all the necessary data, amendments to be made in the specification etc., within a stipulated time frame of another 12 months. The controller may refuse an application based on the examiner's report or suggest for necessary amendments. The controller of patents may suggest for a division of application based on the complete specification, claims indicating more than one invention. The controller has the powers, at the request of the applicant in post-dating an application to such a date not more than six months from the date on which it was actually made subject to the provision of the Act. The controller has the powers, in inclusion of drawings, figures, tables and other data wherever necessary.

The controller of patents may refuse an application where in the specification; claims are anticipated unless necessary changes are made with respect to provisions of the Act in terms of priority date. The controller has the authority to refuse an application under the grounds of substantial risk of infringement of a claim of any other patent and may direct to include the reference in the applicant's complete specification by way of notice to the public and later accept the application based on the grounds that patent was revoked, relevant claim being deleted voluntarily by the other patent holder or on the court's decision indicating the claim is not an act of infringement. The controller has the power in making orders of an equal share of the patent among the co-owners. Where a dispute arises among the joint applicants, the controller has the right to give an opportunity to be heard, and give necessary directions. The controller of patents have the power to assign the survivor or legal heir or as directed by the court as applicant/joint applicant for a patent.

A pre-grant opposition application may be submitted to the controller of patents and after examination, the application may be refused on the grounds of section 3, furnishing false information.

A post-grant opposition may be filed by an interested party at the courts, appellate board with simultaneous notice to the controller of patents within 12 months from the date of publication in the journal, of the invention granted with a patent. Where the controller of patents has received a notice of post-grant opposition being filed at the courts, appellate board, the controller has the right to attend the prosecution.

The controller of patents has received an application for an invention relating to defense of the country, and may direct for prohibiting or restricting the publication in the journal. The controller may direct the invention to the Central government and based on the decision received, a secrecy direction may be revoked. Where an application submitted by the applicant relating to defense and being directed by the controller to the central government, shall be periodically reviewed at six month intervals and if it appears that the invention no longer is prejudicial to the defense of India, the central government may give notice to the controller to revoke the direction.

Residents of India shall not apply for a patent outside India without prior permission received from the controller subject to submission of application within India not less than six weeks before the application outside India.

The controller has the authority to direct an application granted with a patent to be published in the journal and there upon, the relevant documents shall be open for public inspection.

Where a patentee voluntarily offers the surrender of patent, the controller may direct to publish the offer in the prescribed manner and notify every person whose name appears in the register and based on receipt of opposition, the case is heard in front of the controller and finally on valid grounds, directs orders for revoke of a patent.

The controller in general has certain powers of a civil court. He has the powers to enforce attendance of any person, directs for submission of necessary documents, directs for submission of affidavits, directs for examination, awarding costs, reviewing his own decision based on the time provisions, setting aside an order passed, directing for making necessary clerical corrections.

The controller has the powers to grant a compulsory license based on the working status of the patent. He may issue notices to the patentees to regularly submit working status (Annexure 12) of the patents granted. The controller has the powers in revoking the compulsory license. The controller has the authority to revoke a patent granted on the grounds of non-working status, but after following official procedure.

7.12 Patent Agents

Any person who is a citizen of India, completed the age of 21 years and obtained a degree in science, engineering or technology from any university in the territory of India and passed the patent agent examination and paid the required fee to register his/her name shall be deemed as a patent agent. The rights of a patent agent is to practice before the controller, prepare all documents, transact all business and discharge such other functions as may be prescribed in connection with any proceeding before the controller of patents.

A person who has discharged the functions of an examiner, controller for not less than ten years subject to provisions of the Act, shall be deemed as a patent agent.

Even though, the inventor has the provision to file his/her own application for patent, several times the role of patent agent is crucial in legal proceedings. A registered patent agent of Indian patent office is eligible for filing applications either directly or indirectly at international bureau of WIPO.

7.13 International Arrangement

As per the TRIPS agreement, India being a convention country fulfilling reciprocity, has arranged four offices located at Mumbai, Kolkata, Chennai and New Delhi to receive applications for patent. The offices are facilitated with necessary provision of receiving applications for grant of patents at foreign countries through Patent Cooperation Treaty. Indian patent office may receive; a convention application within 12 months from priority date, along with complete specification, necessary documentary proof of multiple priorities. Indian patent office is currently facilitated with all the databases, knowledge resources to conduct prior art search and issue international preliminary examination report, international search reports.

7.14 PENALTIES

A person shall be punishable with an imprisonment to an extend up to 2 years, or with fine or both upon contravening the secrecy directions to be fulfilled for an application of invention relating to defense, nuclear energy.

A person found guilty in false entry of information in the register of patents, shall be punishable with imprisonment to an extend up to 2 years, with fine or both.

A person found guilty in claiming un-authorized exclusive right for a patent shall be punishable with fine which may extent up to one lakh rupees.

A person found guilty in stamping, engraving or impressing a word "patent", or "patented" implying patent for the article has been obtained in India, shall be punishable with fine which may extend up to one lakh rupees.

A person found guilty in stamping, engraving or impressing the words "patent applied for", "patent pending" or some other word on the article, shall be punishable with fine which may extend up to one lakh rupees.

A person found guilty in using his place of business, conducting activities similar to the kind of patent office and wrongly indicating himself connecting to patent office shall be punishable with imprisonment for a term which may extend to six months, or with fine, or with both.

As per the directions of the central government, controller of patents, if a person, company is found guilty in submitting wrong information shall be punishable with imprisonment which may extend to six months, or with fine up to ten lakh rupees, or with both.

A person found guilty, for wrongly representing as a registered patent agent, shall be punishable with fine which may extend to one lakh rupees as first offence and five lakh rupees in case of second or subsequent offences.

Where an employee or a responsible employee or the employer of an organisation found guilty in contravening the provisions of the Act, he shall be punishable with imprisonment, or with fine, or with both.

QUESTIONS

1. What is the basis for enactment of The Patents Act, 1970?

2. Explain in detail inventions not patentable in India?

3. How section 3d, 3e, 3f of The Patents Act, 1970 are critical relating to pharmaceuticals?

4. When inventions are patentable relating to pharmaceuticals?

5. What are the different contents of patent?

6. What are the different types of patent applications?

7. What are the rights of a patentee?

8. What is the term of a patent?

9. What is infringement? Classify different types of infringement and explain in detail?

10. Explain patenting procedure in India with time line?

11. What is compulsory licensing? Explain in detail?

12. What are the different oppositions for a patent? When and where an opposition to be filed?

13. What are the powers of controller of patents?

14. Who are patent agents? What is their eligibility and role in pharmaceuticals?

15. Explain the provisions made by The Patents Act, 1970 when violated?

CHAPTER 8

Surrender, Revocation, Lapse, Restoration of Patent and Register of Patent

In several cases, the current legal status of a patent gives an indication for export of a product to convention countries; develop off-patented products for commercial grounds. In such cases, it is necessary to find out whether any patent was extended, surrendered, revoked, lapsed or restored.

8.1 SURRENDER OF PATENT

A patentee at any time, upon notice to the controller can surrender a patent. The controller may publish to notify other persons whose names were registered for the patent. Upon hearing oppositions, if any, the controller shall revoke the patent. A patentee surrenders a patent on the grounds of infringement of another patent, claiming for an invention that has earlier priority date, patent was obtained wrongly fully, a claim being not an invention, not new, publicly used, does not have inventive step, not useful, not able to enable, lacks disclosure of best method, was secretly used before priority date of the claim, failed to disclose information to the controller ordered to furnish, contravened secrecy direction, the subject matter already known to indigenous community.

8.2 REVOCATION

Several times, patents granted by the patent office were revoked on valid grounds to the provisions of the Act. When a patent was granted and later the central government is satisfied that the patent is for an invention relating to atomic energy, it may direct the controller to revoke the patent after giving notice to the persons whose names were entered in the register and after being heard.

On valid grounds and upon the interest of the public, a patent that was granted may be revoked after notifying the authorized persons as per the register and being heard.

Indian patent office has revoked granted patents relating to traditional knowledge (Annexure 13), etc.

8.3   LAPSE AND RESTORATION

A patent is deemed to have lapsed on the grounds that the maintenance fee was not paid to the patent office. The Act provides a provision of restoration of the lapsed patent within eighteen months from the date on which the patent ceased to have effect. The controller order to publish the application, inviting any opposition to be heard and if the controller finds unintentional grounds of failure to pay the renewal fee, delays, the controller directs for restoration of the patent. Where an infringement suit has been filed with respect to a lapsed patent, and until notice of restoration the controller may not direct for compensation.

8.4   REGISTER OF PATENTS

As per the provisions of the Act, a register shall be maintained at the patent office under the direction of central government assigning the controller to control and manage, wherein details relating to names and addresses of grantees of patents, notification of assignments, transmission of patents, licences under patents, amendments, extension, revocations, validity or proprietorship are included.

An assignment of a patent, title or share of patent, mortgage of licence shall not be valid unless the same in writing the terms and conditions are mentioned in the register. A provision is provided under the Act for rectification of register in terms of omission of an entry, omission of a wrongful entry, rectify an error or defect. Such register is open to the public for inspection wherein prima facie evidence being available.

QUESTIONS

1. Explain the condition when a patent in surrendered?

2. Explain the conditions when a patent is revoked?

3. Explain the condition when a patent is lapsed and conditions that help in restoring?

4. What is the use of register of patents?

CHAPTER 9

Expenditure for Application, Follow Patent Office Procedure, Grant of a Patent

The expenditure incurred for application, filing, and follow patent office procedures until final grant of a patent depends on several factors. The stipulated fee to be paid along with the submission of necessary forms depends on number of pages of complete specification, number of claims, whether the application filed by natural person (inventor), other than natural person, completion of patent office procedures is early when compared to the standard stipulated time frame, changes and amendments by the inventor in specifications etc. The first schedule of The Patent Rules, 2003 is currently amended as 'Patent Amendment Rules, 2014' (Annexure 14) indicating the necessary forms to be submitted and the corresponding fee if any to be paid. Currently, with the minimum provisions being provided to the natural person, the expenditure incurred is atleast Rs. 1, 00,000/- for application filing, follow the patent office protocols and maintain a patent as valid for 20 years. The initial cost of expenditure for filing and getting the grant of a patent may incur a cost of Rs. 5, 000/- to Rs. 10, 000/- (taking into consideration the minimum level) and once a patent is granted, at a later stage the inventor may take a decision in licensing out the invention patented.

QUESTIONS

1. What is the expenditure incurred in filing a patent application?

2. What is the expenditure incurred to maintain a patent until 20 years?

CHAPTER 10

Application Procedure and Time Line for Grant of Patent through PCT

World Intellectual Property Organisation provides a standard time frame to receive application, provide search report and give examination report on patentability to enter from international to national phase and is illustrated in Figure 10.1. When an application is filed initially for a native grant of a patent, the first filing date on which the application was filed is considered as the priority date. Within twelve months, the inventor may take a decision to file application at native patent office (Annexure 15) for grant of patent in the member countries of PCT (Annexure 16). An inventor, of any PCT contracting state/country has the provision in filing application for a patent directly at the International Bureau (IB) of the World Intellectual Property Organisation in any one of the ten international languages recognized i.e., Arabic, Chinese, English, French, German, Japanese, Korean, Portuguese, Russian or Spanish. The date of application through PCT is considered as the international filing date. If the application is submitted in a different language; within one month the translation version(accepted by International Search Authority for examination) has to be furnished. The choice of international search authority and international preliminary examination authority has to be furnished. The required fee with respect to international filing fee, transmittal fee, search fee to be furnished electronically to WIPO bank account along with the application either in Indian rupees, US dollars, euros or Swiss francs. The international bureau transmits all the applications, documents to the international search authority and within 16 months from the priority date, a written opinion is sent to the inventor. With 18 months from the date of priority, the application details are published in international publication. Within 28 months, the application is examined by the International Preliminary Examination Authority (IPEA) and corresponding international examination report on patentability is furnished to the inventor. If the applicant seeks protection of his invention in the PCT contracting states, the application enters from the international phase to the national phase. During the national phase, depending upon the international search report and the international preliminary examination report on patentability, a patent may be granted as per the procedures of the contracting authority. The term of a patent is for 20 years from the date of international filing for an application through PCT. Currently, India has established facility and gained status of ISA (Annexure 17, 18) and IPEA (Annexure 19, 20).

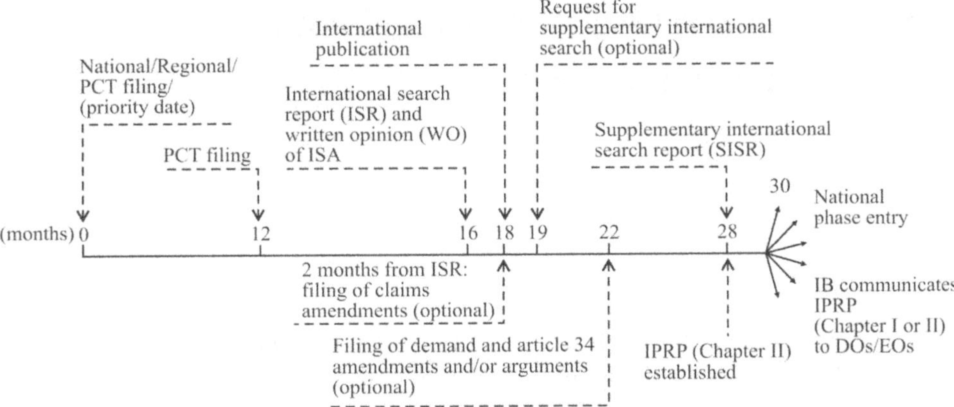

Figure 10.1 Overview of the Patenting Process using the PCT System.

QUESTIONS

1. What are the provisions of PCT?

2. What are the benefits of PCT?

3. Explain in detail for filing a patent application procedure and time line for a grant of patent through PCT?

4. What are the advantages and disadvantages of an application through PCT?

5. What are the advantages and disadvantages of an application through Paris convention and through PCT application?

CHAPTER 11

Non-Patented and Patented Literature Search

Scientific literature search helps in identifying the current status of technology in a field of interest, for a person skilled in the art. Such literature is available as research paper published in journals, thesis books. American Chemical Society provides chemical abstract services where all the scientific literature published is compiled and available in the form of chemical name index, chemical formula index, chemical substance index, patent index. A systematic chronological review updates the information and status of innovations in the field.

In several cases, the literature is available as non-patent or patented. Currently several national and international organisations are maintaining paid databases to retrieve the data. Simultaneously, patent offices of different countries in the World and World Intellectual Property Organisation are maintaining online free databases for applications filed, patents granted and indicating the status of grant, entry from international to national phase. Several times, it is necessary to identify the legal status of a granted patent in terms of whether any patent term has been extended, lapsed for not paying the fee, surrender of patent, and revoke of the patent.

When a generic drug manufacturer wishes to launch an innovator drug product as first generic or a new dosage form, it is necessary to identify the expiry of the product patent. Likewise, a bulk drug manufacturer wishes to identify a particular process of a bulk drug, when it's patent gets expired. It is a common practice in bulk drug manufacturing industry sorting all the existing processes of a bulk drug either as patented or non-patented process, sorting the chemical schemes and finally design a new process that would probably be a non-patented or non-infringing process that is economical when compared to existing technology.

At this point of time, how to identify when a product patent of an innovator drug is expiring? What are the chemical synthetic processes, that are patented, applications filed? For such information, it is necessary to understand the patent office online patent retrieval systems and on what parameters they work.

Every country grants patents in fields of engineering, pharmaceuticals (drugs), chemicals, biotechnology, food, electrical, computer electronics etc. In addition to this, how to distinguish an application, patent belonging to fine chemical industry to chemical belonging to pharmaceutical industry? The patent office, WIPO databases provide a provision of filters and Boolean operators to retrieve data from huge database.

11.1 INTERNATIONAL PATENT CLASSIFICATION

All the applications for a patent are classified based on the field of technology and again further sub-classified. Using the provision of filters along with appropriate codes in the online database, one can retrieve data relating to pharmaceuticals either for new chemical entities, bulk drug process, drug formulations, cosmetics etc.

11.2 DATE OF EXPIRY OF A PATENT

In order to identify what all the patents getting expired in a particular year, the provision of using filing date filter, mentioning a date of 20 years earlier to the expected date of patent expiry retrieves the patents that expired or going to expire.

11.3 TITLE

A title filter helps in knowing about the invention made, patented. Several times, a title is broad and retrieves patents that are of no interest. Several times, the titles given are so misleading and the expected information is no way available in the patents retrieved from the database.

11.4 ABSTRACT

An abstract is a brief discussion about the objective of taking up the invention, invention made and conclusions drawn from the experimental results. In several cases, providing a key word in the abstract filter option retrieves the required patents.

11.5 CLAIMS

The boundary of an invention is known through the claims present in the patent. A patent has independent claims followed by it's dependent claims. If a drug name is indicated in the independent claim, the patent may be concluded for a product patent. If a process, composition is mentioned in the independent claim, the patent is for an invention relating bulk drug process, formulation development respectively. Using appropriate information in the claims filter retrieves patents that are having the key word in the claims.

11.6 Text of the Patent

A text filter helps in searching a word in the entire text of a patent or an application for a patent. Several times, a product patent is for a process of the formulation claiming all the drugs available in the market for the formulation. The drugs may not be included in all, in the claims part of a patent. Such information is available in the text of the patent and such filter provision helps in retrieving the necessary data.

11.7 Name of Patentee

If the name of the first inventor or the company from which the application is made is known and mentioned in the filter, the database retrieves all the patents granted to the inventor or company.

Retrieving data using multiple filters, along with boolean operators such as 'and', 'or' helps in retrieving precise data saving time from retrieving huge data containing both wanted and un-wanted data. Upon searching the individual patent, one may retrieve list of all family patents relating the same invention, get the legal status of the patent term and entry of the application into national phase and grant status in different countries.

Questions

1. What is non-patented literature?

2. What is patented literature?

3. Is it sufficient to search non-patented literature?

4. Is it sufficient to search patented literature?

5. What are the sources for non-patented literature?

6. What are the sources for patented literature?

7. How to plan a technology in pharmaceuticals so as to aim in filing an invention for patent?

8. How you calculate patent expiry and retrieve patents?

9. How you trace out pharmaceutical patents from others?

CHAPTER 12

Comparison of the Principal The Patents Act, 1970 with The Three Amendments (1999, 2002, 2005)

After the TRIPS agreement, during the 10 year transition period, Indian government made necessary changes in The Patents Act, 1970. A total of five amendments were made from 1970 to 2005 and are as follows:

1. The Repealing and Amending Act, 1974 (56 of 1974)
2. The Delegated Legislation Provisions (Amendment) Act, 1985 (4 of 1986)
3. The Patents (Amendment) Act, 1999 (17 of 1999)
4. The Patents (Amendment) Act, 2002 (38 of 2002)
5. The Patents (Amendment) Act, 2005 (15 of 2005)

Post GATT scenario is considered to be the most significant and the amendments are most commonly called as First Amendment for 1999, Second Amendment for 2002 and Third Amendment for 2005. Even though several changes were made, the most prominent changes are discussed.

12.1 THE PATENTS ACT, 1970 (THE PRINCIPAL ACT)

Chapter II of the Act mainly discusses about inventions not patentable. Section 5 under the chapter indicates inventions where only methods or processes of manufacture patentable. In the case of inventions- (a) claiming substances intended for use, or capable of being used as food or as medicine or drug, or (b) relating to substances prepared or produced by chemical processes (including alloys, optical glass, semi-conductors and inter-metallic compounds), no patent shall be granted in respect of claims for the substances themselves, but claims for the methods or processes of manufacture shall be patentable.

The term of every patent granted under this Act shall- (a) in respect of an invention claiming the method or process of manufacture of a substance, where the substance is intended for use, or is capable of being used, as food or as a medicine or drug, be five years from the date of sealing of the patent, or seven years from the date of the patent whichever period is shorter; and (b) in respect of any other invention, be fourteen years from the date of the patent.

12.2 Patents (First Amendment) Act, 1999 Dt. 26-3-1999 w.e.f 1-1-1995

As per TRIPS obligation, a mail box facility is provided to receive the applications for product patents until 2004 and shall be examined and granted from year 2005 upon fulfilling the patentability criteria. A provision of Exclusive Marketing Rights as Chapter IV A was introduced in The Patents Act, 1970 as a first amendment. The exclusive marketing rights are for 5 years for a new drug product to market in India. The provision is limited to transition period until the implementation of product patent regime.

12.3 Patents (Second Amendment) Act, 2002 Dt. 20-5-2003 w.e.f 20-5-2003

As part of second amendment and to harmonize, reciprocate to global scenario, the following changes were made in The Patents Act, 1970:

12.3.1 Patentable Inventions

In Section 2 of the Act, several new terms were introduced and several were replaced. The terms 'non-obvious', 'useful' are considered synonymous to 'inventive step' and 'capable of industrial application' respectively.

12.3.2 Not Inventions

Section 3 of the Act, mainly discusses about subject matter that is not patentable. Plants and animals in whole or any part thereof other than microorganisms but including seeds, varieties and species and essentially biological processes for production or propagation of plants and animals as not inventions.

12.3.3 Term of Patent

To uniform among the countries and to fulfill the TRIPS agreement, the patent protection term was extended from 14 years to 20 years from the date of filing.

12.3.4 Application Requirements

Section 10 of the Act, discusses mainly about the contents of a complete specification. The complete specification must be included with title, abstract, description along with best method, drawings and claims. The date and reference number of deposit of biological materials has to be mentioned.

12.3.5 Compulsory Licence

Chapter XVI of The Patents Act, 1970 deals with working of patents, compulsory licences and revocation. Any interested third party may apply for a compulsory licence for a patented invention after three years from the date of grant of a patent. The similar ground of grant as 'licensing of rights' directly by the central government was omitted.

12.3.6 Right to Import and Parallel Imports

A provision is provided under the Act, wherein a product if imported from an authorized license holder is not an act of infringement.

12.3.7 Bolar Provision

A provision is made in the Act, the act of making or using of a patented product for research development and for submission of information to appropriate authority for market approval is considered as not an act of infringement. A third party may get a market approval for a drug product within three years before the expiration of the term of patent. The provision made in India is based on the case Roche Products vs. Bolar Pharmaceuticals held at US courts. The provision mainly helps the generic drug industry to release the drug product into Indian market soon after expiry of the product patent.

12.3.8 Burden of Proof

A new section 104A in the Act is proposed, that in the case of infringement of process patent, the burden of proof in proving that the patent is not infringed shall be on the alleged infringer. However, the alleged infringer shall not be required by the court to disclose any manufacturing or commercial secrets when such disclosure is found to be unreasonable.

12.3.9 Provision for Traditional Knowledge and Biological Diversity

Subject matters relating to pharmaceuticals and coming under the purview of traditional knowledge shall be identified and a patent shall not be granted or revoked. Prior permission of any resources coming under the purview of The Biological Diversity Act shall be taken from the National Biological Diversity Authority and necessary reference numbers have to be submitted.

12.4 THE PATENTS (AMENDMENT) ORDINANCE, 2004

A provision of depositing of microorganisms as reference for the public under the provision of Budapest treaty was included. Section 5 of the principal The

Patents Act, 1970 relating to process patents was omitted. This indicates that applications containing inventions relating to process as well as product claims are accepted and granted with a patent after fulfilling the patentability criteria. Chapter IV A relating to exclusive marketing rights was omitted indicating product patent grants shall be initiated and henceforth exclusive marketing rights in pharmaceuticals are granted by central drug regulatory authority and not by patent authority.

QUESTIONS

1. Brief about the principal Act of The Patents Act, 1970?

2. What are the provisions made as three amendments in The Patents Act, 1970?

3. How India fulfilled TRIPS agreement with respect to The Patents Act, 1970?

Differences in The Patents Act, 1970 with other Countries

Unlike in India, patents are granted in United States as utility patents, design patents and plant patents. In India, designs and plants are granted with exclusivity by registrations. In United States, exclusivity may be granted for a new use of a known substance, where as in India there are no separate patent grants for a new use. Initially in United States, patents were granted on first to invent basis and to fulfill TRIPS obligation, first to file system has been implemented. Software is patented in United States, where as in India they are copyright protected. Several international applications while entering into national phase in India, there is a likelihood to change the claims so that a patent is granted in India. The reason behind is mainly due to differences in patentability criteria of an individual country.

QUESTIONS

1. How you justify that India "The Patents Act, 1970" is more stringent when compared to US patent system?

CHAPTER 14

Administrative Structure of WTO, Membership and Dispute Settlement as per TRIPS Agreement

The basis of origin, purpose and functions of General Agreement on Tariffs and Trade (GATT), it's conversion to World Trade Organisation (WTO) and it's members complying with TRIPS agreement were discussed earlier. World Trade Organisation is the only global international organisation dealing with the rules of trade between nations after ratification by the parliaments of individual nations. The goal is to help producers of goods and services, exporters and importers conduct their business. The organisation helps in trade negotiations and agreement among nations. The Uruguay round of discussion that led to formation of WTO also brought an agreement among the countries in following the rules and regulations for dispute settlements.

14.1 ADMINISTRATIVE STRUCTURE OF WTO

The topmost decision making body of the World Trade Organisation is the Ministerial Conference that meets every two years. Decisions relating to multilateral trade agreements are taken at the Ministerial Conference. General Council is constituted with a chairman, representatives from all member governments and meets every two years in making decisions and working on behalf of ministerial conference. The General Council has and meets as dispute settlement body and as trade policy review body.

The General Council is supported and facilitated with various committees relating to trade, and separate councils for trade in goods, Trade Related Aspects of Intellectual Property Rights (TRIPS) and trade in services. Secretariat facilitated with director general and staff looks after the administrative aspects of WTO.

TRIPS council, headed by a chairman, is open to all WTO members and administers TRIPS agreement. Members of TRIPS agreement communicate with the council and provide details of the intellectual property legislations, regulations and practices through notifications. Such notifications to the council impart transparency, reviewing those members who delayed in notifying the TRIPS compliance, and providing technical cooperation among countries to bring out laws and implementation.

The organisational structure of World Trade Organisation is as mentioned in Figure 14.1.

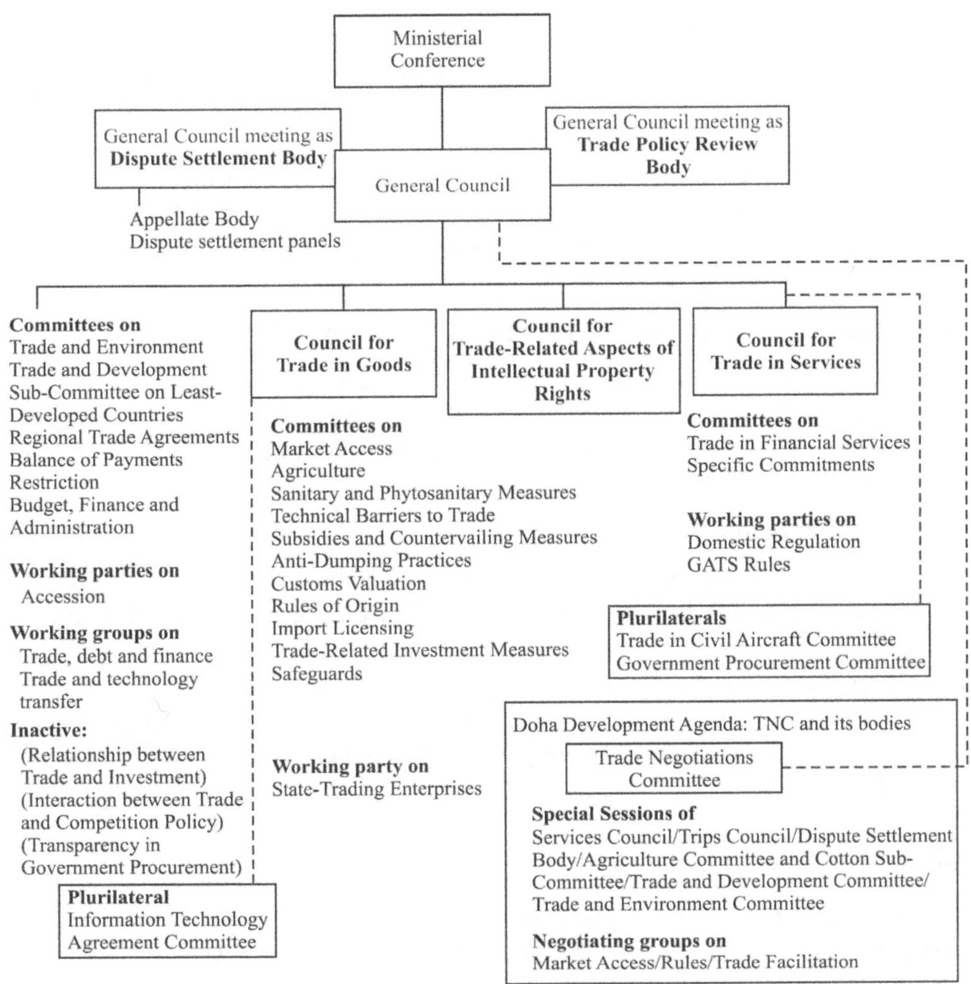

Figure 14.1 Organisational structure of World Trade Organisation.

14.2 Membership

Any country that has the autonomy in the conduct of it's trade policies can join the World Trade Organisation. A four stage protocol is followed.

(a) Voluntary disclosure of the details of the country

The country interested must describe the details of its trade and economic policies especially relating to WTO agreement as a memorandum. The memorandum is examined by the working party dealing with the country's application.

(b) Bilateral talks with non-discrimination rules

The country of interest is provided with a provision of bilateral discussions individually with everymember of WTO so that the trade interests (exports, imports), tariff reductions, policies with respect to goods and services that can be exchanged are identified. Even though the discussion is bilateral, the new member's commitments are non-discrimination rules to all the other members of WTO. Meanwhile, the working party identifies the principles and policies so as to make the new country as a member.

(c) Drafting membership terms (Terms of accession):

Soon after the completion of the examination process, probable bilateral negotiations, the working party finalizes and put forward a report, draft membership treaty (protocol of accession) and lists as schedules of the member and its commitments.

(d) Final decision

The working party's report, package and list of commitments are presented to the WTO's general council or the ministerial conference for majority voting. If two-thirds of the members vote in favour, the applicant country is free to sign the protocol. In some cases, the country's parliament has to ratify the agreement before the membership process is complete indicating the new country is also the member of WTO.

14.3 Dispute Settlement

It was the members after negotiations, authored the agreements and it is the members responsibility to settle disputes, if any. A dispute arises when a member government believes other member government is violating WTO agreement. A dispute relating to non-compliance to TRIPS obligations are subject to WTO's Dispute Settlement Understanding (DSU) comprising rules and regulations for smooth flow of business. The complaining member has to submit a "request for consultations" indicating the issues being violated and seeks Dispute Settlement Body (DSB).The members are expected to enter into consultations within 30 days. Even if after 60 days from the date of request, there is no settlement, the complaining party may request the establishment of a panel. If a third party consultation is denied, alternative means of dispute settlement, including good offices, conciliation, mediation and arbitration may be agreed by the two members. Dispute Settlement Understanding specifies rules and deadlines for deciding the terms of reference and composition of panels. Standard terms of reference will apply unless the parties agree to special terms within 20 days of the panel's establishment. Where the parties do not agree on the composition of the panel within the same 20 days, this can be decided by the Director-General. Panels normally consist of three persons of appropriate background and experience from countries not party to the dispute. The Secretariat will maintain a list of experts satisfying the criteria.

Panel procedures are set out in detail in the DSU. It is envisaged that a panel will normally complete its work within six months or, in cases of urgency, within three months. Panel reports may be considered by the DSB for adoption 20 days after they are issued to Members. Within 60 days of their issuance, they will be adopted, unless the DSB decides by consensus not to adopt the report or one of the parties notifies the DSB of its intention to appeal.

The concept of appellate review is an important new feature of the DSU. An Appellate Body will be established, composed of seven members, three of whom will serve on any one case. An appeal will be limited to issues of law covered in the panel report and legal interpretations developed by the panel. Appellate proceedings shall not exceed 60 days from the date a party formally notifies its decision to appeal. The resulting report shall be adopted by the DSB and unconditionally accepted by the parties within 30 days following its issuance to Members, unless the DSB decides by consensus against its adoption.

Once the panel report or the Appellate Body report is adopted, the party concerned will have to notify its intentions with respect to implementation of adopted recommendations. If it is impracticable to comply immediately, the party concerned shall be given a reasonable period of time, the latter to be decided either by agreement of the parties and approval by the DSB within 45 days of adoption of the report or through arbitration within 90 days of adoption. In any event, the DSB will keep the implementation under regular surveillance until the issue is resolved.

14.4 ISSUES

14.4.1 Anti-Dumping

When a country's industry exports a product to a foreign country at a price lower than the price in the native country, such an export action is called as dumping. The WTO agreement does not regulate the actions of industries engaged in "dumping". Its focus is on how governments can or cannot react to dumping — it disciplines anti-dumping actions, and it is often called the "Anti-dumping Agreement". GATT/WTO has taken necessary measures in terms of inspection of goods, valuating the goods before export, calculating the damage caused by dumped products with respect to domestic industry, extent of exemption if an act of dumping occurred w.r.t percentage of volume, export price, time boundaries in clearing the issues.

14.4.1.1 Issue of India with South Africa

A pharmaceutical company of India has exported ampicillin and amoxicillin 250 mg and 500 mg capsules to South Africa. South African Board on Tariffs and Trade (BTT) imposed anti-dumping duties on India for dumping the pharmaceutical products into the South African Customs Union (SACU). A complaint was lodged by India requesting consultations with South Africa on 1st April, 1999 based on South Africa's initiation of anti-dumping proceeding. India contended that BTT has made an erroneous methodology for determining the normal value and the resulting margin of dumping; however South African authorities established that the evaluation is unbiased. It has been identified that India was not taken into special consideration of a developing nation and hence as a violation.

14.4.1.2 Issue of Chinese Taipei (customs territory of Taiwan, Penghu, Kinmen and Matsu) with India

On 28th October, 2004 Chinese Taipei lodged a complaint on India requesting consultation on the issue of anti-dumping of seven products that include pharmaceuticals and chemicals such as analgin, potassium permanganate, paracetamol, sodium nitrite, caustic soda etc. The products are imported to India and India imposed anti-dumping duties. Chinese Taipei indicates that India violates WTO obligations. Chinese Taipei indicates that India violates with respect to rejection of information provided by Chinese Taipei exporters and lack of satisfaction as to the accuracy and reliability of the information provided by the domestic industry. Chinese Taipei indicates that India has imposed anti-dumping duties with parallel anti-dumping investigation claiming that no import has taken place in India during the period of investigation. India has imposed anti-dumping duties based on best available information on normal value and export price and Chinese Taipei claims that India did not clearly establish the information and determine the normal and export price, and the injury is not based on positive evidence, but on allegations. Moreover, Chinese Taipei claimed that India did not calculate the injury taking into consideration of all the factors legally accepted and did not give enough opportunity to defend. Chinese Taipei finally considered Indian measures are inconsistent.

14.4.2 Hindrance of Import of Pharmaceutical Products

14.4.2.1 Issue of India with Argentina

Argentina government has released Law No. 24.766 and Decree No. 150/92 with two annexures indicating that any drug product that is being imported into Argentinean territory must be registered with the National Administration of Drugs, Food stuffs and Medical Technology, Ministry of Health of Argentina. Annex I of the decree indicates countries and their pharmaceutical products are required to be manufactured in facilities approved by the relevant governmental bodies of these countries or by the Argentinean Ministry of Health and meet the National Health Authority's manufacturing and quality control requirements. Annex II of the decree indicates countries, manufacturing facilities are required to be inspected and approved by the Ministry of Health of Argentina before export of pharmaceutical products into Argentina. India was not figured out in either of the annexes. This discrimination has led to total lack of market access for Indian drugs and pharmaceutical products in Argentina. The Government of India considered that the above Law and Decree of Argentina were in violation of Article 5.1.1 of the Agreement on TBT and violates the fundamental MFN provisions under Articles I and III of GATT 1994. The Government of India considered that the Argentinean Law No. 24.766 and Decree No. 150/92 have also violated obligations under Article 5.2 of the Agreement on TBT, thus constituting unnecessary obstacles to international trade. On 25th May, 2001 India lodged complaint requesting consultations on the issue.

14.4.3 Transit Issue of Pharmaceutical Products

Post WTO agreement brought several advancements in the intellectual property regime in India. Product patent regime is new to India. Several drug products manufactured in India when exported may lead to an act of infringement due to reciprocity. A drug product manufactured in India has to be ensured for existing patents (process or product) in the foreign countries of destination or in the intermittent halting countries. A drug product may be considered as an act of infringement if enter a territory where the patent holder was not intimated or prior permission not taken. Patent holders have a provision of submitting information of their patented products to the regulatory, customs authorities requesting for infringement/seizure if such products enter into the territory.

14.4.3.1 Issue of India with European Union and the Netherlands

A series of pharmaceutical drug product consignments from India were seized by Dutch customs while transit through Netherlands (Schiphol airport). The products were found to be clopidogrel (destination to Columbia), abacavir (destination to Nigeria), olanzapine (destination to Peru), rivastigmine (destination to Peru), losartan (destination to Brazil) and were seized based on act of infringement due to existence of patent by Sanofi-Aventis; Glaxo; Eli Lilly & Co; Novartis AG; E.I. Du Pontde Nemours and Co. Inc., Merck & Co. Inc. and Merck Sharp & Dohme B.V respectively in the territory.

India understands that these seizures were made by applying the so-called "manufacturing fiction" under which generic drugs actually manufactured in India and in transit to third countries were treated as if they had been manufactured in the Netherlands. These consignments were initially detained and later, either destroyed or returned to India. In a few cases, the consignments were permitted to proceed to the destination country after considerable delay. Available evidence confirms that the customs authorities seized at least 19 consignments of generic drugs in 2008 and 2009 while in transit through the Netherlands, 16 of which originated in India. On 11th May, 2010 India lodged complaint requesting consultation.

14.4.4 Implementation of Patent/Intellectual Property System

Even though India has patent system since 1970s as The Patents Act, it was limited to process patents. After India signing WTO agreement, obliged to fulfill TRIPS agreement within the stipulated period. Several issues relating to TRIPS compliance of India were pointed out by member countries.

14.4.4.1 Issue of United States and European Communities with India

As India was only having process patent system, Indian patent office can receive applications only relating to process patents and may reject applications relating to product patents since there is no legislation for grant of product patents in India. Third party countries like United States and the European Community have the rights of exclusivity of their products in India since they are also members of WTO. As there is no mechanism of receiving applications for product patents and grant of exclusive marketing rights for such applications, United States and European community lodged a complaint on India on 2nd July, 1996 for non-compliance to TRIPS agreement. On 29th January, 1997 the dispute settlement body composed a panel and its report indicated clearly that India failed in bringing out a mechanism that preserves novelty and priority in respect of applications for product patents for pharmaceutical and agricultural chemical inventions as well as a mechanism for grant of exclusive marketing rights.

On 15th October, 1997 India as a respondent notified its concern to the legal issues identified by the panel and notified its intension to appeal. After several modifications in the reports of panel and the appellate, the dispute settlement body has finally adopted the report on 16th January, 1998. On 22nd April, 1998 during the meeting conducted by dispute settlement body, the parties agreed for 15 month time from date of adoption. On 14th January, 1999 United States requested consultations with India regarding Patents (Amendment) Ordinance, 1999 promulgated by India to implement the ruling and recommendations of the dispute settlement body. At the DSB meeting on 28 April 1999, India presented its final status report on implementation of the matter which disclosed the enactment.

14.4.4.2   Issue of European Community with Canada and India as Third Party

On 19th December, 1997 the European community lodged a complaint on Canada requesting consultations. The community claims that Canada lacks necessary legislations with respect to protection of inventions in pharmaceuticals, thus non-compliant to TRIPS agreement. The committee claims that Canada does not provide full-fledged time period of patent protection as per TRIPS agreement. On 11th December, 1998 the European Community requested for establishment of a panel at a meeting held by the dispute settlement body held on 25th November, 1998. Due to several reasons the DSB deferred the establishment of panel and later upon second request, a decision to establish a panel was taken on 1st February, 1999. Several countries including India reserved third party rights. On 25th March, 1999 the panel was composed and indicated certain concerns in the report i.e., exception of potential competitors of a patent owner being permitted to use patented invention without prior permission from patent holder during the term of the patent, for the purpose of market approval and release the product into the market soon after patent expires and exception of competitors to stockpile of patented goods during a certain period before patent expires but can be sold after patent expires. The DSB adopted the panel report on 7th April, 2000 and provided a six month period to Canada to fulfill the requirements. Canada informed the members that effective from 7th October, 2000, it has implemented the DSB's recommendations.

14.4.4.3   Issue of United States with Brazil and India as a Third Party

On 30th May, 2000 United States lodged a complaint on Brazil requesting for consultations. United States claims that Brazil's industrial property law establishes local working requirement for enjoyability of exclusive patent rights implying that local production and not importation of the patented product. United States indicated that a patented product in Brazil may be claimed for compulsory licensing provided the patented product is not locally produced. The US considered that such a requirement is inconsistent with Brazil's obligations under Articles 27 and 28 of the TRIPS Agreement, and Article III of the GATT 1994. On 1st February, 2001 DSB established a panel and on 5th July, 2001, the parties to the dispute notified DSB a mutually satisfactory solution on the matter. The mutual understanding was that, if Brazil government wishes to grant a compulsory license based on patents of US origin companies, it will prior hold talks with the United States government within the bilateral mechanism.

14.5 Representation of Indian Government to EU Over the Transit/Border Issue

European Union has proposed a settlement by confirming its principles relating to border enforcement of intellectual property. EU has agreed for necessary changes with respect to interpretation of regulations. India has taken note of the commitment offered and informed that mere transit of goods that intermittently halt at a place other than destination and where patent rights are active may not reflect to act of infringement until unless there are strong grounds of evidence that the goods entered into EU market. India notified EU that it will not request the establishment of a dispute settlement panel at the WTO. With the exchange of letters, India and the EU have reached, an informal settlement of this dispute. India would watch with interest EU's further steps in implementing its commitments. India's options to revive the dispute remain intact in case the EU does not abide by the core principles agreed to in the Understanding. Later, India after witnessing similar kind serial seizures, India and Brazil jointly consulted EU through dispute settlement body, where EU has identified the seizures are a reflection of misinterpretations of the legislations and there after EU showed willingness to resolve this dispute without resorting to the WTO dispute panel.

Thereafter, India engaged in extensive consultations with the EU with the assistance of legal experts. Finally, after several rounds of discussions, India and EU reached an "Understanding" which, inter-alia, contains the principles to guide border enforcement of intellectual property in the EU.

Questions

1. What is the administrative structure of WTO?

2. When disputes arise at WTO?

3. What is the procedure for a country to become a member of WTO?

4. What is the procedure for a country to raise a dispute and settle it?

5. Explain some of the disputes raised at WTO relating to India and how they were settled?

Chapter **15**

Technology Transfer

Technology transfer is a passage of information from giving end to the receiving end. A technology transfer may be from one department to another department within an organisation, from one company to another company, from an educational institution to an industry etc. Technology transfer can be a patented information or non-patented information. Usually a patent discloses all the information relating to performing the technology. In pharmaceuticals, a developed technology from a research and development department is passed to pilot plant department and later to production department. Even though technology transfer involves with clear document transfer, several hurdles arises during the development of the technology at various levels. Hence, a technology transfer involves not only tangible documentation but also with verbal communications.

When a technology is developed especially at the institutional level, it is necessary that the technology developed has to be communicated to the organisations interested to develop on commercial grounds. A platform is necessary to disclose out such technology has been developed. Several government, private organisations give a platform as science conferences, exhibitions, trade fares where developed technologies may be briefly highlighted as poster or oral presentations or one to one discussions.

Indian government in order to increase the economy of the country is simultaneously giving a provision as financial incentives to organizers and technology developers to conduct and bring out awareness of technologies available on hand. Since a technology developed has some commercial value, the developer expects some commercial benefits as he has invested money and spent time. So, it is necessary for a technology developer to disclose what the technology developed and explain the benefits out of his technology. It is a thumb rule that the developer of the technology has to ensure all legal and financial matters and later transfer the technology.

A technology transfer (Annexure 21) may have to fulfill information relating to scientific, regulatory, quality control, quality assurance etc. Qualified and responsible personnel from R&D, regulatory, quality control, quality assurance, legal departments etc., involve in several rounds of discussions in developing documents individually fulfilling all the needs and later compiled by all departments at one place, finally the documents being validated to ensure that the documentation has been made proper as per guidelines and finally being transferred to the receiving end.

Several times companies merge and technology has to be transferred relating to a drug product that was approved based on country's guidelines, ICH guidelines etc. It is necessary to transfer technology by the giving company in terms of process developed, data developed and submitted to regulatory for approval of the process, validation protocol followed and approved, analytical methods developed and validated, cleaning methods developed and validated, all kinds of data developed and furnished to regulatory. It is necessary that all the personnel responsible and involved in the technology transfer from various departments in the pharmaceutical industry have clear knowledge and communication skills to transfer all the crucial or secret information of the company relating to the drug product. Circumstances may arise where the technology transfer agreement may be withdrawn where the giving company objects in providing the crucial information to the giving company. Hence, it is necessary that a legal agreement should be made before hand in terms of financial share if the product is brought into the market on commercial grounds.

For instance, at the institutional level the process developed for a bulk drug, drug product and written step by step process in the bench records to be transferred to the receiving end.

QUESTIONS

1. What is technology transfer in pharmaceuticals?

2. Explain in detail various aspects of technology transfer that arise in pharmaceuticals?

3. Explain in detail technology transfer in pharmaceuticals?

Hatch-Waxman Act of United States-A Relation to Drug Discovery, Regulatory and Market Approval

Forecast strategies have to be developed by the professionals relating to pharmaceuticals in such a way that to launch a drug product into the market, when a project has to be started keeping in view when a patent, market and data exclusivity of the innovator expires for a bulk drug, drug product. A forecast strategy means by knowing when exclusivity term expires, indicates when a particular project has to be started in the pharmaceutical industry to release the drug as first generic in the market. Too early starting a project may lead to a loss to the company and too late starting a project may lead the pharmaceutical company with fewer margins of profits. Releasing the drug product as a first generic indicates that the product has no competition except the innovator's product. As the product is available from fewer manufacturers, the first generic manufacturer enjoys better margins and later on both the profits of innovator and first generic manufacturer significantly comes down as the number of manufacturers releasing the drug product into the market increases. United States drug regulatory system is one of the well-established systems among the countries in the World. Understanding drug discovery process, patent approval and expiry process, market exclusivity approval and expiry process of United States helps in better understanding of launch of drug products by back ward calculations to meet the objective of launch of drug product as first generic into the market. The chapter discusses the provisions made in US to launch drug products into the market with a complete balance mechanism among innovator, generic manufacturer and end user of medicines and the link between drug discovery, drug approval keeping in mind patent and market exclusivity.

16.1   Origins of US Drug Law

It was in 1848 "The Drug Importation Act" was established in US and since then authorities for possible adulterations inspected imported drugs. In 1906, the Food and Drugs Act was passed to inhibit interstate business of misbranded and adulterated drugs. The Sherley Amendment in 1912 prohibited labeling with false therapeutic claims. In 1927, the Food, Drug and Insecticide Administration was formed from Bureau of Chemistry, and later in 1930 shortened to Food and Drug Administration (FDA). In 1933, FDA recommended the revision of the Food and Drugs Act. It was in 1937, poisonous solvent diethylene glycol of Elixir Sulfanilamide that killed 107 persons and made to realize the necessity of drug safety before marketing. In the following year the Food and Drugs Act was re-named as "The Federal Food, Drug and Cosmetic Act" with new provisions i.e., control of cosmetic and therapeutic devices, drug safety prior marketing, setting of tolerances of unavoidable poisonous substances, authorizing factory inspections etc. Despite several changes in the Act, in 1962 a sleeping pill Thalidomide found causing birth defects led to further stringent drug regulations. With "Fair Packing and Labeling Act" FDA enforced honest and informative labeling system for drugs.

16.2   Drafting the Hatch Waxman Act

In 1978 President Carter asked a team to review industrial innovation and the team suggested patent term restoration for pharmaceuticals and other products that required regulatory review. Later, President Reagan supported the proposal and later turned to a bill S.255. The bill failed due to lack of majority. Congressman Henry A. Waxman, chairman of the Health Sub-Committee took the issue and the patent term restoration bill changed to The Patent Term Restoration and Drug Price Competition Bill. This in turn enhanced further complications. In 1984, Public Law 98-417 (the Hatch Waxman Act) was enacted.

16.3   Overview of Drug Discovery, Regulatory and Market Approval Process

16.3.1   Investigational New Drug (IND) Application

Soon after the inventor company is with the new chemical moiety, the immediate step is to proceed further for the animal studies during which the moiety is preliminarily tested for the pharmacological activity and toxicity. Once the moiety is found promising, the inventor company gets permission from FDA through Investigational New Drug Application for use for testing in humans. This helps the inventor company to send to various places, the new moiety not for sale but for further studies.

It is in the IND application, the inventor specifies all the necessary pre-clinical data to say that the moiety is safe, details of manufacturing process including stability, controls so that the moiety is reproduced consistently and finally including protocols and plans in conducting the clinical studies so that the moiety is exposed to unnecessary risks in subjects.

As part of the process, the inventor is asked to wait for 30 days during which the FDA reviews the safety and later asks to proceed for further investigations.

16.3.2 New Drug Application (NDA)

It is through the New Drug Application the inventor company proposes the FDA for approval of new chemical entity for marketing and sale. As part of the New Drug Application, the inventor has to submit all the data obtained during the animal and human studies. In other way to say, the IND becomes a part of the NDA. The purpose and goal of the NDA is to review and make decision regarding safety, efficacy, benefit outweighing the risks, label contents, method of manufacturing, quality, strength and purity by the FDA Authority. To fulfill the authority, the inventor company has to provide all the necessary documentation. Usually, the inventor who is the first to develop the new drug and who gets an FDA approval to manufacture, sell the drug as a branded drug with a brand name. Since the inventor company has dedicated time, money, naturally during the 5-year exclusivity period of marketing the prices of the drug are usually high.

16.3.3 Hatch Waxman Act and Abbreviated NDA

Before 1962, the older well established innovator and brand name drugs were approved in abbreviated process as generics. Unlike only safety prior to 1962, with Kefauver-Harris amendments to the Federal Food, Drug and Cosmetic Act, the drugs should fulfill safety as well as efficacy. The Drug Price Competition and Patent Term Restoration Act (commonly known as the Hatch Waxman Act) of 1984 extended for the approval of generics those including prior 1962 and post 1962.

The Hatch Waxman Act established the Abbreviated New Drug Application and eliminated repetition of pre-clinical and clinical testing that was necessary for NDA. The provision helped the generic applicant to depend on the previously available data at the FDA. It is to be understood that the provision is to provide drugs that were earlier made available as brands. To fulfill as an abbreviated, the generic product must possess the same active ingredient(s), the same dosage form and same route of administration as that of the brand drug. Additionally, the label of the generic that has to be approved must contain all the necessary information like brand.

Since the pre-clinical and clinical data of the brand applicant is made available to the generic applicant, the Hatch Waxman Act provided incentives in the form of Patent term extensions as well as market exclusivity (5 years) for the brand applicant. To the generic applicant the Act provided a 180-day exclusivity to market his product provided being a first applicant.

Hatch Waxman Act on one side provides a provision of availability of high quality, low price, off patent generics to consumers and on the other side encouraging innovative drug development therapies.

16.3.4 Impact of Hatch Waxman Act on Patent system: The Bolar Amendment

According to the present patent law, the life span of the patent is 20 years from the date of first filing or 17 years from the date of grant which ever was longer. In order to release a generic drug, the individual has to wait until the patent expires. It is also time consuming to develop a generic off patent. If anyone tries to use the patented information for the development of generic drug, the act was considered as infringement. With the case of Roche vs. Bolar, an amendment called as Bolar Amendment brought a provision (through the Hatch Waxman Act) of lead time to develop, perform necessary testing and seek US regulatory approval so that they can be ready for release soon after expiration of the patent of the innovator.

16.3.5 Role of Filing Patent Information

Once the FDA approves an innovator drug, the innovator has to submit all the necessary related patent information so that it is published in the "Orange Book" of the FDA. The objective of the FDA is that, in future an ANDA applicant utilizes some of the critical data for his generic drug approval. This information helps an ANDA applicant regarding inventor's patent number, patent expiry that is claiming drug, method, composition of use and any other patents pending. Additionally, it is the responsibility of the innovator to include in the "Orange Book' regarding the patents granted after the approval of NDA. The "Orange Book" provision mainly helps the ANDA applicant to predict when to start developing his generic product, when it would be likely able to market the drug.

16.3.6 Patent Term Extension

The Hatch Waxman Act provided a provision to the NDA holders in Patent Term Extension. This provision is to compensate the time loss during the testing and approval process of the FDA. The testing phase is considered from the time the IND application is filed and the approval phase is considered from the date of NDA application to the FDA review. From this, the patent extension term is calculated based on the formula that allows half of testing phase and the entire approval phase to a maximum of 5 years patent extension but no more than 14 years from NDA approval.

16.3.7 Certification and Notification Requirement of the Act

With the regulations, the FDA publishes all the necessary NDA patent information in the Orange Book. The ANDA applicant for the generic has to submit the reference-listed drugs (RLD) i.e., the NDA related patents for the approval. The FDA cannot approve the ANDA application until the NDA listed patents are expired.

In order to get approved for a generic, the ANDA applicant has to make certifications as per the provisions of the Hatch Waxman Act [21 USC §355 (j)(2)(A)(vii)(I)-(IV)] and regulations [21 CFR 314.94(A)(12)(i)]. The ANDA applicant has to choose the 4 certifications in addressing each patent. The four certifications are commonly referred as paragraph I, II, III and IV.

Paragraph I Certification: An ANDA applicant chooses Paragraph I certification when there is no patent listed in the Orange Book. Even though the NDA holder possess a patent and decided not to list as an RLD, the FDA approves immediately an ANDA provided the holder meets the approval requirements.

Paragraph II Certification: An ANDA applicant chooses Paragraph II certification when there is a patent listed in the Orange Book, but expired. If the applicant meets the approval criteria, the FDA approves immediately for a generic.

Paragraph III Certification: An ANDA applicant chooses Paragraph III certification when there is a patent listed as RLD but not expired and plans to market the product prior patent expiration. In such cases the law inhibits the FDA from approval until the patent expires.

Paragraph IV Certification: An ANDA applicant chooses Paragraph IV certification when he wishes to challenge one or more patents listed and intends to market the generic product before the patent expires. The ANDA holder would challenge by saying that the patent is invalid, unenforceable, or will not be infringed by the manufacture, use or sale of the generic product. Soon after receiving the certification IV and on accepting for a review, the FDA sends acknowledgement for review. Soon after the ANDA applicant receives the notice from the FDA, he has to bring to the notice of the patent holder with the ANDA application number, description of the proposed drug product and the patent numbers with expiration dates that are being challenged. In addition to these, the ANDA applicant must describe the facts that the patent is not infringed, is invalid or unenforceable. If within 45 days of receipt of the notice from the ANDA holder, the NDA holder files a lawsuit at the federal district court, the FDA is inhibited in approving the ANDA for a period of 30 months. During this 30 months stay, both the NDA and ANDA applicants can litigate.

16.3.8   Market Exclusivity Provision by Hatch Waxman Act

Market Exclusivity is an exclusive concept from patent protection. Perhaps both patent protection and Market Exclusivity overlap each other; it is the Hatch Waxman Act that provided exclusivity for brand drugs. The three provisions that are provided as Market exclusivity are, firstly a five year period of market exclusivity for the New Chemical Entity to the NDA applicant. The New Chemical Entity is the drug moiety and not its salt or ester. The New Chemical Entity exclusivity blocks exclusivity so that no generic application is filed while the exclusivity is in force. The FDA can accept an ANDA application after 4 of 5 years of market exclusivity provided the ANDA applicant certifies paragraph IV certification challenging a patent. The provision saves one year of the ANDA applicant to litigate provided the innovator sued the ANDA applicant.

Secondly, three - year market exclusivity is granted by the FDA for a change in drug in terms of a new dosage form, new salt or ester, new usage or indication, strength etc. Since the drug product is in force of Market exclusivity, an ANDA application may be accepted by the FDA but may not be approved if the change has been approved earlier. This exclusivity conveys when the FDA may approve generic for the changed product.

Thirdly, for a generic, the FDA grants 180-day exclusivity to the first ANDA applicant. This provision blocks any ANDA filed later for a period of 6 months and may be approved by the FDA after the exclusivity has expired. This 6 months period helps the generic firms to develop non-infringing formulations of patented products. This 180-day period is valuable for an ANDA applicant in order to gain and retain substantial share of the generic market.

16.3.9   Market Exclusivity Provision not under the Provision of Hatch Waxman Act

Two provisions of Market exclusivity are in force in United States of America but not under the provision of Hatch Waxman Act. The first provision is the Orphan drug exclusivity. Orphan drugs are those that are used for the treatment of rare diseases i.e., diseases caused to a population of about 2,00,000 or fewer. Since rare diseases are for a fewer population, the innovator company cannot have much benefits due to less market. In order to encourage the innovator in the development of the Orphan drugs, an exclusivity of 7 years was enacted under the Orphan Drug Act. This provision blocks the approval of generics by the FDA during the exclusivity period.

The second provision is the Pediatric exclusivity. The drug moiety that was approved by the NDA for market exclusivity of 5 years (or 3 years of Hatch Waxman Act) and found use as pediatric, an additional period of 6 months is granted as market exclusivity. Thus the provision inhibits the FDA in granting a generic until full term of exclusivity is completed. The main feature of this 6 months exclusivity is that it not only protects main drug and formulation of the innovator but also prevents other formulations having the same drug ingredient. This special provision is an incentive to the innovator (NDA applicant) to study and develop proper use and labeling to the pediatric population. NDA products with no existing patent or exclusivity protection are not eligible to take advantage of the pediatric exclusivity.

16.3.10   Provisions for Antibiotics

Prior to Hatch Waxman Act, there existed abbreviated approval for the antibiotics. Thus there are no provisions of patent and exclusivity for antibiotics. To provide provisions of the Hatch Waxman Act to antibiotics, the FDA defined as old antibiotics those applications pending with effect from November 20, 1997 or any application containing antibiotic submitted after November 20, 1997 that contains an old antibiotic. New applications that contains completely new antibiotic that was not earlier reviewed or approved by the FDA after November 20, 1997 would be eligible for the Hatch Waxman patent and exclusivity provisions.

16.4   CASE STUDIES

16.4.1   Barr Laboratories vs. Eli Lilly

Barr Laboratories launched a generic version of Prozac (fluoxetine hydrochloride) in 20-mg capsules challenging Eli Lilly's patents. Being first to file, the company gained exclusivity for six months.

Details

In December 1995, Barr Laboratories Inc filed an ANDA application for fluoxetine hydrochloride to market as an anti-depressant. The same ingredient is an active ingredient in Eli Lilly's drug Prozac. Eli Lilly on April 10, 1996 brought an infringement action against Barr's ANDA application. Barr argued saying the claims of Eli Lilly's patents does not comply with the best mode and invalid for double patenting. The district court decision was in favour of Eli Lilly. However, being Barr first to file, the company gained exclusivity for 6 months.

16.4.2   Glaxo Smith Kline vs. Apotex

Glaxo Smith Kline the innovator company launched Paxil (paroxetine hydrochloride) as an anti-depressant. A Canadian company, Apotex filed an ANDA under paragraph IV certification for a generic version of the same on March 1998. GSK sued an act of infringement. GSK later listed additional patents in the "Orange Book" and then further acts of infringements. The suits created automatic stay on FDA approval for more than five years. This brought benefit to GSK in having more business for Paxil.

16.4.3 Teva vs. Pfizer

Ivax is the first company to file an ANDA for the active ingredient of Zoloft. Teva filed the second ANDA. Teva certified that the proposed formulation either infringe Pfizer's US Patent No: 5,248, 699 or the patent is invalid. Pfizer had sued Ivax, but settled out of court for a duopoly to begin on June 20, 2006 and potentially last 180 days past the patent expiration in 2010. Thus FDA could not approve Teva's generic drug until 180 days of exclusivity of Ivax expired.

By settling with Ivax, Pfizer insulated through Hatch-Waxman exclusivity the validity of the US Patent No: 5,248,699. The insular effect also extended the term of the US Patent No: 4,356, 518, which expires on June 30, 2006 to coincide with the Patent No: 5,248,699 expiration in 2010. Thus Teva can think about the release of the generic after 2010.

16.4.4 Mova vs. Upjohn

Mova Pharmaceutical Corp. first filed an ANDA to market a generic version of micronized glyburide. Upjohn sued against Mova for an act of patent infringement. Meanwhile, the FDA approved an ANDA for the generic drug submitted by Mylan Pharmaceuticals. Mova filed case in the United States District Court for the District of Columbia. Finally, the Court decided that it was Mova's first filing and not Upjohn's patent infringement suit that required the FDA to withhold approval from paragraph IV filers. The Court granted preliminary injunction requiring the FDA to suspend its approval of Mylan's ANDA.

16.4.5 Inwood Laboratories Inc. vs. Young

Inwood filed a generic drug application with paragraph IV certification and proposed that their product do not infringe any Orange Book listed patent. Inwood was the first to file an ANDA under the certification and the patent holder elected not to sue. The FDA approved and Inwood claimed 180 days exclusivity. The FDA's conclusion was that 180 days exclusivity commences only when the First applicant has been sued for patent infringement. The District court ruled that the statute is clear on its face, no successful defense was needed and finally the complaint was dismissed.

16.4.6 Purepac, Teva vs. FDA

Roche Laboratories Inc sold Ticlopidine hydrochloride under the brand name Ticlid. Purepac filed an ANDA containing a paragraph IV certification. However, the first applicant was TorPharm and Roche did not sue TorPharm within 45 days provided as statute. Purepac's application could not be made effective until at least 180 days after FDA received notice of first commercial launch of the drug. Following first commercial launch, Purepac received the approval.

Like Purepac, Teva filed a paragraph IV certification for the same drug and was also not sued by Roche. Like Purepac, Teva also received tentative approval pending the expiration of TorPharm's 180-day exclusivity period. Teva filed a suit against Roche saying that Roche's Orange Book listed patent was not infringed and finally the case was dismissed due to lack of jurisdiction regarding the subject matter. The dismissal was brought into the attention of FDA and the FDA did not agree with the Teva's interpretation. Teva sued FDA.

TorPharm still did not have the approval for the generic drug product when Teva filed an appeal at the District Court decision. Since the FDA regulates from the statute on a case-by-case basis, it was not able to convince and distinguish the case from Granutec from that in Teva. The District Court found that the FDA decisions were arbitrary and capricious. Finally, FDA approved all tentatively approved ANDAs to ticlopidine hydrochloride.

QUESTIONS

1. What is the drug approval process in United States?

2. What is the role of Hatch Waxman Act of United States?

3. How Hatch Waxman Act of US influence in India?

4. How you relate drug discovery, drug approval process, marketing and data exclusively in US and in India?

5. How Bolar provision helps in pharmaceuticals?

Intellectual Property Validation

In pharmaceutical regulatory affairs, a commonly listened term is Validation. Validation is defined as a documentation process which implies that a process was conducted as per the defined standards. In case of patent system, validation is a process of patent application filed through PCT, Regional patent office and granted with a regional (or international) patent and ensuring whether the invention had undergone the process of national phase entry in the region and was granted with a patent by the specific country. At this phase it is necessary to remind that there is no one single global patent protecting an invention in entire countries of the World but a single patent application applied through PCT or regional patent office being forwarded to several countries falling within the region (or PCT member states) being granted with patent by each and every specific country, provided the inventor enters the national phase.

An invention filed through PCT undergoes initially international phase scrutiny and at a later stage a national phase. An international phase application when enters the national phase undergo several changes (or already made) due to variations in the country legislations. For instance, a US patent application may contain an invention claiming a use, whereas the same application through PCT when enters national phase of India, it needs changes where in claims for uses are not granted with patent.

Like international phase and national phase for a PCT application, one can expect regional route (phase) and national route (phase) entry of an application that was submitted at regional patent office. This implies that like PCT members being with WIPO administration (IB-International Bureau) at the international phase, several regional countries with an internal understanding have an administrative body to receive one application and minimize duplication processes so that a patent is granted in every country of the region upon entry into the national (route) phase.

Some of the regional patent offices are as follows:

Table 17.1 List of Treaties/Conventions/Agreements

Name of Regional Patent Office	List of Member Countries
African Intellectual Property Organization (OAPI) (http://www.oapi.int/)	Benign, Burkina Faso, Cameroon, Central African Republic, Union of the Comoros, Congo Brazzaville, Ivory Coast, Gabon, Guinea, Guinea Bissau, Equatorial Guinea, Mali, Mauritania, Niger, Senegal, Chad, Togo
African Regional Intellectual Property Organization (ARIPO) (http://www.aripo.org/)	Botswana, The Gambia, Ghana, Kenya, Lesotho, Malawi, Mozambique, Namibia, Sierra Leone, Liberia, Rwanda, São Tomé and Príncipe, Somalia, Sudan, Swaziland, Tanzania, Uganda, Zambia and Zimbabwe (Observers-Angola, Algeria, Burundi, Egypt, Eritrea, Ethiopia, Libya, Mauritius, Nigeria, Seychelles, South Africa and Tunisia)
Eurasian Patent Organization (EAPO) (https://www.eapo.org/en/)	Turkmenistan, Republic of Belarus, Republic of Tajikistan, Russian Federation, Republic of Kazakhstan, Azerbaijan Republic, Kyrgyz Republic, Republic of Armenia, Republic of Moldova
European Patent Organisation (EPO) (https://www.epo.org/index.html)	Albania, Austria, Belgium, Bulgaria, Switzerland, Cyprus, Czech Republic, Germany, Denmark, Estonia, Spain, Finland, France, United Kingdom, Greece, Croatia, Hungary, Ireland, Iceland, Italy, Liechtenstein, Lithuania, Luxembourg, Latvia, Monaco, Former Yugoslavia Republic of Macedonia, Malta, Netherlands, Norway, Poland, Portugal, Romania, Serbia, Sweden, Slovenia, Slovakia, San Marino, Turkey
Patent Office of the Cooperation Council for the Arab States of the Gulf (GCC Patent office) (http://www.gccpo.org/DefaultEn.aspx)	United Arab Emirates, Kingdom of Bahrain, Kingdom of Saudi Arabia, Sultanate of Oman, State of Qatar, State of Kuwait
The ASEAN Patent Examination Co-operation (ASPEC) is the first regional patent work-sharing programme (not a regional patent office but an understanding for patent examination) (https://www.aseanip.org/)	IP Offices of Brunei Darussalam, Cambodia, Indonesia, Lao PDR, Malaysia, The Philippines, Singapore, Thailand, and Viet Nam

EUROPEAN PATENT PROSECUTION AND VALIDATION PROCEDURE

In brief, an inventor from India can protect his invention through Paris convention or through PCT application. Several times, an inventor may plan to submit direct application in a country or a regional application, but upon taking permission from the Controller of Patents (under certain conditions). The strategy behind being selective is based on nature of invention, potential markets, expenditure etc.

In case of European Patent Office (EPO), the application may be submitted at one of the branch office located at Munich, The Hague or Berlin. At EPO, an application may be submitted within 12 months with respect to an earlier national application or within 31 months of that priority as regional phase through PCT application.

Applications submitted at EPO are officially prosecuted (Figure 17.1) in either one of the languages i.e., English, French or German (as per London Agreement). The application is ensured for formal compliance, and is examined for absolute patentability, invention, novelty, inventive step, sufficiency, clarity and support. Upon fulfilling the objections (official, oppositions etc.,), fees, translations, the EPO grants a patent and publishes.

Upon regional patent grant, it is mandatory to enter into national level, which is called as validation. As the European regional patents are granted with respect to European Patent Convention (EPC), individual country cannot reject a patent grant. Hence, within three months (Figure 17.2) of regional patent grant, a validation filing is necessary either individually or through patent attorney (or agent). Several of the European Patent Convention Countries are not on par with London agreement and accept "English" language applications for submission, which is beneficial to Indian inventors. There upon, with the individual country protocol and time lines, a patent is granted by the country.

Yet another approach of utilization of the word 'validation' is with respect to knowing the legal status of the patent in various countries of the World. Supplementary Protection Certificates (SPC), an extension of patent term is usually observed at the level of delayed patent grants, patent prosecutions, product approvals etc. Such review of validation helps to plan the development of the products neither too early nor too late.

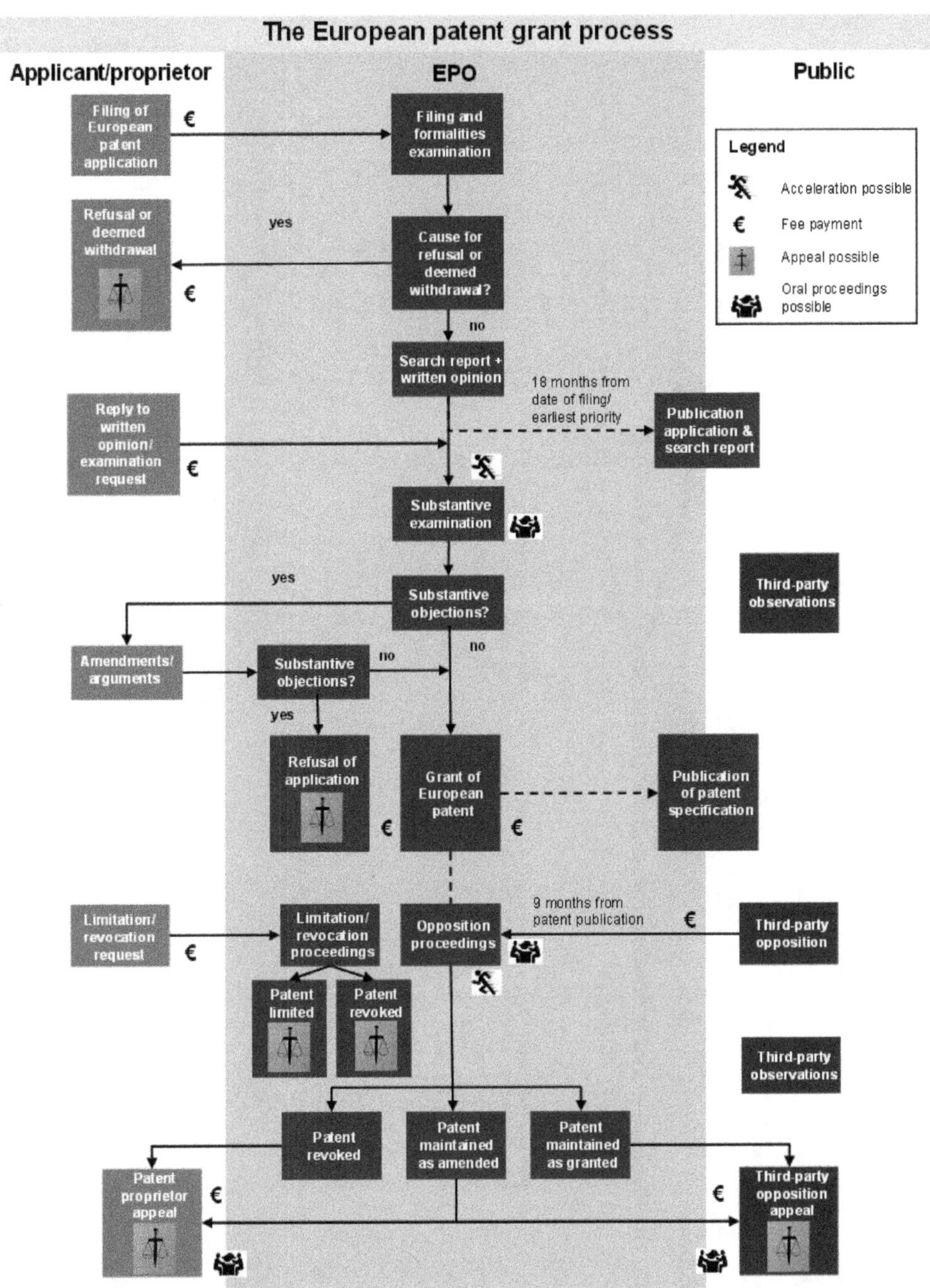

Figure 17.1 Overview of the Procedure for the Grant of a European Patent.

European patent validation timeline

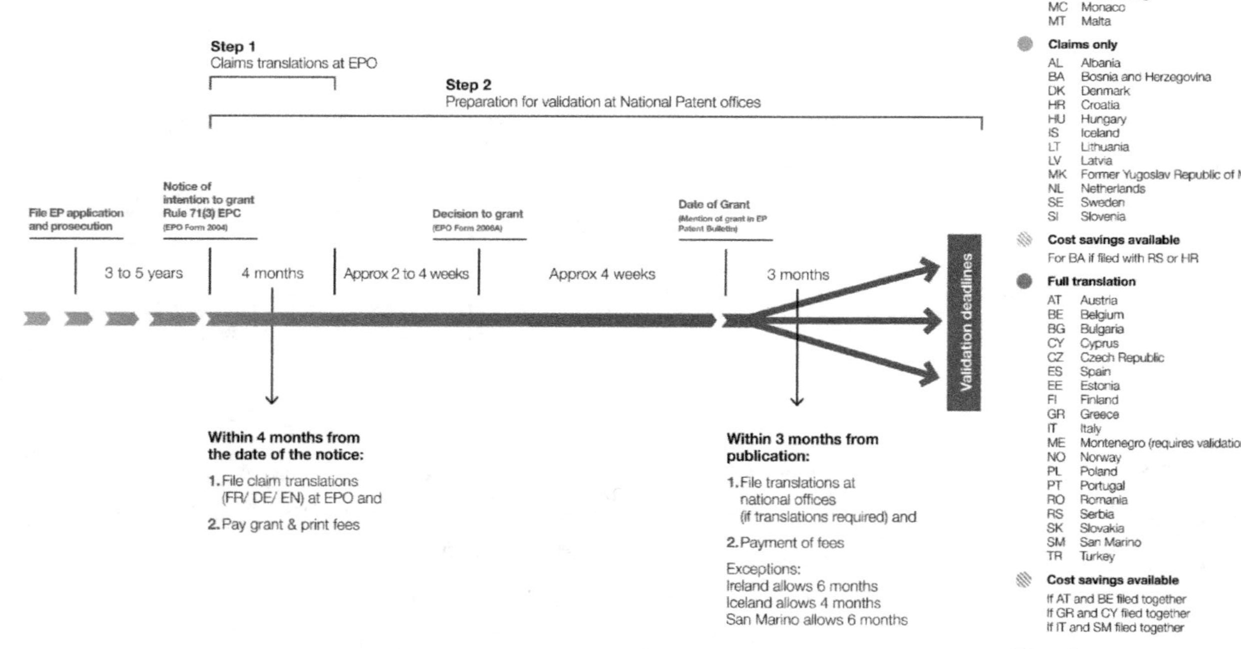

Figure 17.2 European Patent Validation Timeline.

QUESTIONS

1. What is meant by validation with respect to pharmaceutical regulatory and intellectual property systems?

2. Explain the validation protocol when a patent application is filed through PCT, regional patent offices?

Intellectual Property Audits

Intellectual Property Audits (usually called as IP Audits) gained their prominence very recently. The reason behind is that, a company has both tangible and in-tangible assets. It is the in-tangible assets of the company (like trade secrets, business methods etc.,) that usually enhance the growth of the company to higher levels. An IP auditor (usually a patent agent, attorney) assesses the Strengths, Weakness, Opportunities and Treats (SWOT) of a company with respect to intellectual property. The auditor assesses the market potential of the existing trademarks, designs of the company as well as helps the organisation in right planning with IP related product development. In certain circumstances, the auditor assesses the current status of IP of the company and directs for protection and immediate business. An IP audit leads to either license, sell away, buy or launch a product by the company. An appropriate IP audit, may lead to appropriate working status of a company's inventions, develop forecast strategies of when current active patents expire and how early to plan so as to launch the product into the market soon after patent expiry. In certain circumstances of mergers and acquisitions, IP audits helps in taking right decisions. Assessing possible infringements and developing products that are non-infringing needs thorough literature search. IP audits are gaining importance where an innovator has product patents with limited process patents and approaching patent licensing with other inventors having economical different process patents for the same product. Where a situation of IP litigation arose, the damage of business is assessed for claiming the damages. Overcoming of data exclusivity issues and benefiting with Bolar provision is tricky and needs IP auditing. As a whole IP auditing is a management strategy that helps the employer, employee possess with appropriate rights of knowledge, business share. Benefits of compulsory licensing mechanism, launching of a product in a country where no legislations exists, but with monopoly kind of business environment can be understood by IP auditing. Yet another aspect of IP auditing is to have the updated legal status of a patent whether active, expired or extended with extra time of protection. Such extended patent term is usually observed for delayed patent grants, delayed product approvals, less business of geriatric, pediatric, orphan drug products. IP auditors help in developing agreements to export products where there is no patent in India infringing, but third country wishes to import under compulsory licensing mechanism upon discussion among patent holder/s, importer and exporter.

QUESTIONS

1. What is meant by IP Auditing?

2. Explain in detail the applications of IP Auditing relating to pharmaceuticals?

National Phase Entry for IP Protection

When a patent application has been filed as regional or PCT application, the application's entry into individual country for patent grant is called as national phase entry. Even though several international and regional conventions/ treaties/agreements help in minimizing application submissions, costs, translations, examinations, certain aspects are not uniform among the global countries. This clearly indicates that there exists difference in the intellectual property legislations. Such differences may lead to some modifications in protection of claims but if the invention fulfills the patentability criteria, the invention may be granted with patent in all the countries of the World. It is the national phase entry of an application that usually requires the changes in the specifications. But, it is necessary to understand that the patentability criteria, prosecution timelines, procedures are almost similar but definitely not identical. Hence, it is necessary to understand the prosecution protocol of each and every country. Even though it is beyond the scope of the book to explain each and every prosecution, Figure 19.1, provides the fundamental prosecution protocol such as filing provisional, complete specifications, publication, request for examination, pre-grant opposition, release of First Examination Report (FER), fulfilling the FER objections, order of grant, publication, waiting for any post-grant oppositions and final issue of patent certificate. Hence national entry of any international application undergoes the protocol with respect to the country's. This implies that the patent office procedure of India is followed for all international applications received either through PCT or Paris Convention.

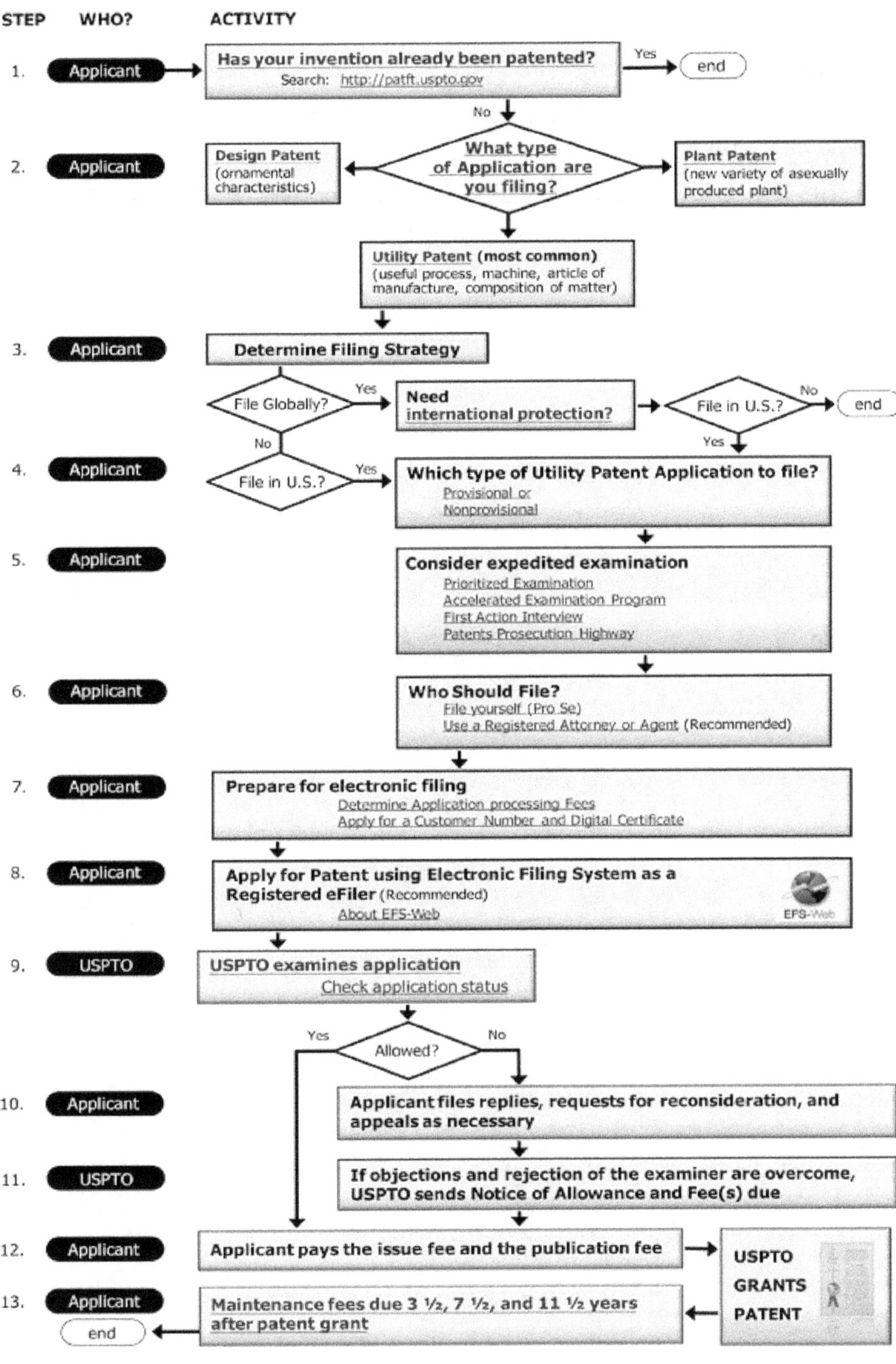

Figure 19.1 Prosecution Procedure for obtaining US Utility Patent.

Questions

1. What is meant by international phase and national phase entry?

2. Write in detail about national phase entry of an IP protection, especially for a patent application?

3. Write in detail the national phase entry protocol for any two countries?

CHAPTER 20

Intellectual Property Litigation Prosecution

Prosecution is a term being used in several circumstances. To the current context, a prosecution is the legal proceeding and debate among plaintiff and defendant upon an issue in the courts, in front of judge. Relating to pharmaceuticals, several infringements, para-IV challenges, product patent grants oppositions, patentability criteria issues were witnessed. Especially, in Indian legal system, the courts are categorised into District, High and Supreme Courts. A case filed by a plaintiff is usually at the jurisdiction of the issue occurred. Depending on the nature of issue, a case can be either a civil or a criminal. In order to clear off the pending cases at the courts, Intellectual Property Appellate Board (IPAB), equivalent to High Courts was established to handle issues relating to creations (intellectual property). Several third parties such as social welfare organisations, individuals file cases on intellectual property issues, for the benefit of the society. In certain circumstances individual/company cases are witnessed.

For instance, a case was filed in Indian court where in the petitioner clearly indicated the innovators negligence of not submitting complete information regarding the working status of patented inventions. This led to a final judgment of furnishing appropriate and correct information by the patent holders. According to the legal system, a judgment that is objectionable at the lower courts may be re-initiated at the higher courts and to the extremes, the Supreme Court of India judgment as the final. When a litigation is in another country, it is necessary to understand the court hierarchy system of that country. In brief, in the United States, the courts are categorised into District Courts, Court of Appeals and the Supreme Court.

For instance, the US patent litigation time line as follows, Figure 20.1.

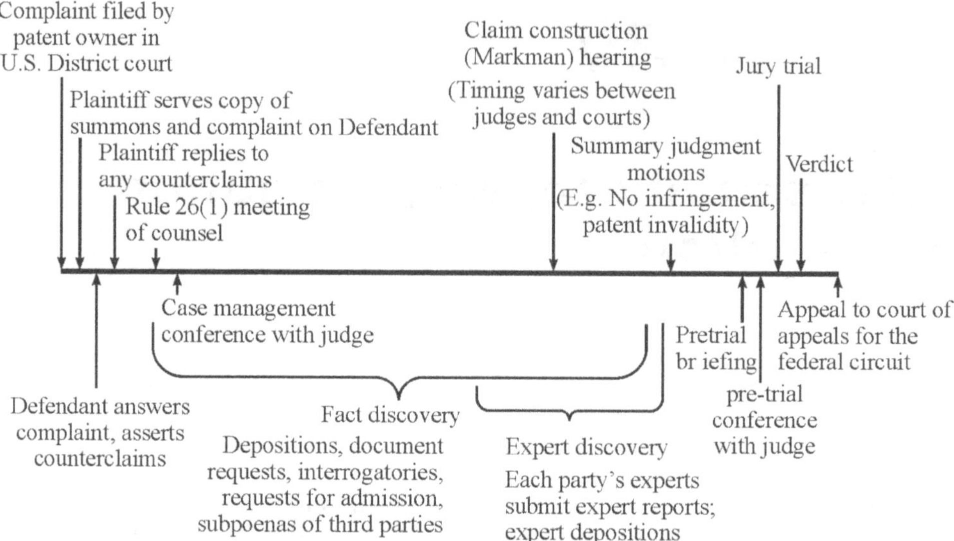

Figure 20.1 US Patent Litigation Timeline

Questions

1. Write in detail about litigation prosecution?

2. Write the various contexts a prosecution is involved with respect to intellectual property system?

CHAPTER 21

FAQs in Pharmaceuticals on Patents – Regulatory – Marketing

1. What is Intellectual Property Right?

Creations of brain are called as intellectual. Since these creations have commercial value are called as property. As intellectual property belongs to an individual, they are rights of an individual. Hence, the word coined as intellectual property rights.

2. Why intellectual property rights came suddenly into lime light?

It is believed that an economy of a country depends directly or indirectly on creations that are generated by the intellectual of nationals. It is the responsibility of the government to safe guard intellectual property of its nationals. India has intellectual property system since 1950s (Copyrights), 1970s (Patents), Harappa civilizations (Trade marks), but soon after India signing WTO agreement (1995), a transition period of 10 years was given under TRIPS obligation of WIPO/WTO. Since then, India has to safeguard intellectual property of the citizens with amending already existing laws and vesting new laws.

3. How intellectual property rights are classified? What are the governing bodies/legislations of intellectual property rights?

Intellectual property rights are classified into two categories i.e., Industrial property rights, Copyrights.

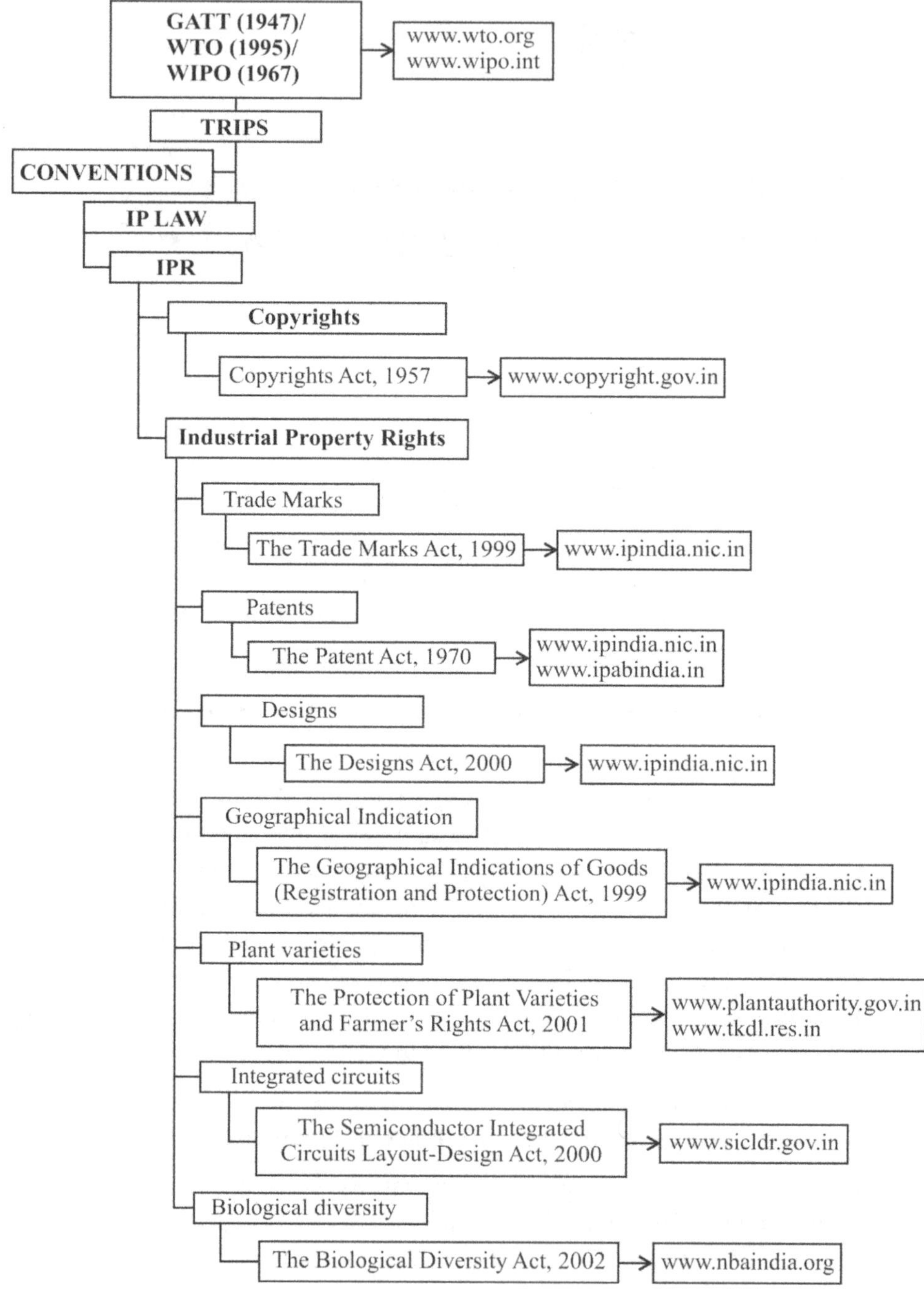

Figure 21.1 Classification of Intellectual Property Rights.

4. What is the objective and role of GATT/WTO?

The role of General Agreement on Tariff and Trade (GATT) is to provide a stable and predictable international trade system. It acts as a mediator in settling the disputes between countries regarding trade. It holds frequent negotiations, encourages reductions in tariffs so that expansion in world trade becomes possible.

In 1970s despite, GATT's success in trade growth through tariff reductions, global competition led a series of economic recessions leading to high rate unemployment, factory closures. To overcome this, Governments were driven to devise other forms of protection i.e., bi-lateral market sharing agreements within competitors and embark subsidies to maintain holds on agricultural trade. In addition to this, advancements in science, individual needs, world trade became complex. Trade services were found promising globalization of world economy, but rules not covered in GATT. These changes undermined the credibility and effectiveness of GATT. Together, these and other factors influenced among GATT members and concluded to vest multilateral system. This led to Uruguay round of negotiations; the last and largest round of GATT converting to World Trade Organization (WTO).

5. What is the objective and role of WIPO?

The role of World Intellectual Property Organization (WIPO) is to promote international cooperation with respect to creation, dissemination, use and protection of works of the human mind for economic, social, cultural progress of all mankind. It enhances a worldwide balance of the creation i.e., by protecting moral, material interests of the creators and providing access to the socio-economic and cultural benefits to others. Thus, WIPO promotes protection of intellectual property and bring out cooperation among the union.

In addition to these, WIPO sets norms, standards and execute legal technical assistance, registration activities for intellectual property protection to member countries. It is the WIPO; which is responsible for the formation of Patent Co-operation Treaty (PCT).

6. What is a patent?

Patent is a document granted by government to the inventor as an exclusive right to sell, make, use, import upon disclosure of the invention by the inventor for a certain period of time. Patent is a limited time monopoly. However, patents are not compared as monopoly.

7. What is the life time of a patent?

A patent is granted for an invention for 20 years from date of first filing. However, certain patents are extended beyond 20 years especially for pediatric, orphan drugs. Several patents other than these are indirectly extended on new inventive step of earlier patent, new use (in some countries) etc.

8. How patents are classified based on pharmaceutical products?

Patents are basically classified into:
  (i)   Product Patents
  (ii) Process Patents
  (iii) Platform Patents (Industry terminology)

9. How application filings for a patent are classified at patent office?

Patent applications are classified into:

A.
  (i)   Provisional specification
  (ii) Complete specification
  (iii) Patent of Addition
  (iv) Divisional patent

B. Convention Application

C. PCT Application
  (i)   International phase
  (ii) National phase

10. When an invention patentable?

Inventions that are novel, non-obvious, useful and enabled are eligible for patentability. In other words, the subject matter should be eligible for patentability.

11. When inventions are not patentable?

Subject matter that is frivolous, natural law, intended for commercial exploitation, contrary to public order or morality, serious prejudice to human, animal, plant life or health or the environment, mere discovery, scientific discovery, abstract theory, mere discovery of new form of known substance, mere admixture, mere arrangement or re-arrangement or duplication of known devices, method of agriculture, process for the medicinal, surgical, curative, prophylactic or treatment of human beings/ animals, whole plant, whole animals, mathematical methods, business methods, computer program, literary, dramatic, musical, artistic, cinematography, television productions, mere scheme, method of performing mental act, method of playing game, presentation of information, topography of integrated circuits, traditional knowledge, invention relating to atomic energy are not patentable.

12. When an application has to be filed for a patent?

When the inventor is sure that his subject matter of innovation is novel, non-obvious, useful, the inventor can file an application for a patent. However, an application filed by an inventor may be rejected for a patent provided the subject matter is not novel, obvious and has no industrial applicability.

13. Does an invention process to be completed before filing for a patent?

No, the invention process need not be complete. If the work results fulfill patentable subject matter, the inventor can file for a patent.

14. What is the best option to save an invention?

An invention usually need not be the best mode at the initial stage. If the subject matter is novel, non-obvious and useful, it is advised that the inventor file his provisional patent application so as to have the benefit of priority date under Paris convention.

15. Through whom inventions are filed for a patent?

Inventions are usually filed through patent attorneys and patent agents. It is only the patent attorneys and patent agents who can argue the patentability at the courts. However, inventors can file a patent.

16. What is Paris Convention?

Basically, under the traditional patent system, the inventor has to file applications in each and every country where he wishes to possess a patent. The Paris Convention provided a great opportunity in claiming the priority date of an earlier application for the subsequent filings in foreign countries if the parent and foreign countries are members of the Convention. The advantage with the Paris Convention is that, the inventor after filing a patent in his own country can decide within a period of 12 months whether to file patent applications among Paris Convention countries. This in turn means that the inventor if wishes to file patent application in foreign countries; within a period of 12 months he has to make all the necessary arrangements of language translations, filing of patent applications in all the countries, bare fees of patent offices, attorney's. Suppose that, the inventor has filed patent applications in several countries of Paris Conventions Union and later if the patent office does not grant a patent or the invention found not useful, it is a big damage to the inventor.

17. Is there a provision for World patent?

There is no world patent. However, an inventor has a provision through Paris convention, PCT where he can file in a particular member country and within stipulated time can protect his invention in other member countries.

18. What is a member country?

Several countries in the world are members to Paris convention, WIPO, PCT. It is necessary to be a member to safe guard intellectual property rights in other member countries covered under Paris convention, WIPO, PCT. It is several times necessary to find out when a country in the world became a member to Paris convention, WIPO, PCT.

19. Is it necessary to have a law background?

No, it is not necessary to have a law background. Practice of law relating to intellectual property rights is by authorized patent attorneys, patent agents who have taken examinations both written and oral conducted by Government of India.

20. Is it necessary to have science background?

Inventions usually have science background and it is necessary to decide an invention is novel, non-obvious, useful and enabled. Several science graduates are qualified Patent attorneys, patent agents.

21. What is advisable for a better practice of intellectual property rights?

It is always advisable to have intellectual property right law, science background and being qualified as patent attorney or patent agent. Several lawyers and scientists have mutual understanding that helps the patent attorneys to prosecute cases.

22. What should an inventor do, if he does not want to protect his invention as patent and such invention is not patented by others in future?

If the inventor has a novel, non-obvious, useful invention that has potential patentability and not wishing to patent or let others not to patent such invention in future, it is necessary to bring in to public domain through journal publications. Such publications bring obviousness to the invention. Such publications still safeguard the inventor for certain period of time in having a second thought and file for a patent within stipulated period of time.

23. What is the cost of patent filing and protection for the entire 20 years?

The following is the minimum cost incurred for a application filing and maintaining a granted patent.

S. No	On what Payable	For Natural Person (Rs.)	For other than natural person(s) either along or jointly with natural person(s)-(Rs.)
1	On application for a patent-provisional/complete	1600	8000
2	Renewal of Patent for 3rd year	800	4000
3	Renewal of Patent for 4th year	800	4000
4	Renewal of Patent for 5th year	800	4000
5	Renewal of Patent for 6th year	800	4000
6	Renewal of Patent for 7th year	2400	12000
7	Renewal of Patent for 8th year	2400	12000
8	Renewal of Patent for 9th year	2400	12000
9	Renewal of Patent for 10th year	2400	12000
10	Renewal of Patent for 11th year	4800	24000
11	Renewal of Patent for 12th year	4800	24000
12	Renewal of Patent for 13th year	4800	24000
13	Renewal of Patent for 14th year	4800	24000
14	Renewal of Patent for 15th year	4800	24000
15	Renewal of Patent for 16th year	8000	40000
16	Renewal of Patent for 17th year	8000	40000
17	Renewal of Patent for 18th year	8000	40000
18	Renewal of Patent for 19th year	8000	40000
19	Renewal of Patent for 20th year	8000	40000

24. What does a patent contains?

A patent contains an invention giving details the differences in prior art, describing in detail the invention process with best mode and finally the claims made by the inventor.

25. What is a product patent?

If the active ingredient (drug) is present in the independent claim, it gives an indication that the patent claims for the molecule as such indicating a product patent.

26. What is a process patent?

Bulk drugs, formulations are developed by different methods involving series of steps. A process patent explains how the bulk drug, formulation developed.

27. Does a patent can be for a product and process?

Yes, there are several patents claiming for a molecule and process involved in developing bulk drug, formulation. However, a patent usually contains only one invention. If more than one invention, it may be necessary to file for individual inventions.

28. What are the different parts in a patent?

A patent contains the following parts:

Title

Bibliography

Abstract

Prior art

Summary

Description of invention

Tables

Figures

Claims containing independent and dependent claims

29. What is an infringement?

Infringement is an act which falls under the claims of a patent. In other words, during the developing of innovations, the process involved may fall, may act same to the claims in a patent.

30. What are the different types of infringement?

Infringement is three types:

(i) Direct infringement (Literal infringement)

(ii) Doctrine of Equivalence

(iii) Prosecution history estoppel

31. What is the importance of claims in a patent?

It is the claims that are present in the patent that decides the boundaries of the innovation. Drafting claims in a patent is crucial and any minor flaws may give a lead to another person for a new invention leading to a new patent.

32. Can we rely completely on the title of a patent for expected information during patent search?

Usually a title of a patent should reflect complete details that are present in a patent. Several times, a title of the invention mislead and divert attention of the patent to meet our objective of search. It is not mandatory that all the family patents have same title.

33. What is a family patent?

One single invention, filed and granted with patents of several countries is called as a family patent.

34. How to identify that first filing country and country of origin of innovation among family patents?

Date of filing of an application for a patent is the first clue to identify the country of origin of innovation among the family patents. In other words, first filings indicates priority date. This first filing usually indicates country of origin of innovation, innovator. However, it is not a thumb rule to say that an innovation first originated in a particular country. This deviation can be due to filing through PCT/WIPO, individual country filing. It is not mandatory that an innovation is first filed and granted in country of origin of innovation. It is upto the discretion of innovator to decide filing application for a patent in the member countries.

35. What is a platform patent?

Industry terminology of platform patent is especially for formulation patents. The speciality of such patents is that a formulation is designed and in addition the active ingredients/therapeutic classes available in market are all claimed for that formulation. This is an indication of a product patent.

36. What is prior art?

All the inventions made in the past are available in journals, which is a prior art of a particular subject of innovation. A prior art may be an article in a journal or a patent or several times both. Several times a prior art may not be present in a journal but available and known to public as a public domain.

37. What are the sources of prior art search?

Innovations are published in journals. All the journals are indexed and compiled based on topic of innovation documented by Chemical Abstract

Services, Belstein etc. Currently, chemical abstract services are widely used for prior art search for an invention, patent. American Chemical Society as chemical abstract service publishes abstracts which gives details of inventions published in journals. American Chemical Society publishes this compiled information in the book, CDROM, online search form.

38. What are the sources for prior art search relating to patents?

Innovations that are granted with patents are published as a document and are available at patent office of every country. Currently, several patent offices provide online retrieval of patents from database established by country's patent office on free/paid basis. However, several countries still do not have softcopies/online version and it is necessary to communicate with a country's patent office.

39. What are the best resources for prior art, patent search, patent expiry, market potential, market demands?

Information relating to these are available through costly online databases such as STN, Scifinder, Dialog Pro, Questel orbit, Thomson Reuters etc., in addition to free databases related by country's patent offices.

40. Which is the ultimate online paid database?

STN is the world's leading database. The advantage with STN is that it is a network of several individual databases. An individual can login a particular database and fulfill the objective of search. The disadvantage with STN is the search is very expensive in terms of time and type/amount of data downloaded. If wisely used, search becomes very fast and saves time and money when compared to manual search.

41. How patent filings are considered in different countries?

Several patent offices follow first to file while some first to invent (USA) basis. Currently, USA is practicing first to file system.

42. What is patent mapping?

Patent mapping mainly deals with identifying by hierarchy from innovator to current status of technology available by means of patents for a particular drug product. In addition to this, identifying drugs going off patent as pipeline drugs.

43. What are the different stages involved from filing an application to grant of a patent?

Filing and grant of patent involves the following:

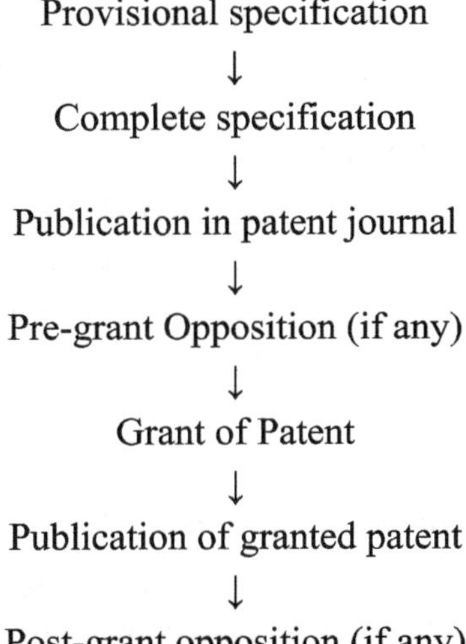

44. What is Compulsory licensing?

When a patented invention is not in use for the public or if the cost of innovation available to public is very high or not fare or a patented invention is not directly manufactured in the country or life care drug or a condition of national emergency gives a provision to apply for a compulsory license for a patented invention. Such provision can be requested only after certain period of grant of a patent. It is necessary to prove the strong grounds on which compulsory license to a patent has to be granted.

45. What are the strategies necessary to have patents?

The following are the strategies necessary to have patents:

(i)   Innovation bent of mind

(ii) Establishing resources financially, infrastructure

(iii) Dedicated research personnel

(iv) Lead identification for initiating research

(v)   Overcome lag phase in developing products through research and development until releasing into the market

(vi) Dedicated investment to research and development

46. What is Freedom to operate?

With globalization, export of a drug (bulk drug/formulation) to a foreign country may be an act of infringement. It is necessary to identify the patents available in that particular country where the product is intended to be exported and analyze whether such products are free from act of infringement. Such analysis results to freedom to operate.

47. What is the legal status of a patent?

A patent is usually granted for a period for 20 years from date of filing. Several patents are discontinued by inventor by not paying the renewal fee. In certain cases, the patent period is extended due to additional patents relating to advancement of innovations. It is always necessary to know the legal status of a patent so as to release a drug product into the country's market.

48. How to search legal status of a patent?

Databases operated by different country's patent offices update the legal status of a patent application, granted patent. Several paid databases like STN, Dialog Pro, Thompson Reuters etc., regularly update such information country wise.

49. What is Novelty?

A subject matter that is new and not existing earlier in any means. Such subject matter may be novel to the inventor but may be obvious to person skilled in the art. Hence, a decision on novelty is very critical for a subject matter to be patentable.

50. What is meant by obviousness?

A subject matter that is already known to the public is obvious. A decision relating to obviousness can be decided by a person skilled in the art.

51. What is meant by Usefulness?

A subject matter invented should have use especially to the industry or the public. If such use is not available for the subject matter, patentability is lost.

52. What is meant by enabling for patentable subject matter?

An invention is clearly described and mentioned in the patent document. In addition to providing the methodology of achieving such invention, there is a necessity to indicate the best method of achieving such invention among the information established by the inventor in the patents. This is called as enabling the patentable subject matter. In other words, disclosing clearly the methods of achieving the invention.

53. What is PCT?

Patent Cooperation Treaty brings out several benefits for the users of patent system i.e., brings one application filing with one single language which in turn is valid in PCT member countries, provides single time examination of the patent instead each member country, provides international search rather than each country search so that prior art can be easily judged in order to get a patent, provides international publication of international publications with related international search reports, bring down one single communication to all designated offices, provides any person from the member country to file single opposition regarding the patentability of the invention, provides uniform procedure and economical benefit to the inventor in all mentioned aspects.

In addition to these the main objective of PCT is to facilitate and accelerate access by industries and other sectors to technical information relating to inventions and to assist developing countries in gaining access to technology.

54. What is TRIPS?

The wide variation in the standards and protection of intellectual property, lack of multilateral frame of principles, rules and disciplines dealing with international trade led to tensions in international economic relations. In order to solve these tensions, an agreement i.e., Trade Related Aspects of Intellectual Property Rights was framed addressing basic GATT principles and those of international intellectual property agreements. This brought a provision of adequate intellectual property rights, effective enforcement measures of those rights, multilateral dispute settlements and transitional arrangements. TRIPS guidelines are set forth for the minimum standards of intellectual property rights. The extent of stringency and waiver is at the discretion of individual country needs.

55. What is a branded drug?

Drugs released into the market by the innovator are basically called as branded drugs.

56. What is a generic drug?

Drug formulations released by companies under the similar grounds of the branded formulation are called as generics.

57. What is New Chemical Entity?

A molecule that was invented and undergone the process of preclinical and clinical studies, finally approved by regulatory authority to release into the market through NDA.

58. What is New Molecule Entity?

A molecule that was approved by drug regulatory authority in other countries and available in the market, while the molecule was first time approved by the US Food and Drug Administration. New Chemical Entities that are not analogs to existing drugs, new combinations of drugs, are also considered under the category of NMEs.

59. What is a first generic?

A generic drug that was approved and released into the market for the first time after the patent and market exclusivity expiry of the branded drug is called as first generic.

60. What is a tentative approval?

A generic drug approved by the regulatory authority and under the waitlist into the market until the patent and market exclusivity expiry occurs. New indications, use of innovator drug lead to tentative approvals.

61. What is Data exclusivity?

An innovator company that has developed new chemical entity and applied for an NDA application submits all the data relating to pre-clinical, pharmacodynamic and pharmacokinetic studies both for the bulk drug and formulations. Such data is established by the innovator company investing money and time. Such information is crucial and Hatch Waxman act provides a provision to the generic companies to utilize such data for releasing generic. As a benefit to the innovator company such data is protected currently by data exclusivity in several countries.

62. What is Bolar provision?

In United States a provision called as Bolar amendment was established by which, use of patented drugs is not an act of infringement for Research and Development. Such provision helps the generic industries to develop generic drug products during the patent term and not at any cost for commercial purpose.

63. What is Market Exclusivity?

Innovator companies, who's New Chemical Entities, were approved under NDA is released into the market as branded drugs. Since the innovator company invested money and time, a provision is provided as a benefit to the branded company as market exclusivity for a certain period of time (varies in different countries).

64. What is an NDA application?

A New Drug Application is filed usually by a innovator company for study and approval of New Chemical Entity. If the New Chemical Entity is approved by the drug authorities, it is released into the market as new drug. Several drugs in the new dosage form are filed through NDA.

65. What is an ANDA application?

An abbreviated new drug application is filed for release of a generic formulation into the market. Such formulations should fulfill the minimum criteria of bioequivalence studies as per the regulations of the country.

66. How generic drugs are certified during filing for approval by generic drug companies as ANDAs?

In order to get approved for a generic, the ANDA applicant has to make certifications as per the provisions of the Hatch Waxman Act [21 USC §355 (j) (2) (A) (vii) (I) - (IV)] and regulations [21 CFR 314.94(A) (12)(i)]. The ANDA applicant has to choose the 4 certifications in addressing each patent. The four certifications are commonly referred as paragraph I, II, III and IV.

Paragraph I Certification: An ANDA applicant chooses Paragraph I certification when there is no patent listed in the Orange Book. Even though the NDA holder possess a patent and decided not to list as an RLD, the FDA approves immediately an ANDA provided the holder meets the approval requirements.

Paragraph II Certification: An ANDA applicant chooses Paragraph II certification when there is a patent listed in the Orange Book, but expired. If the applicant meets the approval criteria, the FDA approves immediately for a generic.

Paragraph III Certification: An ANDA applicant chooses Paragraph III certification when there is a patent listed as RLD but not expired and plans to market the product prior patent expiration. In such cases the law inhibits the FDA from approval until the patent expires.

Paragraph IV Certification: An ANDA applicant chooses Paragraph IV certification when he wishes to challenge one or more patents listed and intends to market the generic product before the patent expires. The ANDA holder would challenge by saying that the patent is invalid, unenforceable, or will not be infringed by the manufacture, use or sale of the generic product. Soon after receiving the certification IV and on accepting for a review, the FDA sends acknowledgement for review. Soon after the ANDA applicant receives the notice from the FDA, he has to bring to the notice of the patent holder with the ANDA application number, description of the proposed drug product and the patent numbers with expiration dates that are being challenged. In addition to these, the ANDA applicant must describe the facts that the patent is not infringed, is invalid or unenforceable. If within 45 days of receipt of the notice from the ANDA holder, the NDA holder files a lawsuit at the federal district court, the FDA is inhibited in approving the ANDA for a period of 30 months. During this 30 months stay, both the NDA and ANDA applicants can litigate.

67. What is Orange book of USFDA?

Orange book is a list of all approved formulations by USFDA to market in United States. Orange book contains approved drugs for human use. The list includes patent and market exclusivity expiry.

68. What is Green book of USFDA?

Green book is a list of all approved formulation by USFDA to market in United States. Green book contains approved drugs for veterinary use.

69. What is Yellow book of USFDA?

Yellow book is a compiled list of industries in United States of America.

70. What is a DMF?

Drug Master Files are usually filed by bulk drug companies who have manufactured a bulk drug complying USFDA rules and regulations. Filing a DMF by a manufacturing company does not mean the drug is approved by USFDA.

71. What is the benefit of DMF?

Drug master files help the manufacturer in recommending by the US client for the approval of the drug that has been manufactured in a place other than United States. Upon recommending the manufacturer by the client to the USFDA, the authorities initiate the inspection process for approval of drug and the manufacturing facility.

72. What are the different types of DMFs?

Drug master files are classified into five types and are as follows as per USFDA:

Type I: Manufacturing Site, Facilities, Operating Procedures, and Personnel (no longer applicable)

Type II: Drug Substance, Drug Substance Intermediate, and Material Used in Their Preparation, or Drug Product

Type III: Packaging Material

Type IV: Excipient, Colorant, Flavor, Essence, or Material used in their preparation

Type V: FDA accepted reference information

At USFDA, DMF filings are classified as "I"-Inactive, "A"-Active, "N"-Not an assigned number, "P"-DMF Pending Filing Review

73. What is eCTD?

Electronic common technical document is the electronic version of submission of applications relating to drug master files, drug approval applications. The provision is part of ICH guidelines to make the application submission and approval process easier and faster. There is no compulsion that an application is submitted only through eCTD.

74. What is a chemical abstract?

Research work of scientists is explained in brief as a whole in as an abstract in a research paper published in a journal. Such information from various journals is compiled by American Chemical Society as Chemical abstract service.

75. How are the databases relating to chemical abstract services available?

All the abstracts in journals are compiled in different volumes titled as 'Abstracts' by chemical abstract service. All the abstracts of journals are again indexed by American Chemical Society as follows:

(i) General Subject index

(ii) Chemical formula (Molecular formula) index

(iii) Chemical name index

As a routine practice, subject, formula, name index were checked year/ volume wise to identify the abstract number. In the Abstract books of American Chemical Society, the abstract number is identified and the corresponding abstract on referring will indicate the name of the journal, volume number and page number in which the research paper is published.

76. What is the time plan and patenting process through PCT?

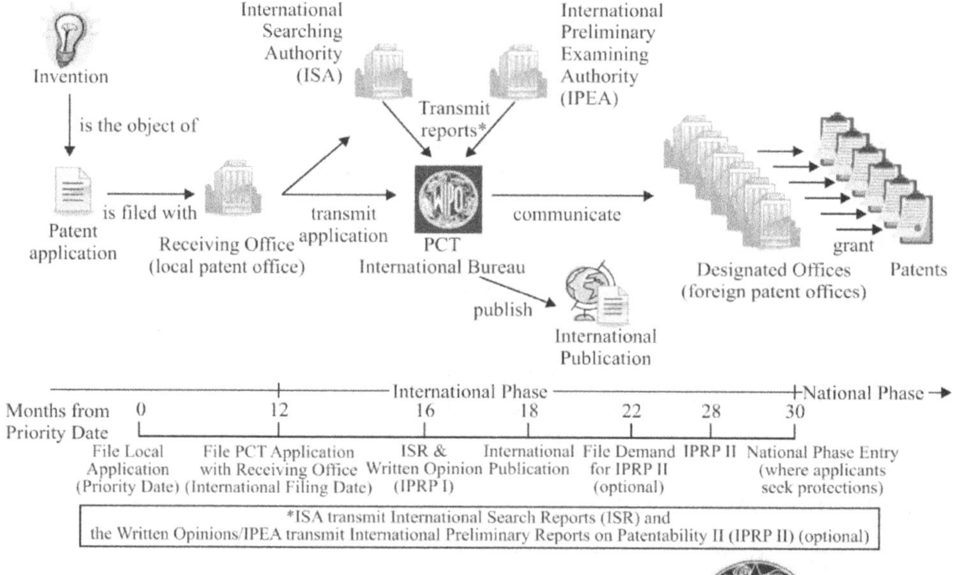

Figure 21.2 Overview of the Patenting Process using the PCT System.

77. What is the time plan and patenting process in India?

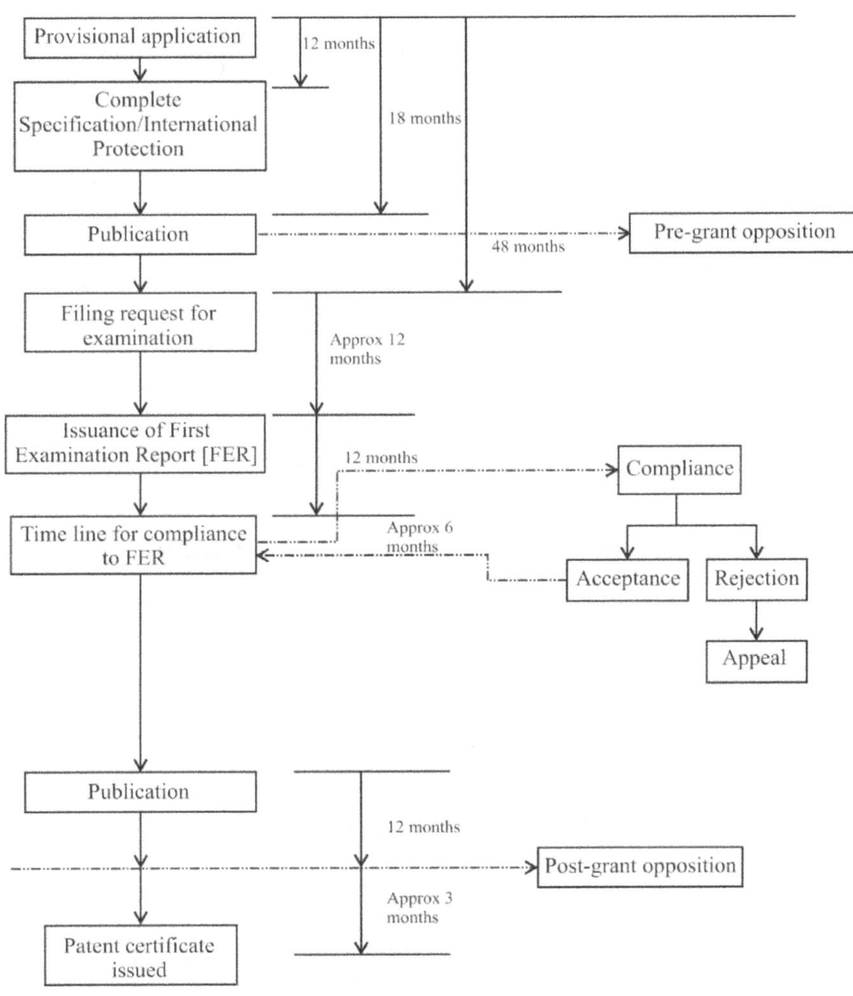

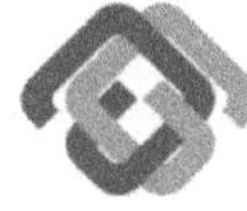

Figure 21.3 Indian Patent Procedure.

78. What is the pricing trend of innovator and generic drugs (copyright protected)?

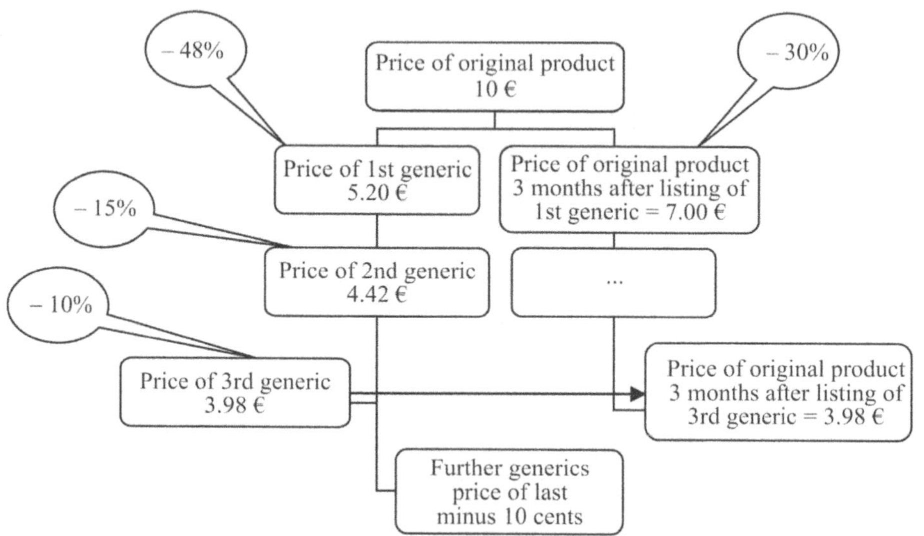

79. What are the top 10 countries as per Global Innovation Index?

Top 10 Countries as per GII, 2011	
Rank	**Country**
1	Switzerland
2	Sweden
3	Singapore
4	Hong Kong (SAR)
5	Finland
6	Denmark
7	United States
8	Canada
9	Netherlands
10	United Kingdom

80. How is Global Innovation Index, Innovation Efficiency Index calculated?

The Global Innovation Index is computed as an average of the scores across inputs pillars (describing the enabling environment for innovation) and output pillars (measuring actual achievements in innovation). Five pillars constitute the Innovation Input Sub-Index: 'Institutions,' 'Human capital and research,' 'Infrastructure', 'Market sophistication' and

'Business sophistication'. The Innovation Output Sub-Index is composed of two pillars: 'Scientific outputs' and 'Creative outputs'. The Innovation Efficiency Index, calculated as the ratio of the two Sub-Indices, examines how economies leverage their enabling environments to stimulate innovation results.

81. What is the data exclusivity period of different countries (indicative)?

Exclusivity Period	Country
10 Years	Belgium (BE)
	France (FR)
	Germany (DE)
	Italy (IT)
	Luxembourg (LU)
	Netherlands (NL)
	Sweden (SE)
	United Kingdom (UK)
6 Years	Austria (AT)
	Bulgaria (BG)
	Cyprus (CY)
	Czech Republic (CZ)
	Denmark (DK)
	Estonia (EE)
	Finland (FI)
	Greece (GR)
	Hungary (HU)
	Iceland (IS)
	Ireland (IRL)
	Latvia (LV)
	Lithuania (LT)
	Malta (MT)
	Norway (NO)
	Poland (PL)*
	Portugal (PT)
	Romania (RO)
	Slovakia (SK)
	Solvenia (SI)
	Spain (ES)

82. What is the time scale of Drug discovery, Patent and Regulatory process?

Time Scale of Drug Discovery, Patent & Regulatory Process

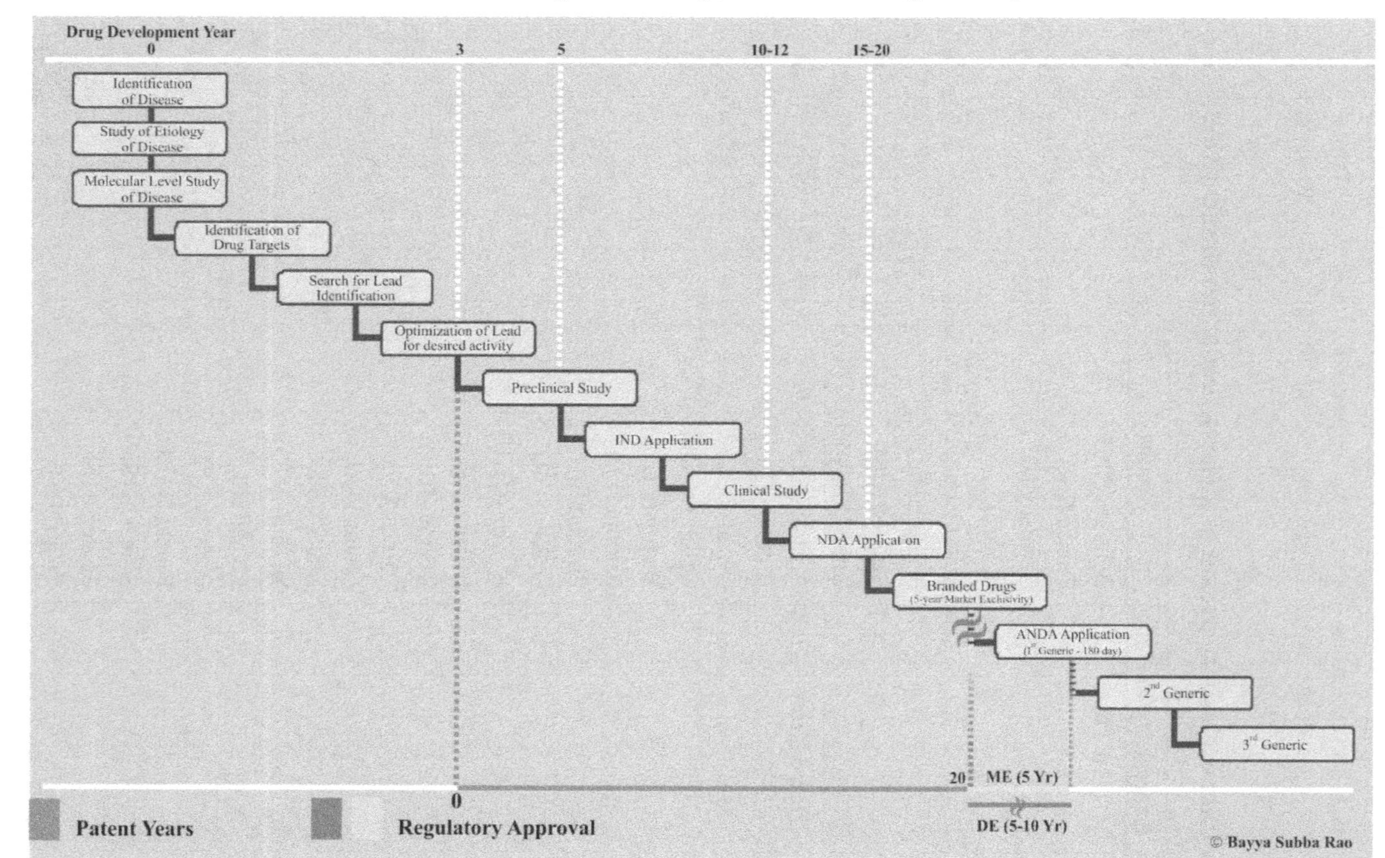

83. What is a block buster drug?

When a popular drug has an annual sale of at least $ 1 bn, it is called as block buster drug.

84. What is an orphan drug?

Drugs that are useful for rare diseases (orphan diseases) is called as orphan drug. A rare disease occurs in less than 2,00,000 individuals in United States or less than 5 per 10,000 individuals in European Union.

85. What are the International patent searching authorities?

The international patent searching authorities are as follows:
   (i)   Austrian Patent Office
   (ii) Australian Patent Office
   (iii) European Patent Office
   (iv) China Intellectual Property Office
   (v)   United States Patent and Trademark Office
   (vi) Swedish Patent Office
   (vii) Indian Patent Office

86. What are the international preliminary examining authorities?

The international preliminary examining authorities are as follows:
   (i)   Austrian Patent Office
   (ii) Australian Patent Office
   (iii) European Patent Office
   (iv) China Intellectual Property Office
   (v)   United States Patent and Trademark Office
   (vi) Swedish Patent Office
   (vii) Indian Patent Office

87. How to calculate patent expiry date?

Patent expiry is calculated from the date of first filing. If an application is though PCT, the patent expiry date is calculated from date of filing the application to PCT.

88. What are the different exclusivity regimes in United States?

   (a) 5 year exclusivity regime: The regime is for innovator companies for the approved new drug application.

(b) **4 year exclusivity regime:** The regime is for innovator companies for the approved new drug application where a generic company has filed a ANDA with a certification of patent invalidity or non-infringement (Paragraph IV certification).

(c) **3 year exclusivity regime:** The regime is for innovator/other companies for the approved new drug application that has been identified with new use/indication. Such application contains reports of new clinical investigations conducted or sponsored by the sponsor that were essential to the approval of the application or the supplement.

In addition to this, US has orphan drug exclusivity, pediatric drug exclusivity, generic drug exclusivity, drugs approved between 1982 and 1984, medical devices exclusivity. The exclusivity period starts from the date of approval by the FDA.

89. What are the different exclusivity regimes in European Union?

In European Union, a 8 + 2 + 1 formula is applied to all the member states i.e., eight years of data exclusivity, two years of market exclusivity, one year exclusivity provided, the drug is identified with a new use/indication. However, the tenure of exclusivity is not uniform and there is a necessity to monitor by individual countries.

90. When market exclusivity, data exclusivity starts?

Market exclusivity is a term widely used in United States, while data exclusivity term is used in European Union. The exclusivity rights starts from the date of approval to market the products. In common the start date and end date of exclusivity provided indicates for both marketing and protecting the innovators data.

91. What are the high lights of amendments of The Patent Act, 1970?

The Patent Act, 1970 was amended thrice to fulfill the obligations of TRIPS. The key important aspects are as follows:

(i) **First Amendment, 1999:** For inclusion of Exclusive Marketing Rights, Mail box facility for accepting applications relating to product patents.

(ii) **Second Amendment, 2002:** Increase in term of patent from 14 to 20 years, compulsory licensing, right to import and parallel imports, bolar provision.

(iii) **Third Amendment, (Ordinance), 2004:** Inclusion of process as well as product patent regime.

92. What are parallel imports?

It is a right to import patented products from an authorized license holder indicating that the provision is not an act of infringement.

93. How to monitor regularly patent applications filed, published, granted, pre grant opposition, post grant opposition and rejected?

Indian patent office regularly publishes such information in a journal relating to patents. Such journal is available online with the Indian patent office. The journal is released by the patent office in every week.

94. What are the main differences in patent system among United States and India?

In United States, patents are granted as plant, utility and design patents. In addition to this, patents are granted for new indication/use. Computer programming is patented in United States.

In India, patents are granted for inventions. Plants and designs are protected by registration. Computer programming is protected by copyright in India.

95. How to identify patent agents?

The list of patent agents registered is available online at Indian patent office at www.ipindia.nic.in

96. Why are the forecast strategies necessary in pharmaceuticals?

It is necessary to plan well in advance an economical drug process development, a generic drug so that the product developed reaches the market soon after the product patent/market exclusivity of an innovator's drug expires. Reaching the drug product into the market soon after the innovator's patents expires requires information when a patent, market exclusivity expires. Several companies that are involved in contract bulk drug manufacturing, generic drug development have to plan their projects at least 5 years in advance so that the product is developed, filed for drug master filing, filed for drug approval so that the drug product is approved on time and can be reached to the market soon after the patent, market exclusivity expires.

97. What are the parameters usually necessary as forecast strategies so that drug products are developed and reached into the market?

Parameters like, when a drug product patent is expiring? What is the market end date of innovator's products? What is the data exclusivity period? What is the volume of bulk drug consumed globally? What is the current demand? What is the shortage? How many companies are filing DMFs in various countries? How many molecules/formulations/ formulation strengths/combinations/dosage forms/route of administrations available in the market? What is the export potential? What is the import potential? What is the capacity of the country in producing the drug product? How many companies have developed the products and filed for drug approval at the drug regulatory? etc., are some of the parameters to develop forecast strategies.

98. What are the resources for developing forecast strategies?

IMS health is one of the most reliable data providers relating to drug product consumptions, sales, and patent expiry. Currently, several organisations are providing such crucial information.

99. How to calculate when to start a project so that the product reaches the market at the earliest?

A project initiation should not be too early or too late to meet the objective of releasing the product into the market. To develop project start strategies, parameters like How long a drug process (economical) can be developed? How long a generic drug product is developed? How long bio-equivalence/bio-availability studies? How long filing an application and for drug approval from country's drug regulatory authority? When is the patent and market exclusivity expiry for the innovator's drug product? are some that helps the company in developing drug product projects.

100. How should a pharmaceutical company aim?

A contract bulk drug manufacturing company should aim in developing drug products of demand keeping in view of when a product patent is getting expired. A generic drug manufacturer intending to export has to aim in developing drug products that can be released as first generics, new dosage forms, new routes of administration so that the company has less competition and better margins. As the competition increases, prices come down leading to fewer margins of profits. It is necessary to understand that drug regulatory authority of different countries provide detailed information online for information and companies should maintain dedicated personnel for compiling such information.

101. **What are the territorial jurisdiction of various regional Indian patent offices?**

The territorial jurisdiction of appropriate office for the applicants are as follows:

Office	Territorial Jurisdiction
Patent Office Branch, Mumbai	The States of Maharashtra, Gujarat, Madhya Pradesh, Goa and Chhattisgarh and the Union Territories of Daman and Diu & Dadra and Nagar Haveli
Patent Office Branch, Chennai	The States of Andhra Pradesh, Karnataka, Kerala, Tamil Nadu and the Union Territories of Pondicherry and Lakshadweep, Telangana
Patent Office Branch, New Delhi	The States of Haryana, Himachal Pradesh, Jammu and Kashmir, Punjab, Rajasthan, Uttar Pradesh, Uttarakhand, Delhi and the Union Territory of Chandigarh.
Patent Office, Kolkata	The rest of India.

102. **What is meant by sequence listing?**

Especially relating to bio-technology inventions, sequence of nucleotides and amino acids are determined. Such sequence is listed in a standard format as prescribed by WIPO Standard ST.25. European Patent Office with the collaboration of European Bio-informatics Institute has developed Biological Sequence Submission Application for Patents (BiSSAP) so as to make sequencing in a harmonized manner. BiSSAP is a computer program, free to download, helps in creating, amending, verifying and validating sequences while submitting patent applications. It is mandatory to submit sequence listing of biotechnology related inventions even at Indian patent office or through PCT.

103. **What strategy and approach to be followed while filing patent applications?**

For an inventor, the first approach to decide is that he can apply either individually or through a patent agent or an attorney. The second approach is firstly applying application in India for local patent and simultaneously planning either direct application in a country through Paris Convention or for several countries through PCT (or regional application through Paris Convention). The strategies the inventor to keep in mind is how early to apply, how to minimise procedures, how to get patents granted at the earliest, how to minimize expenditure. This can be achieved based on company's policy of financing and expenditure. It is necessary to understand that an application through PCT is the best for economic reasons as well as minimizing protocols, but it is necessary to wait at least 30 months to enter national phase. An inventor, based on potentiality of invention with respect to business, he may select potential market countries for patent protection. Under such circumstance, the inventor may plan for selected countries by direct application provided the countries are members of Paris Convention. This aspect looks simple theoretically, but is complex while practical implementation.

ANNEXURE 1

ANATOMY OF A US PATENT

Engineering & Science Library

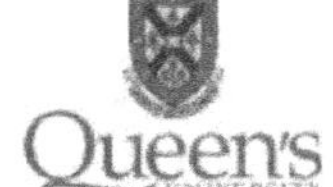

Anatomy of a U.S. Patent Document

Document number: The prefix US indicates that this is a U.S. patent. The B2 code indicates that this patent has a previously published application.

Source: Country that issued the patent.

Date of Issue

INID codes

Title of the invention

Inventor

Assignee/Owner

Application number and date

Prior publication data: Number and date of previously published application.

Related U.S. application data: Number and date of prior application(s) related to this patent.

International Patent Classification

U.S. Patent Classification: USPC codes represent the subject matter of the invention. 36/3A is the code for shoe and boot ventilated uppers.

Field of search: USPC codes consulted by the patent examiner during the prior art search.

Drawing: Representative drawing selected from the drawing sheets.

References: U.S. and foreign patent documents and other publications cited as related prior art by the inventor and patent examiner.

Patent examiner: Official who examined the application.

Patent attorney: Legal counsel hired by the inventor to prosecute the application.

Abstract: Simple, non-technical description of the invention.

Term adjustment: Additional days added to the term of the patent to make up for processing delays.

Front page: the first page of a patent document containing bibliographic data.

INID codes: Patent offices use INID codes to identify bibliographic data on the front page of patent documents. (See sidebar.) These two-digit codes, which may be enclosed in parentheses, brackets or circles, came into general use in the 1970s. INID is an acronym for Internationally agreed Numbers for the Identification of (bibliographic) Data.

The USPTO publishes unexamined applications 18 months after the earliest filing date. Prior to 2001, applications were kept secret until a patent issued.

Selected INID Codes

10 Patent number
12 Document type
21 Application number
22 Date of application
45 Date of patent
51 IPC classification
52 National classification
54 Title of the invention
56 References
57 Abstract
58 Field of search
60 Related application data
65 Published application data
72 Inventor(s)
73 Assignee (owner)
74 Attorney or agent

Document number and date printed at the top of every sheet.

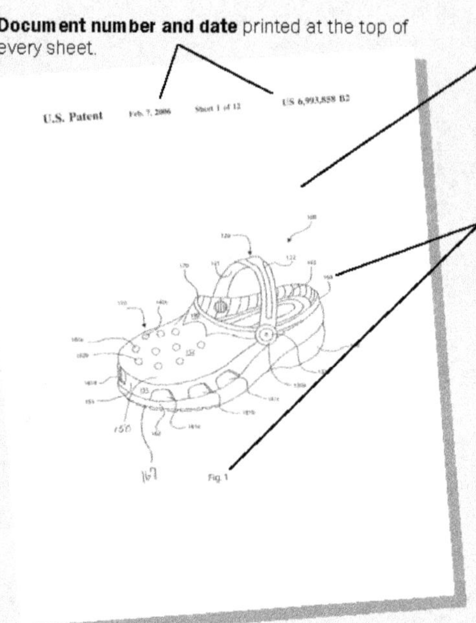

Drawing sheets: Located after the front page. Drawings are common in patents for electrical and mechanical devices as well as articles of manufacture; chemical and biotechnology patents may or may not include drawings. The patent office selects one representative drawing to appear on the front page of the patent.

Drawings must confirm to drafting guidelines set by the patent office. They must be labeled clearly and provide enough detail for the reader to understand the invention's design and use.

Types of U.S. patents:
1. Utility patent - protects new and useful:
   - Products (tool, shoe, toy, etc.)
   - Compositions (chemical compound, alloy, etc.)
   - Machines
   - Processes
2. Design patent - protects new and original:
   - Ornamental designs for articles of manufacture
3. Plant patent - protects distinct and new.
   - Varieties of asexually propagated plants. (Reproduced by means other than seeds, such as grafting, budding, etc.)

Document number   **Column and line numbers**

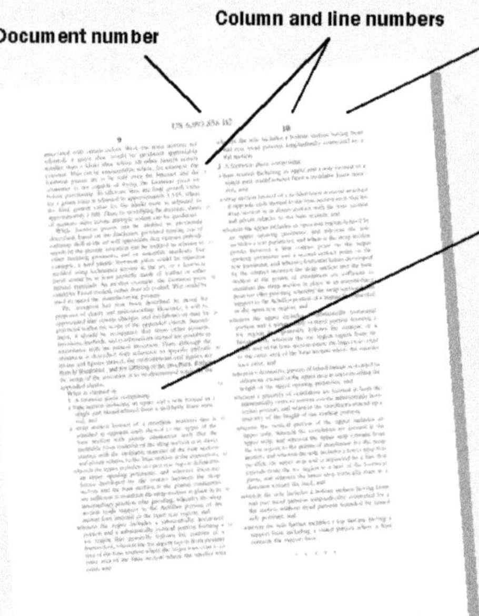

Specification: Written description of the invention that precedes the claims. Includes a discussion of the related prior art (previously issued patents and other publications), a description of the drawings (if any) and the preferred embodiment of the invention. The specification must describe the invention in sufficient detail so that anyone of ordinary skill in the same technical field can understand it.

Claims: Paragraphs located at end of the specification that define the scope of protection of a patent. The phrases "I claim" or "What is claimed" precedes the numbered claims. Patents must have at least one claim, but most usually have several and some hundreds of claims. The claims define the legal boundaries of the invention in the way a property deed defines the physical boundaries of an area of land.

Limitations of Patent Documents
Unlike journal articles, patent applications are not peer-reviewed and experimental proof is not required in order to obtain a patent. Although patents contain detailed technical information, they can also be frustratingly vague (especially older patents) and written in an arcane technical-legal jargon often called "patentese."

Term: Twenty years from the date of application. In some cases, the term of the patent may be extended due to delays in the processing of the application. After the patent has expired, the invention becomes public domain. In addition, patent owners must pay a maintenance fee at 3.5, 7.5 and 11.5 years after issue or else the patent will expire.

Michael White
Librarian for Research Services
May 2008

ANNEXURE 2

TRADEMARKS REGISTERED

Trade Marks Journal No: 1636   14/04/2014

Reg. No. TECH/47-714/MBI/2000
Registered as News Paper

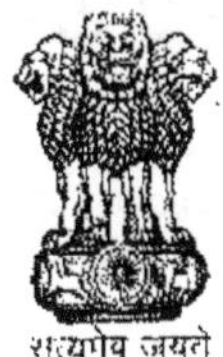

व्यापार चिन्ह पत्रिका

TRADE MARKS JOURNAL

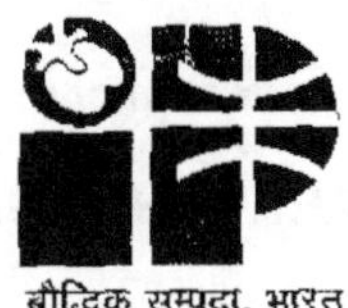

बौद्धिक सम्पदा, भारत
Intellectual Property India

भारत सरकार
व्यापार चिन्ह रजिस्ट्री

Government of India
Trade Mark Registry

प्रकाशन ঃ भारत सरकार व्यापार चिन्ह रजिस्ट्री
एस. एम. रोड एंटॉप हिल के पास पोस्ट ऑफिस के पास पडाला मुंबई 400037
दुरभाष ঃ 022 24101144 , 24101177 , 24148251 , 24112211.
फैक्स ঃ 022 24140808
Published by: The Government of India, Office of The Trade Marks Registry,
Baudhik Sampada Bhavan (I.P. Bhavan)
Near Antop Hill, Head Post Office, S.M. Road, Mumbai-400037.
Tel:022-24140808

Trade Marks Journal No: 1636 ,   14/04/2014   Class 5

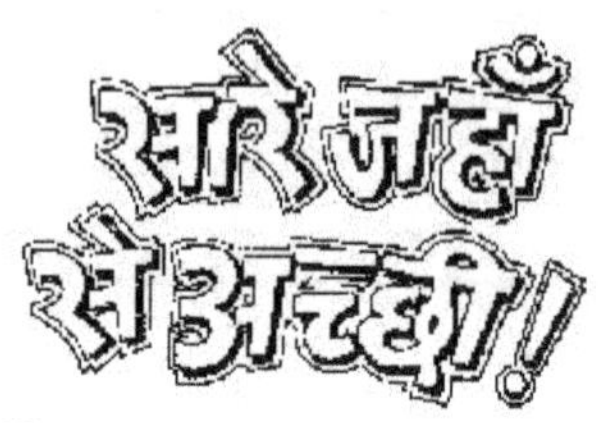

Advertised before Acceptance under section 20(1) Proviso
810788   17/07/1998
DABUR INDIA LIMITED.

Trading as DABUR INDIA LIMITED.

22 - SITE - IV, SAHIBABAD, GHAZIABAD, UTTAR PARDESH.
MANUFACTURERS.
A COMPANY INCORPORATD UNDER THE COMPANIES ACT,

Address for service in India/Agents address:
THE ACME COMPANY
B-41, JAIPUR ESTATE, NIZAMUDDIN EAST, NEW DELHI - 110 013.
Used Since :01/01/1996

DELHI

AYURVEDIC MEDICINAL AND PHARMACEUTICAL PREPARATIONS.

TRANSLITERATION: SARE JAHAN SE ACHHI !

Trade Marks Journal No: 1636 ,   14/04/2014   Class 5

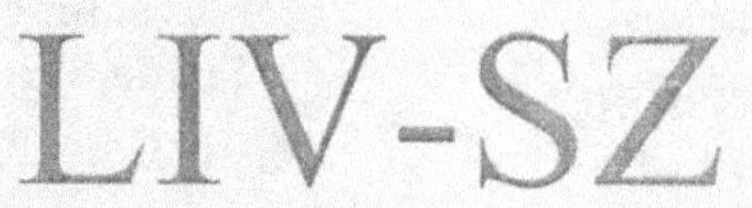

Advertised before Acceptance under section 20(1) Proviso
2121847   28/03/2011
SMD REMEDIES PVT. LTD.
30, KIRTI NAGAR, SANWER ROAD, UJJAIN (M.P).
MERCHANTS AND MANUFACTURERS
A PRIVATE LIMITED COMPANY REGISTERED UNDER THE COMPANIES ACT, 1956.

Address for service in India/Attorney address:
S. SINGH & ASSOCIATES
213, 3RD FLOOR PARMANAND COLONY, DR. MUKHERJEE NAGAR DELHI-9
Used Since :01/04/2007

MUMBAI

MEDICINAL AND PHARMACEUTICAL PREPARATIONS; INCLUDED IN CLASS 5

Trade Marks Journal No: 1636 ,   14/04/2014   Class 5

DANOPAR

Advertised before Acceptance under section 20(1) Proviso

2143728   13/05/2011

MR. SAIFUDDIN DANISH

trading as DANISH LABORATORIES

13, DADABHAI NAOROJI MARG, UJJAIN |(M.P.)

MANUFACTURERS AND MERCHANTS

A SOLE PROPRIETORSHIP FIRM

Address for service in India/Attorney address:

S. SINGH & ASSOCIATES

213, 3RD FLOOR PARMANAND COLONY, DR. MUKHERJEE NAGAR DELHI-9

Used Since :01/05/2011

MUMBAI

MEDICINAL AND PHARMACEUTICAL PREPARATIONS; INCLUDED IN CLASS 5

Trade Marks Journal No: 1636 ,   14/04/2014   Class 5

METRONAZOLE

Advertised before Acceptance under section 20(1) Proviso

2287188   22/02/2012

ABARIS HEALTHCARE PVT. LTD.

Trading as ABARIS HEALTHCARE PVT. LTD.

406, SAFFRON, PANCHWATI, AHMEDABAD - 380015. (GUJARAT STATE) INDIA

MANUFACTURER, MERCHANT & TRADERS

01/05/2005

Address for service in India/Attorney address:

RAVAL & CO.,

A-1, 1ST FLOOR, SATYAMEV-1, OPP. GUJARAT HIGH COURT, SOLA, S.G.ROAD, AHMEDABAD - 380 060

Used Since :20/09/2001

AHMEDABAD

MEDICINAL & PHARMACEUTICAL PREPARATIONS INCLUDED IN CLASS - 05.

Trade Marks Journal No: 1636 , 14/04/2014   Class 5

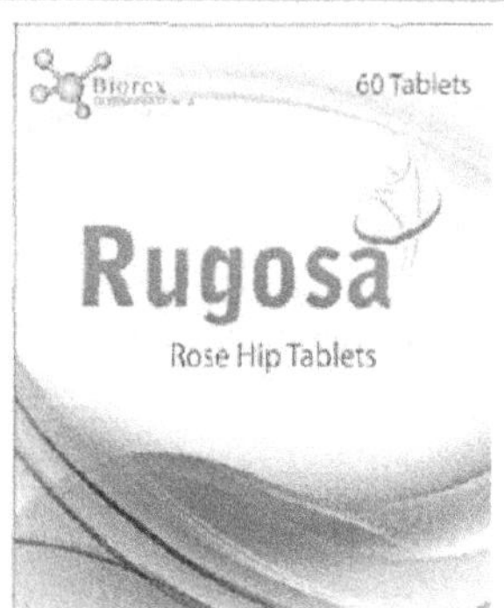

Advertised before Acceptance under section 20(1) Proviso

2441353   12/12/2012

BIOREX HEALTHCARE PVT LTD

A-1/85-A ,MAA SHAKTI APARTMENTS, PASCHIM VIHAR, NEW DELHI-110063

MANUFACTURER, TRADER & MERCHANTS

Address for service in India/Agents address:

DUA ASSOCIATES.

202 - 206, TOLSTOY HOUSE 15, TOLSTOY MARG, NEW DELHI - 110 001.

Used Since :31/10/2012

DELHI

MEDICINAL AND PHARMACEUTICAL PREPARATIONS

ANNEXURE 3

GEOGRAPHICAL INDICATIONS REGISTERED AND GUIDELINES

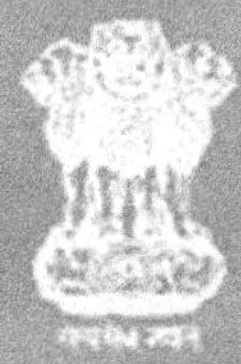

GEOGRAPHICAL INDICATIONS JOURNAL

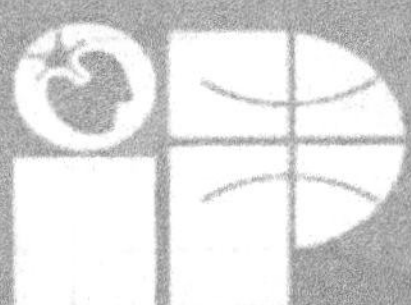

NEW G.I APPLICATION DETAILS

App.No.	Geographical Indications	Class	Goods
405	Makrana Marble	19	Natural Goods
406	Salem Mango	31	Horticulture
407	Hosur Rose	31	Agricultural
408	Payyanur Pavithra Mothiram	14	Handicraft
409	Kodali Karuppur Saree	24 & 25	Textile
410	Thammampatti Wood Carvings	20	Handicraft
411	Rajapalayam Lock	6	Manufactured
412	Chamba Painting	16	Handicraft
413	Kangra Paintings	16	Handicraft
414	Punjabi Jutti	25	Handicraft
415	Aipan	16	Handicraft
416	Lahaul & Spiti Wool Weaving	23	Handicraft
417	Lacquer Ware Furniture	20	Handicraft
418	Jhajjar Pottery	21	Handicraft
419	Tamta Copperware Craft	6	Handicraft
420	Rewari Jutti	25	Handicraft
421	Hoshiarpur Wood Inlay	20	Handicraft
422	Kandangi Sarees	24	Textile
423	Thanjavur Pith Works	20	Handicraft
424	Karupur Kalamkari Paintings	24	Handicraft
425	Thanjavur Cut Glass Work	20	Handicraft
426	Mahabalipuram Stone Sculpture	19	Handicraft
427	Nagercoil Temple Car	20	Handicraft
428	Kannyakumari Stone Carving	19	Handicraft
429	Arumbavur Wood Carving	20	Handicraft

Table *Contd...*

430	Namakkal Makkal Stone Works	21	Handicraft
431	Kallakurichi Wood Carving	20	Handicraft
432	Kinnauri Kala Zeera	31	Agriculture
433	Bandar (Machilipatanam) Laddu	30	Food Stuff
434	Ratlami Sev	30	Food Stuff
435	Assam Karbi Anglong Ginger	30	Agriculture
436	Tripura Queen Pineapple	31	Agriculture
437	Memong Narang	31	Agriculture
438	Tezpur Litchi	31	Agriculture
439	Joha Rice of Assam	30	Agriculture
440	Sathebari Bell Metal Crafts	6	Handicraft
441	Karbi Textiles Products	24 & 25	Textile
442	Sital Pati Mats & Crafts of Goalpara	20	Handicraft
443	Larnai Clay Pottery	21	Handicraft
444	Bamboo Shang Trop	6	Handicraft
445	Stone Carving Craft	21	Handicraft
446	Kauna Reed Craft	21	Handicraft
447	Manipur Dolls and Toys Craft	21	Handicraft
448	Solapith Crafts of Birbhum District	16	Handicraft
449	Burdwan Natungram Wood Craft	21	Handicraft
450	Naga Angami Shawl	24	Textile
451	Naga Ao Shawl	24	Textile
452	Naga Sumi Shawl	24	Textile
453	Bankura Panchmura Terracotta Craft	21	Handicraft
454	Monpa Wooden Mask	21	Handicraft
455	Sherdukpen Handlooms & Textiles	21	Handicraft
456	Monpas Handlooms & Textile Goods	24 & 25	Textile

Table Contd...

457	Varanasi Wooden Lacquer Wear & Toys	27	Handicraft
458	Mirzapur Handmade Dari	27	Handicraft
459	Nizamabad Black Clay Pottery	27	Handicraft
460	Machilipatnam Imitation Jewellery	14	Handicraft
461	Indian Thangka Paintings	16	Handicraft
462	Wood Craft of Sikkim	20	Handicraft
463	Sikkim Lepcha Handloom	24	Handicraft
464	Sirsi Siddapur Yellapur Arecanut	31	Agriculture
465	Khasi Mandarin	31	Agriculture
466	Kachai Lemon	31	Agriculture

Advertised under Rule 41(1) of Geographical Indications of Goods (Registration & Protection) Rules, 2002in the Geographical Indications Journal 56 dated 21st January 2014

Authorised User Application No. - 1610 in respect of Kashmir Pashmina
Registered GI Application No. - 46

Application is made by, **Mr. Mohammad Saleem Sofi**, Village & Post: Rathpora, Eidgah, SafaKadal, District: Srinagar - 190002, Jammu & Kashmir, India, dated for June 25, 2013 Registration in Part-B for Authorised User in respect of Registered Geographical Indication **Kashmir Pashmina** under Application No - 46 in respect of Yarns and Threads, for textile use, Textiles and Textiles goods, not included in other classes; bed and table covers & Clothing, falling in Class 23, 24 & 25 is hereby advertised as accepted under sub-section (1) of Section 13 of Geographical Indications of Goods (Registration and Protection) Act, 1999.

(A)	**Applicant**	:	Mr. Mohammad Saleem Sofi
(B)	**Address**	:	Mr. Mohammad Saleem Sofi, Village & Post: Rathpora, Eidgah, Safa Kadal, District: Srinagar - 190002, Jammu & Kashmir, India
(C)	**Date of Authorised User Application**	:	June 25, 2013
(D)	**Registered Geographical Indication**	:	**Kashmir Pashmina**

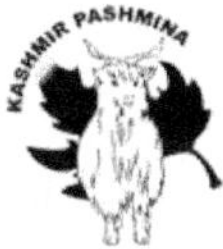

(E)	**Registered Proprietor**	:	TAHAFUZ, Srinagar
(F)	**Address**	:	TAHAFUZ, (Registered Under the J & K Societies Act, Registration Number: 5611-S/2007) Nowshera, Zadibal, Post Office: Nowshera, District: Srinagar - 190 011, Jammu & Kashmir, India.
(G)	**Class**	:	23, 24 & 25
(H)	**Goods**	:	**Class 23, 24 & 25** - Yarns and Threads, for textile use, Textiles and Textiles goods, not included in other Classes; bed and table covers & Clothing.

*________*_______*________*

THE GEOGRAPHICAL INDICATIONS OF GOODS
(REGISTRATION AND PROTECTION) ACT, 1999

(To be filled in triplicate alongwith the Statement of Case accompanied by five additional representation of the Geographical indication)
One representation to be fixed within the space and five others to be send separately

FORM GI-1

A	Application for the registration of a geographical indication in Part A of the Register Section 11 (1), Rule 23(2) Fee: Rs.5,000 (See entry No.1A of the First Schedule)	
B	Application for the registration of a geographical Indication in Part A of the Register from a convention country Section 11(1), 84(1), Rule 23(3) Fee : Rs.5,000 (See entry No.1 B of the First Schedule)	

1. Application is hereby made by for the registration in Part A of the Register of the accompanying geographical indication furnishing the following particulars : -
   - Name of the Applicant :
   - Address :
   - List of association of persons/producers/organization/authority:
   - Type of goods:
   - Specification:
   - Name of the geographical indication [and particulars]
   - Description of the goods :
   - Geographical area of production and map :
   - Proof of origin [Historical records] :
   - Method of Production :
   - Uniqueness :
   - Inspection Body :
   - Other:

Along with the Statement of Case in Class[b] ..... [b] .... in respect of [c] .... in the name(s) of[d] ...... whose address is .... Who claims to represent the interest of the producers of the said goods to which the geographical indication relates and which is in continuous use since in respect of the said goods.

2. The Application shall include such other particulars called for in rule 32(1) in the Statement of Case.
3. All communications relating to this application may be sent to the following address in India.
4. In the case of an application from a convention country the following additional particulars shall also be furnished.
   (a) Designation of the country of origin of the Geographical Indication.
   (b) Evidence as to the existing protection of the Geographical Indication in its country of origin, such as the title and the date of the relevant legislative or administrative provisions, the judicial decisions or the date and number of the registration, and copies. of such documentation.

[e]SIGNATURE
NAME OF THE SIGNATORY
(IN BLOCK LETTERS)

C	Application for the registration of a geographical indication In Part A of the Register for goods falling in different classes Section 11 (3), Rule 23(5) Fee: Rs.5,000 for each class (See entry No.1C of the First Schedule)	
D	A single application for the registration of a geographical Indication in Part A of the Register for goods falling in different classes from a convention country Section 11(3), rule 23(4) Fee : Rs.5,000 for each class (See entry No.ID of the First Schedule)	

1. Application is hereby made by for the registration in Part A of the Register of the accompanying geographical indication furnishing the following particulars : -
    - Name of the Applicant :
    - Address :
    - List of association of persons/producers/organization/authority:
    - Type of goods:
    - Specification:
    - Name of the geographical indication [and particulars]
    - Description of the goods :
    - Geographical area of production and map :
    - Proof of origin [Historical records] :
    - Method of Production :
    - Uniqueness :
    - Inspection Body :
    - Other:

along with the Statement of Case in Class

    i)   Class^b ……….. in respect of^c………..
    ii)   Class^b ……….. in respect of^c………..
    iii)   Class^b ……….. in respect of^c………..

In the name(s) of ^{d} …………… Whose address is ……. Who claim (s) to represent the interest of the producers of the goods to which the geographical indication relates and which geographical indication is used continuously since …… in respect of the said goods.

2. The Application shall include such other particulars called for in rule 32(1) in the Statement of Case.
3. All communications relating to this application may be sent to the following address in India.
4. In the case of an application from a convention country the following additional particulars shall also be furnished.
    a. Designation of the country of origin of the Geographical Indication.
    b. Evidence as to the existing protection of the Geographical Indication in its country of origin, such as the title and the date of the relevant legislative or administrative provisions, the judicial decisions or the date and number of the registration, and copies. of such documentation.

^{e}SIGNATURE
NAME OF THE SIGNATORY (IN BLOCK LETTERS)

For instruction please see overleaf

G1-1A to 1D

The Registrar of Geographical Indications,

The office of Geographical Indications Registry.

    (a) Strike out whichever is not applicable.

    (b) The Registrars' direction may be obtained if the class of the goods is not known.

    (c) Here specify the goods. Only goods included in one and the same class to be specified.

    (d)   Insert legibly the full name, description (occupation and calling and nationality of the applicant).   In the case of a body corporate or firm the country of incorporation or the registration, if any, as   the case may be, should be stated, See rule 15.

    (e) Signature of the applicant or his agent.

Procedure for Filing G.I Application

I.   Form and signing of application

1.   Every application for the registration of a geographical indication shall be   made in the prescribed form (GI-1A to ID) accompanied by the prescribed fee (Rs.5,000).

2.   It shall be signed by the applicant or his agent.

3.   It must be made in triplicate along with three copies of a Statement of Case accompanied by five additional representations.

II.   Fees

1.   Fees may be paid in cash or sent by money order or by a bank draft or by a cheque.

2.   Bank Drafts or cheques shall be crossed and be made payable to the Registrar at the appropriate office of the Geographical Indication Registry.

3.   It should be drawn by a scheduled bank at the place where the appropriate office of the Geographical Indications Registry is situated.

4.   Where a document is field without fee or with insufficient fee such document shall be deemed to have not been filed.

III.   Sizes

1.   All applications, shall   be typewritten, lithographed or printed in Hindi or in English.

2.   It should in large and legible characters with deep permanent ink upon strong paper, on one side only.

3.   The size should be a approximately 33 cms by 20 cms and shall have on the left and part thereof a margin of not less than 4 centimeters.

IV.   Signing of documents

1.   In case of

   i.   An association of persons or producers shall be signed by the authorized signatory.

  ii. A body corporate or any organization or any authority established by or under any law for the time being in force shall be signed by the Chief Executive, or the Managing Director or the secretary or other principal officer.

  iii. In case of partnership it shall be signed by at least one of the partners.

2. The capacity in which an individual signs a document shall be stated below his signature.

3. Signatures shall be accompanied by the name of the signatory in English or in Hindi and in capital letters.

V. Principal place of business in India

1. Every application for registration of a G.I shall state the principal place of business in India.

2. A body corporate should state the full name and nationality of the Board of Directors.

3. Foreign applicants and persons having principal place of business, in their home country should furnish an address for service in India.

4. In the case of a body corporate or any organization or authority established by or under any law for the time being in force, the country of incorporation or the nature of registration, if any, as the case may be shall be given.

VI. Convention Application should contain the following

1. A certificate by the Registry or competent authority of the Geographical Indications Office of the convention country.

2. The particulars of the geographical indication, the country and the date or dates of filing of the first application.

3. The application must be the applicants' first application in a convention country for the same geographical indications and for all or some of the goods.

4. The application must include a statement indicating the filing date of the foreign application, the convention country where it was filed, the serial number, if available.

VII.   Statement of user in applications

An application to register a geographical indication shall contain a statement of user alongwith an affidavit.

VIII.   Content of Application

Every application shall be made in the prescribed forms and shall contain the following :

1. A statement as to how the geographical indication serves to designate the goods as originating form the concerned territory in respect of specific quality, reputation or other characteristics.

2. The three certified copies of class of goods to which the geographical indication relates

3. The geographical map of the territory.

4. The particulars of the appearance of the geographical indication words or figurative elements or both;

5. A statement containing such particulars of the producers of the concerned goods proposed to be initially resisted. Including a collective reference to all the producers of the goods in respect of which the application is made.

6. The statement contained in the application shall also include the following:

An affidavit as to how the applicant claim to represent the interest of the association of persons or producers or any organization or authority established under any law.

The standards benchmark for the use of the geographical indication or the industry standard as regards the production, exploitation, making or manufacture of the goods having specific quality, reputation or other characteristic of such goods that is essentially attributable to its geographical origin with the detailed description of the human creativity involved, if any or other characteristic;

The particulars of the mechanism to ensure that the standards, quality, integrity and consistency or other special characteristic are maintained by the producers, or manufacturers of the goods.

Three certified copies of the map of the territory, region or locality;

The particulars of special human skill involved or the uniquess of the geographical environment or other inherent characteristics associated with the geographical indication.

The full name and address of the association of persons or organization or authority representing the interest of the producers of the concerned goods;

Particulars of the inspection strucsture ;

In case of a homonymous indication, the material factors differentiating the application from the registered geographical indications and particulars of protective measures adopted.

IX. Acknowledgement of receipt of applications:

1. Every application of the registration of a geographical indication in respect of any goods shall, on receipt be acknowledged by the Registrar.

2. The acknowledgement shall be by way of return of one of the additional representations with the official number of the application duly entered thereon.

ANNEXURE 4

DESIGNS REGISTERED

DESIGN NUMBER	245241
CLASS	24-02
1)KONINKLIJKE PHILIPS ELECTRONICS N.V., A COMPANY ORGANIZED AND EXISTING UNDER THE LAWS OF THE KINGDOM OF THE NETHERLANDS, RESIDING AT EINDHOVEN, WHOSE POST-OFFICE ADDRESS IS GROENEWOUDSEWEG 1, 5621 BA, EINDHOVEN, THE NETHERLANDS	
DATE OF REGISTRATION	10/05/2012
TITLE	PATIENT INTERFACE ASSEMBLY

PRIORITY

PRIORITY NUMBER	DATE	COUNTRY
001945833-0001	10/11/2011	OHIM

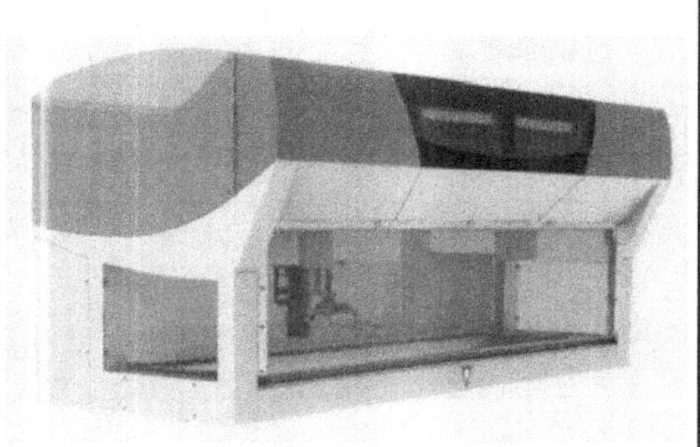

DESIGN NUMBER	242265
CLASS	24-01
1)TECAN TRADING AG SEESTRASSE 103, 8708 MANNEDORF, SWITZERLAND	
DATE OF REGISTRATION	16/01/2012
TITLE	AUTOMATED LABORATORY DEVICES

PRIORITY

PRIORITY NUMBER	DATE	COUNTRY
CH 138182	19/07/2011	SWITZERLAND

DESIGN NUMBER	244785
CLASS	15-09
1)M/S. PROCUT ELECTRONICS 48, V.K. ESTATE, B/H. MANGLAM CINEMA, ODHAV, AHMEDABAD-382415, GUJARAT, INDIA	
DATE OF REGISTRATION	24/04/2012
TITLE	WOOD CUTTING MACHINERY

PRIORITY NA

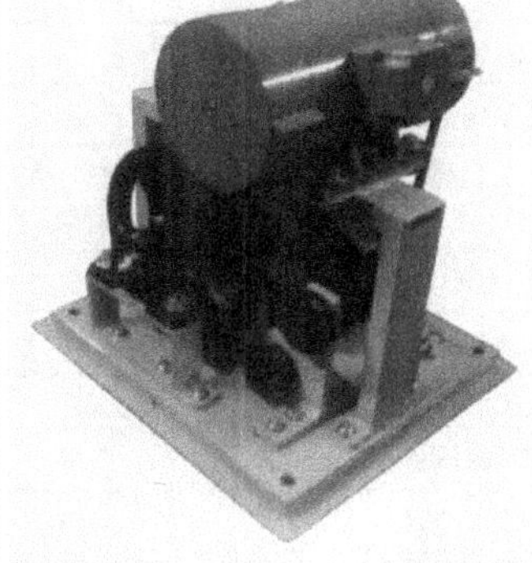

DESIGN NUMBER	243618
CLASS	31-01
1)M/S J. B. EQUIPMENTS A-3, KHASRA NO. 61/21, NARESH PARK EXTN., NANGLOI, NEW DELHI, INDIA	
DATE OF REGISTRATION	05/03/2012
TITLE	CHAPATI MAKER
PRIORITY NA	

DESIGN NUMBER	243627
CLASS	24-03
1)SANTEN PHARMACEUTICAL CO., LTD. 9-19, SHIMOSHINJO 3-CHOME, HIGASHIYODOGAWA-KU, OSAKA-SHI, OSAKA 5338651, JAPAN	
DATE OF REGISTRATION	05/03/2012
TITLE	INTRAOCULAR LENS

PRIORITY

PRIORITY NUMBER	DATE	COUNTRY
29/401, 063	06/09/2011	U.S.A.

DESIGN NUMBER	240226
CLASS	24-01
1)ETHICON ENDO-SURGERY, INC., 4545 CREEK ROAD, CINCINNATI, OH 45242, USA.,	
DATE OF REGISTRATION	13/10/2011
TITLE	SURGICAL GENERATOR
PRIORITY	

PRIORITY NUMBER	DATE	COUNTRY
29/389, 531	13/04/2011	U.S.A.

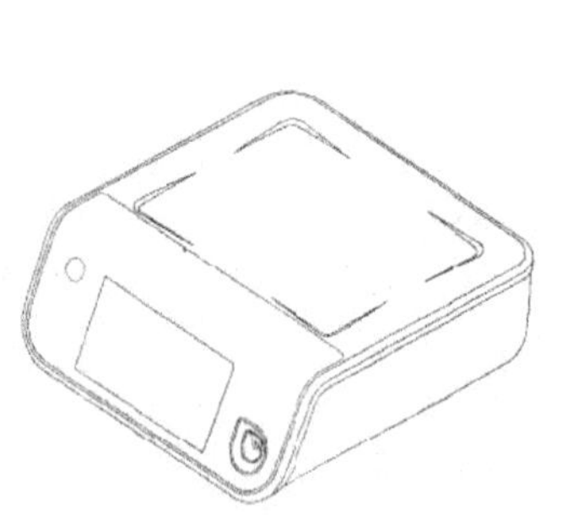

DESIGN NUMBER	240396
CLASS	24-04
1)3M INNOVATIVE PROPERTIES COMPANY DELAWARE, 3M CENTER, SAINT PAUL, MINNESOTA 55133-3427, USA	
DATE OF REGISTRATION	24/10/2011
TITLE	HYDROCOLLOID FIRST AID DRESSING

PRIORITY

PRIORITY NUMBER	DATE	COUNTRY
29/390, 380	25/04/2011	U.S.A.

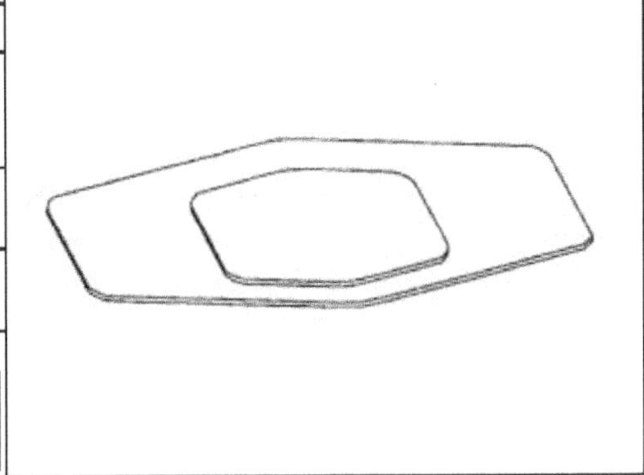

DESIGN NUMBER	245947
CLASS	07-06
1)MA DESIGN INDIA PRIVATE LIMITED, A COMPANY INCORPORATED IN INDIA HAVING ITS PRINCIPAL PLACE OF BUSINESS AT A-41, SECTOR-80, PHASE-II, NOIDA-201305, U.P.	
DATE OF REGISTRATION	14/06/2012
TITLE	NAPKIN HOLDER
PRIORITY NA	

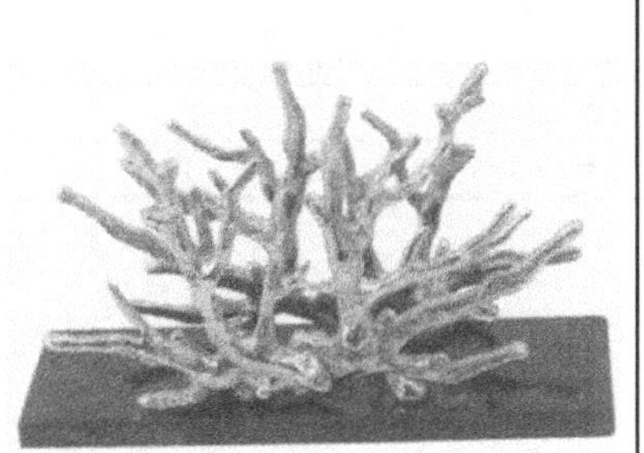

DESIGN NUMBER	256028
CLASS	24-01
1)ANALYTICA LIMITED A COMPANY ORGANIZED AND EXISTING UNDER THE LAWS OF AUSTRALIA, HAVING ITS OFFICE AT 320 ADELAIDE STREET, BRISBANE QUEENSLAND 4000, AUSTRALIA	
DATE OF REGISTRATION	23/08/2013
TITLE	PERINEOMETER

PRIORITY

PRIORITY NUMBER	DATE	COUNTRY
12210/2013	14/05/2013	AUSTRALIA

DESIGN NUMBER	256734	
CLASS	15-01	
1)YANMAR CO.,LTD., A CORPORATION ORGANIZED AND EXISTING UNDER THE LAWS OF JAPAN, OF 1-9, TSURUNOCHO, KITA-KU, OSAKA-SHI, OSAKA 5308311, JAPAN		
DATE OF REGISTRATION	24/09/2013	
TITLE	INTERNAL COMBUSTION ENGINE	
PRIORITY		
PRIORITY NUMBER	DATE	COUNTRY
2013-6641	26/03/2013	JAPAN

DESIGN NUMBER	255933
CLASS	09-05
1)NAVA HEALTH CARE PVT. LTD SITUATED AT 1105, 11TH FLOOR, KIRTI SHIKHAR BUILDING, DISTT. CENRE, JANAK PURI, NEW DELHI-110058 (INDIA) A COMPANY INCORPORATED UNDER THE INDIAN COMPANIES ACT, OF ABOVE ADDRESS	
DATE OF REGISTRATION	21/08/2013
TITLE	BLISTER PACK
PRIORITY NA	

ANNEXURE 5

PLANT VARIETY REGISTERED

भारतीय पौधा किस्म जरनल

PLANT VARIETY JOURNAL OF INDIA

खण्ड – 08, अंक – 04, अप्रैल 01, 2014
Vol. - 08, No. – 04, April 01, 2014

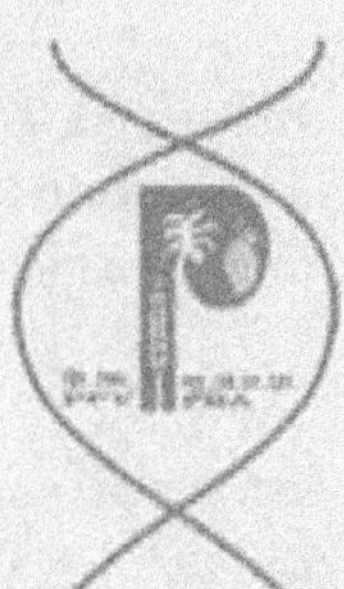

पौधा किस्म और कृषक अधिकार संरक्षण प्राधिकरण
एनएएससी काम्प्लैक्स, डीपीएस मार्ग, निकट टोडापुर गांव, नई दिल्ली–110012

PROTECTION OF PLANT VARIETIES & FARMERS' RIGHTS AUTHORITY

NASC COMPLEX, DPS MARG, Opp. Todapur Village, New Delhi-110012

Acid lime (*Citrus aurantifolia* Swingle)

I   Subject

These test guidelines shall apply to all the varieties of acid lime (*Citrus aurantifolia* Swingle)

II.   Materials required

1. The Protection of Plant Varieties and Farmers' Rights Authority (PPV & FRA) shall decide on the quantity and quality of the planting materials required for testing the varieties and where it is to be delivered for registration under the Protection of Plant Varieties and Farmers' Rights (PPV & FR) Act, 2001.
2. Applicants submitting such materials from a country other than India shall make sure that all customs and pre and post quarantine requirements stipulated under relevant national legislations and regulation are complied with.
3. The materials are to be raised as nucellar seedlings and a minimum of ten plants to be supplied by the applicants or his/her nominee during the month of June- July for each DUS Centre. Planting materials supplied shall be healthy and free from pests, diseases and mechanical injury. Age of the plants shall be above six months from the date of transplanting in secondary nursery and raised in the black polythene bags 300 μ thickness UV stabilized (12cm x 6cm size) with potting mixture (soil, FYM and sand in 1 : 1: 1 ratio).
4. The plants should not have undergone any treatment which would affect the expression of the characters of the variety, unless the competent authority allows or requests for any such treatment.
5. The planting material shall not have undergone any chemical and bio-physical treatment unless the competent authority or applicant specifically request for such treatment. If it has been treated, full details of the treatment must be mentioned explicitly.

III.   Conduct of test

1. The minimum duration of the DUS tests shall normally be at least for two independent identical fruiting seasons in different years.
2. The test should be carried out under conditions ensuring satisfactory growth for the expression of the relevant characteristics of the variety and for the conduct of the examination. In particular, it is essential that the tree produces a satisfactory crop of fruit in each of the fruiting seasons in two consecutive years. In case of any climatic vagaries data from third fruiting season may also be considered.

3. Test Design

The design of the tests should be such that plants or parts of the plant may be removed for measurement or counting without prejudice to the observations which may be made up to the end of the vegetative /fruiting season as the case maybe. Unless otherwise indicated, all observations are to be recorded on five plants.

Additional Tests

Additional tests, for examining special characteristics, may be established by the PPV&FR Authority.

4. On- site testing :

The guidelines developed by PPV&FR Authority for on- site testing will be followed with the specific requirement for acid lime.

- The age of the plants for on-site shall be minimum of five years from the date of planting in the field.
- A minimum of two plants must be made available for field gene bank. For inspection and examination even single tree could be considered only for farmers' varieties. The trees should be healthy, free from pests and diseases and raised under standard management practices.
- On-site examination shall be arranged during vegetative and fruiting seasons.

IV. Methods and observations

1. The characteristics described in the Table of Characteristics (see section VII) shall be used for the testing of candidate varieties.
2. For the assessment of DUS characters, observations shall be made on five plants.

Observations

(a)Leaf: Observations on the leaf should be made on the fully expended leaves of spring flush.

(b) Fruit: Observations on the fruit should be made at the stage of harvest maturity. Fruits should be sampled from the periphery of the tree

(c) Fruit rind: Observations on the fruit rind should be made at the middle, between the base and apex of the fruit.

(d) Number of spines per 30 cm length from basal bud on one year old shoot.

V. Grouping of varieties

1.The candidate varieties of DUS testing shall be divided into groups to facilitate the assessment of distinctiveness. Characteristics, which are known from experience not to vary, or to vary only slightly within a variety and in which their various states are fairly evenly distributed across all the varieties in the collection are suitable for grouping purpose.

2. Characteristics for grouping are those in which the documented states of expression, even when produced at different locations. These can be used, either individually or in combination with other such characteristics to (a) select varieties of common knowledge that can be excluded from the growing trials used for examination of distinctiveness; and (b) organize the growing trials so that similar varieties are grouped together.

The following characteristics are to be used for **grouping** of acid lime varieties :

(a) Tree growth habit (characteristic - 1)
(b) Spine density (characteristic - 2)
(c) Fruit diameter (characteristic - 8)

VI. Characteristics and symbols

1   To assess Distinctiveness, Uniformity and Stability, the characteristics and their states as given in the Table of Characteristics (Section VII) shall be used.

2   Notes (1 to 9) shall be given for each state of expression for different characteristics for the purpose of electronic data processing.

3.   Legend

(*) Characteristics that shall be observed during every growing season in all the varieties and shall always be included in the description of the variety. In exceptional cases wherein the state of expression of any of these characters is not recorded due to environmental vagaries, adequate explanation may be provided.

(+) See Explanation on the Table of characteristics in Section VIII. It is to be noted that for certain characteristics, the plant parts on which observations are to be taken are given in the explanation or figure (s) for clarity and not the colour variation.

4. A code number given in the sixth column of Table of characteristics indicates the optimum stage for the observation of each characteristics during the growth and development of the plant. The relevant growth stages corresponding to these code numbers are described below:

Decimal Code for the growth stages :

Growth stage	Code
Full grown bearing tree	100
One year old spring flush shoots	30
Fully expanded leaves of spring flush shoots	30
Harvest maturity	95

4. Observations on fully expanded leaf on the middle portion of the spring flush.

5. The mature/ripe fruit is the fruit at the stage ready for consumption. This stage is   reached when the segment is juicy and fruits developed characteristic colour.

6. The colour expression must be recorded using RHS colour chart

5. Type of assessment of characteristics indicated in column seven of Table of Characteristics is as follows:

MG : Measurement by a single observation of a group of plants or parts of plant
MS : Measurement of a number of individual plants or parts of plant
VG : Visual assessment by a single observation of a group of plants or parts of plant
VS : Visual assessment by observation of individual plants or parts of plant

VII.   Table of Characteristics

S. No	Characteristics	States	Note	Example varieties	Stage of observation (Code)	Type of assessment
1	2	3	4	5	6	7
1 (*) (+)	Tree growth habit	Erect	1	Chakradhar	Full grown bearing tree (100)	VG
		Spreading	2	Sai Sharbati, Vikram, Pramalini, Balaji, Phule Sharbati.		
		Drooping	3	-		
2. (*)	Spine density on the adult tree (No. of spines on one year old spring shoot, 30cm length)	Low (< 10)	3	Chakradhar	Full grown bearing tree (100)	MG
		Medium (10-15)	5	Sai Sharbati, Vikram, Pramalini, Balaji, Phule Sharbati		
		High (>15)	7	--		

Table *Contd...*

3.	Spine length (mm)	<5	1	Chakradhar	One year old spring flush shoots (30)	MS
		5 -15	2	Sai Sharbati, Vikram, Pramalini, Balaji, Phule Sharbati		
		>15	3	--		
4 (+)	Leaf lamina length [mm]	Short(<60)	3	Chakradhar	Fully expanded spring flush leaves (30)	MG
		Medium(60-70)	5	Sai Sharbati, Vikram, Pramalini, Balaji, Phule Sharbati,		
		Long(>70)	7	--		
5. (+)	Leaf lamina width [mm]	Narrow(<35)	3	Chakradhar	Fully expanded spring flush leaves (30)	MG
		Medium(35 -40)	5	Sai Sharbati, Vikram, Pramalini, Balaji, Phule Sharbati,		
		Broad(>40)	7	--		
6. (+)	Petiole wings	Absent	1	Chakradhar	Fully expanded spring flush leaves (30)	VG
		Present	9	Sai Sharbati, Vikram, Pramalini, Balaji, Phule Sharbati		
7.	Fruit weight (g)	Light (<40)	1	Vikram, Pramalini, Chakradhar	Harvest maturity (95)	MG
		Heavy (> 41)	2	Sai Sharbati, Balaji, Phule Sharbati		
8 (*) (+)	Fruit diameter (mm)	Small (<40)	3	Chakradhar,	Harvest maturity (95)	MG
		Medium (41 -45)	5	Vikram, Pramalini, Balaji		
		Large(>45)	7	Sai Sharbati, Balaji, Phule Sharbati		
9	Fruit length	Short (<40)	3	Chakradhar	Harvest	MG

Table Contd...

(+)	(mm)	Medium (40 -45)	5	Vikram, Pramalini, Balaji	maturity (95)	
		Long(>45)	7	Sai Sharbati, Phule Sharbati		
10	Albedo colour	Greenish	1	--	Harvest maturity (95)	VS
		White	2	Sai Sharbati, Vikram, Pramalini, Balaji,Chakradhar, Phule Sharbati		
		Yellow	3	---		
11	Fruit axis	Solid	1	Sai Sharbati, Vikram, Pramalini, Balaji, Phule Sharbati	Harvest maturity (95)	VS
		Hollow	2	Chakradhar		
12	Number of segments per fruit	8-10	1	Sai Sharbai, Vikram, Pramalini, Balaji,Chakradhar, Phule Sharbati	Harvest maturity (95)	VS
		>10	2	--		
13	Fruit rind (epicarp) thickness (mm)	Thin (<2)	3	Sai Sharbati, Vikram, Pramalini, , Balaji,Chakradhar, Phule Sharbati	Harvest maturity (95)	MS
		Thick(>2)	5	--		
14	Fruit juiciness (%)	Low (<40)	3	--	Harvest maturity (95)	MS
		Medium (40 to 50)	5	Vikram, Pramalini, Chakradhar		
		High (>50)	7	Sai Sharbati, , Balaji, ,Phule Sharbati,		
15 (+)	Total Soluble Solids	Low (<6)	3	-	Harvest maturity (95)	MS
		Medium (6 to7)	5	--		

Table *Contd…*

	(TSS, ^{0}Brix)	High (>7)	7	Sai Sharbati, Vikram, Pramalini, Balaji, Chakradhar, Phule Sharbati		
16 (+)	Titratable acidity (% citric acid)	Low (<5)	3	--	Harvest maturity (95)	MS
		Medium (5 to 6)	5	Chakradhar		
		High (>6)	7	Sai Sharbati, Vikram, Pramalini, Balaji, Phule Sharbati		
17	Seediness (Number of seeds/ fruit)	<4	1	Chakradhar	Harvest maturity (95)	MS
		4-10	2	Sai Sharbati, Vikram, Pramalini, Balaji, Phule Sharbati, Niboo		
		>10	3	--		

VIII. Explanation on the Table of Characteristics :

Characteristic 1. Tree growth habit

Recorded on the tree not less than 5 years age in natural state just after fruit harvesting

Characteristic 4. Leaf lamina length [mm]

Recorded from petiole base to lamina tip

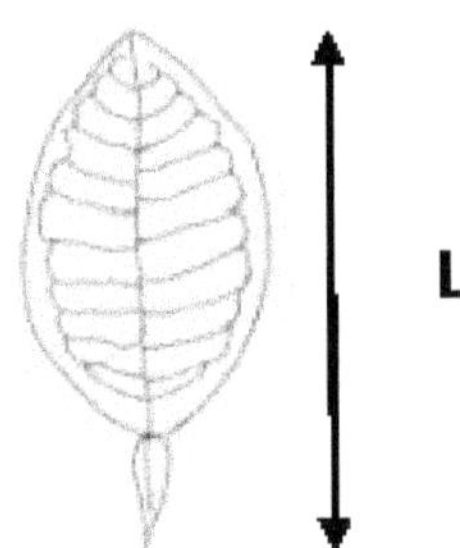

Characteristic 5. Leaf lamina width [mm]

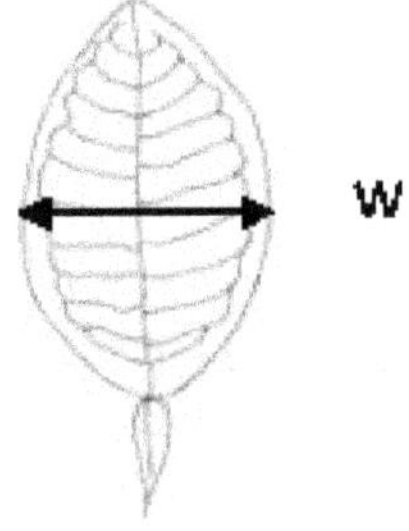

Characteristic 6. Absence/presence of petiole wings

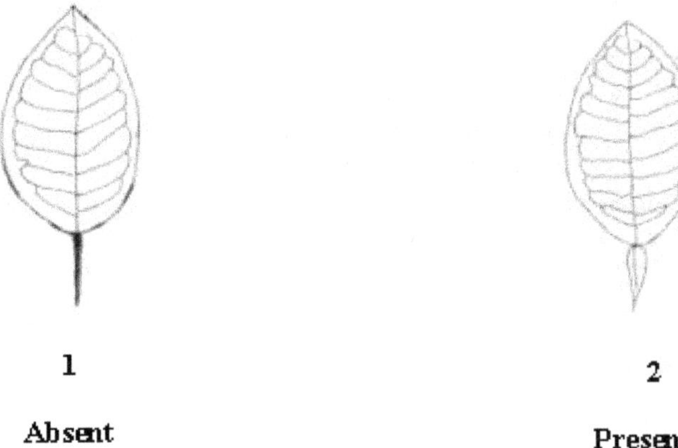

Characteristic 8. Fruit diameter

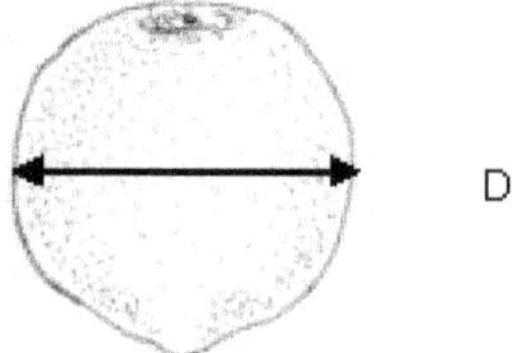

Characteristic 9. Fruit length

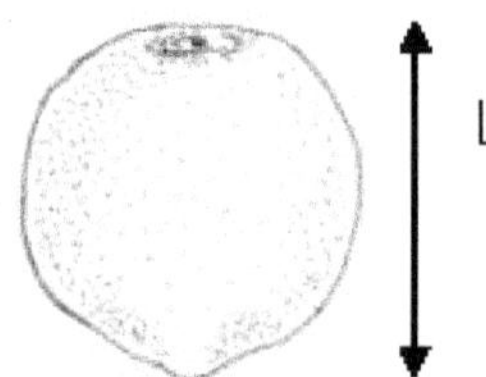

Characteristic 16. Fruit juice TSS (^{0}Brix)

The fruit samples were harvested as per maturity standard. The juice will be extracted by juicer or electronic juicer machine and total soluble solids (TSS) determined. The hand held/ digital refractometer should be used to measure the TSS ^{0}brix in juice sample. One or two drops of the juice should be placed on refractometer and per cent TSS on the scale should be recorded. The reading are to be taken at room temperatures.

Characteristic 17. Titratable acidity (% Citric acid)

The juice acid content of the samples should be recorded by visual titration method as suggested by Ranganna(1986). The titration sample prepared with 5ml of juice mixed with 20 ml of distilled water put in volumetric flask to makeup the volume to 25 ml. Thereafter 5 ml mixed sample should be taken for further titration using phenolphthalein as an indicator against 0.1 N sodium hydroxide. The titrated acidity expressed as percentage citric acid.

$$\text{Acidity}(\%) = \frac{\text{Titre value x Normality of alkali x Volume made up x Equivalent weight of acid (i.e. 64 x100)}}{\text{Volume of aliquot taken for estimation x Weight or volume of sample taken x1000}}$$

X. Working Group details

Theese Test Guidelines developed by the NRC for Citrus, Nagpur, the Nodal Officer, DUS Center and finalized by the Task Force (1/2013) constituted by the PPV & FR Authority.

The Members of the Task Force (1/2013)

Dr. V. A. Parthasarathy -   Chairman

Dr B.M.C. Reddy -

Dr S. N. Pandey -

Dr H. Ravishankar –

Dr Umesh Srivastava -

Dr I. P. Singh -

Dr. Tejbir Singh -   Member Secretary

Nodal Officer

Dr I.P. Singh, Principal Scientist (Hort.) and Nodal officer DUS project

National Research Centre for Citrus (NRCC), Amravati Road, Nagpur

Co-Nodal Officer

Dr R.K. Sonkar, Principal Scientist (Hort.)

National Research Centre for Citrus (NRCC), Amaravati Road, Nagpur

IX. DUS testing centers

Nodal DUS Test Centre	Other DUS Test Centres
National Research Centre for Citrus (NRCC), Amravati Road, Nagpur (Maharashtra)- 440010	Horticultural Experiment Station, Indi /Bijapur, Karnataka.

ANNEXURE 6

PATENT APPLICATION
FORMS 1, 2, 3, 5, 28 (SME)

<table>
<tr>
<td>

FORM 1
THE PATENTS ACT 1970
(39 of 1970)
&
The Patents Rules, 2003
APPLICATION FOR GRANT OF PATENT
(See section 7,54&135and rule20 (1))

</td>
<td>

(FOR OFFICE USE ONLY)

Application No:
Filing Date:
Amount of Fee Paid:
CBR No:
Signature:

</td>
</tr>
</table>

1. APPLICANT (S)

Name	Nationality	Address

2. INVENTOR (S)

Name	Nationality	Address

3. TITLE OF THE INVENTION

4. ADDRESS FOR CORRESPONDENCE OF APPLICANT/AUTHORIZED PATENT AGENT IN INDIA	Telephone No. Fax No. Mobile No. E-mail:

5. PRIORITY PARTICULARS OF THE APPLICATION (S) FILED IN CONVENTION COUNTRY

Country	Application Number	Filing Date	Name of the Applicant	Title of the Invention

6.   PARTICULARS FOR FILING PATENT COOPERATION TREATY (PCT) NATIONAL PHASE APPLICATION

International application number.	International filing date as allotted by the receiving office.

7.   PARTICULARS FOR FILING DIVISIONAL APPLICATION

Original (first) application number.	Date of filing of Original (first) application

8.   PARTICULARS FOR FILING PATENT OF ADDITION

Main application/patent Number.	Date of filing of main application

9. DECLARATIONS:

(i) Declaration by the Inventor(s)
  I/We, the above named inventor(s) is/are the true & first inventor(s) for this invention and declare that the applicant(s)herein is/are my/our assignee or legal representative.

(a) Date___________
(b) Signature(s)
(c) Name(s)

(ii) Declaration by the applicant(s) in the convention country
  I/We, the applicant(s) in the convention country declare that the applicant(s)herein is/are my/our assignee or legal representative.
(a) Date___________
(b) Signature(s)
(c) Name(s) of the signatory

Table Contd...

(iii) Declaration by the applicant(s):
I/We, the applicant(s) hereby declare(s) that: -

- ☐ I am /We are in possession of the above-mentioned invention
- ☐ The provisional/complete specification relating to the invention is filed with this application.
- ☐ The invention as disclosed in the specification uses the biological material from India and the necessary permission from the competent authority shall be submitted by me/us before the grant of patent to me/us.
- ☐ There is no lawful ground of objection to the grant of the Patent to me/us.
- ☐ I am/ We are the assignee or legal representative of true & first inventors.
- ☐ The application or each of the applications, particulars of which are given in Para - 5 was the first application in convention country/countries in respect of my/our invention.
- ☐ I/We claim the priority from the above mentioned application(s) filed in convention country/countries and state that no application for protection in respect of the invention had been made in a convention country before that date by me/us or by any person from which I/We derive the title.
- ☐ My/our application in India is based on international application under Patent Cooperation Treaty (PCT) as mentioned in Para - 6.
- ☐ The application is divided out of my/our application particulars of which are given in Para - 7 and pray that this application may be treated as deemed to have been filed on _________ under sec.16 of the Act.
- ☐ The said invention is an improvement in or modification of the invention particulars of which are given in Para - 8.

10. Following are the attachments with the application:

- (a) Provisional specification/Complete specification
- (b) Complete specification (in conformation with the international application)/as amended before the International Preliminary Examination Authority (IPEA), as applicable (2 copies), No. of pages _____ No. of claims________
- (c) Drawings (in conformation with the international application)/as amended before the International Preliminary Examination Authority (IPEA), as applicable (2 copies),No. of sheets_________
- (d) Priority documents
- (e) Translation of priority document/Specification/International Search Report
- (f) Statement and undertaking on Form 3
- (g) Power of Authority
- (h) Declaration of inventorship on Form 5
- (i) Sequence listing in electronic form
- (j) ....

Fee Rs............... ....in Cash./ Cheque / Bank Draft bearing no.........................
Date...........................on ....Bank.

I/We hereby declare that to the best of my/our knowledge, information and belief the fact and matters stated herein are correct and I/We request that a patent may be granted to me/us for the said invention.

Dated this .,....................day of.................20............

Signature:-
Name:

To, The Controller of Patent
The Patent Office, at...........

Note: -*Repeat boxes in case of more than one entry.
*To be signed by the applicant(s) or by authorized registered patent agent otherwise where mentioned.
*Tick (√)/cross (×) whichever is applicable/not applicable in declaration in para-9.
*Name of the inventor and applicant should be given in full, family name in the beginning.
*Complete address of the inventor and applicant should be given stating the postal index no./code, state and country. *Strike out the column which is/are not applicable * For fee: See First Schedule

FORM 2
THE PATENT ACT 1970
(39 of 1970)
&
The Patents Rules, 2003
PROVISIONAL/COMPLETE SPECIFICATION
(See section 10 and rule13)

1. TITLE OF THE INVENTION

2. APPLICANT (S)
(a) NAME:
(b) NATIONALITY:
(c) ADDRESS:

3. PREAMBLE TO THE DESCRIPTION

PROVISIONAL	COMPLETE
The following specification describes the invention.	The following specification particularly describes the invention and the manner in which it is to be performed.

4. DESCRIPTION (Description shall start from next page.)

5. CLAIMS (not applicable for provisional specification. Claims should start with the preamble — **"I/we claim"** on separate page)

6. DATE AND SIGNATURE (to be given at the end of last page of specification)

7. ABSTRACT OF THE INVENTION (to be given along with complete specification on separate page)

Note: -
 *Repeat boxes in case of more than one entry.
 *To be signed by the applicant(s) or by authorized registered patent agent.
 *Name of the applicant should be given in full , family name in the beginning .
 *Con.plete address of the applicant should be given stating the postal index no./code, state and country.
 *Strike out the column which is/are not applicable

FORM 3

THE PATENTS ACT, 1970
(39 of 1970)
&
The Patents Rules, 2003
STATEMENT AND UNDERTAKING UNDER SECTION 8
(See section 8, rule 12)

1. Namely of the applicant(s).

I/We.[1]..______________________

____

____

hereby declare:

2. Name, address and nationality of the joint applicant:

(i) that I/We have not made any application for the same/substantially the same invention outside India.
   Or

(ii) that I/We who have made this application
No.______________ Dated________ alone/jointly
   with [2] ....,
   made for the same/substantially same invention,
   application(s) for patent in the other countries, the
   particulars of which are given below:

Name of the country.	Date of application	Application No.	Status of the application	Date of publication	Date of grant

3. Name and address of the assignee

(iii) that the rights in the application(s) has/.have been assigned to. [3]

____

that I/We undertake that upto the date of grant of the patent, by the Controller, I/We would keep him informed in writing the details regarding corresponding applications for patents filed outside India within three months from the date of filing of such application.

Dated this .... day of 20

4. To be signed by the applicant or his authorised registered patent agent.

Signature [4]..

)[5]

5.Name of the natural person who has signed.   (

To
The Controller of Patents,
The Patent Office, At

<u>Note: Strike out whichever is not applicable.</u>

F O R M 5
THE PATENTS ACT, 1970
(39 of 1970)

&

The Patents Rules, 2003
DECLARATION AS TO INVENTORSHIP
[See section 10(6) and rule 13(6)]

1. NAME OF APPLICANT (S)

hereby declare that the true and first inventor(s) of the invention disclosed in the complete specification filed in pursuance of my /our application numbered dated is/are

2. INVENTOR (S)
(a) NAME
(b) NATIONALITY
(c) ADDRESS

Dated this ....day of..................20............

Signature: -
Name of the signatory: -

3. DECLARATION TO BE GIVEN WHEN THE APPLICATION IN INDIA IS FILED BY THE APPLICANT (S) IN THE CONVENTION COUNTRY: -

We the applicant(s) in the convention country hereby declare that our right to apply for a patent in India is by way of assignment from the true and first inventor(s).

Dated this ....day of..................20............

Signature: -
Name of the signatory: -

4. STATEMENT (to be signed by the additional inventor(s) not mentioned in the application form)

I/We assent to the invention referred to in the above declaration, being included in the complete specification filed in pursuance of the stated application.

Dated this ....day of..................20............

Signature of the additional inventor(s): -

Name: -

To, The Controller of Patent

The Patent Office, at...........

Note
*Repeat boxes in case of more than one entry.
*To be signed by the applicant(s) or by authorized registered patent agent otherwise where mentioned.
*Name of the inventor and applicant should be given in full, family name in the beginning .
*Complete address of the inventor should be given stating the postal index no./code, state and country.

*Strike out the column which is/ are not applicable

FORM 28

THE PATENTS ACT, 1970
(39 of 1970)
AND
THE PATENTS RULES, 2003

TO BE SUBMITTED BY A SMALL ENTITY
[See rules 2(fa) and 7]

Insert name, address and nationality.	I/We ....
	....
	....
	applicant/patentee in respect of the patent application no. ....or patent no............
	hereby declare that I/we am/are a small entity in accordance with rule 2(fa) and submit the following document(s) as proof:
State the particulars of the documents.	(i.) Evidence of registration under the Micro, Small and Medium Enterprises Act, 2006 (27 of 2006 (in case of Indian entities).
	(ii.) Any other document (in case of foreign entities).
To be signed by the applicant(s) / patentee (s) / authorised registered patent agent.	The information provided herein is correct to the best of my/our knowledge and belief.
Name of the natural person who has signed.	
Designation and official seal, if any, of the person who has signed.	Dated this ....day of .... 20...
	Signature ....
	(Name) ....
	(Designation) ....

To
The Controller of Patents,
The Patent Office,
At...................................

Note: Indian entities shall submit the evidence mentioned above to be eligible for claiming the status of a small entity.".

ANNEXURE 7

DOCTRINE OF EQUIVALENCE
CASE STUDY

United States Court of Appeals
for the Federal Circuit

DURAMED PHARMACEUTICALS, INC.
(NOW KNOWN AS TEVA WOMEN'S HEALTH, INC.),
Plaintiff-Appellant,

v.

PADDOCK LABORATORIES, INC.,
Defendant-Appellee.

2010-1419

Appeal from the United States District Court for the Southern District of New York in Case No. 09-CV-1905, Senior Judge Leonard B. Sand.

Decided: July 21, 2011

CHARANJIT BRAHMA, Kirkland & Ellis, LLP, of Washington, DC, argued for plaintiff-appellant. With him on the brief were COREY J. MANLEY and J. JOHN LEE; and ALEXANDER F. MACKINNON, of Los Angeles, California. Of counsel was ROBERT G. KRUPKA, of Los Angeles, California.

EDGAR H. HAUG, Frommer Lawrence & Haug, LLP, of New York, New York, argued for defendant-appellee. With him on the brief was DAVID A. ZWALLY.

Before LOURIE, GAJARSA, and DYK, *Circuit Judges.*

LOURIE, *Circuit Judge.*

Duramed Pharmaceuticals, Inc. ("Duramed") appeals from the decision of the United States District Court for the Southern District of New York granting summary judgment of noninfringement to Paddock Laboratories, Inc. ("Paddock"). *Duramed Pharms., Inc. v. Paddock Labs., Inc.*, 715 F. Supp. 2d 552 (S.D.N.Y. 2010). Because the district court did not err in holding that prosecution history estoppel bars Duramed's allegations of infringement under the doctrine of equivalents, we affirm.

BACKGROUND

Duramed owns U.S. Patent 5,908,638 ("'638 patent"), which claims conjugated estrogen pharmaceutical compositions for use in hormone replacement therapies. The claimed conjugated estrogens are extremely water sensitive and thus highly susceptible to moisture degradation during storage. *See* '638 patent col.6 ll.46-56. Accordingly, Duramed developed a formulation for conjugated estrogens that includes a moisture barrier coating ("MBC") to inhibit the absorption of moisture and reduce storage-related degradation. *See id.* col.6 ll.36-45.

Duramed filed a patent application on its formulation on July 26, 1995. Original independent claim 1 recited a conjugated estrogen pharmaceutical composition "coated with a moisture barrier coating." J.A. 254. Original dependent claim 7 limited "said moisture barrier coating" to one that "comprises ethylcellulose." J.A. 255. The examiner rejected both claims as obvious, but during an interview advised that he would allow the application if Duramed amended claim 1 to include, *inter alia*, the limitations of claim 7. In a response received December 3, 1998, Duramed amended claim 1 to recite pharmaceutical compositions with "a moisture barrier coating comprising ethylcellulose." J.A. 304. Claim 1 of the issued '638 patent, the patent's only independent claim, accordingly reads as follows:

> 1. A pharmaceutical composition in a solid, unit dosage form capable of oral administration for the hormonal treatment of peri-menopausal, meno-pausal and post-menopausal disorders in a woman comprising:
>
> conjugated estrogens coated onto one or more organic excipients forming a powdered conjugated estrogen composition where said composition is substantially free of inorganic excipients and further comprises about 30-70% gel-forming organic excipient and about 30-70% non-gel forming organic excipient by weight and having less than about 2.5% free water by weight and greater than 2.5% total water wherein said solid unit dosage form is coated with *a moisture barrier coating comprising ethylcellulose.*

'638 patent claim 1 (emphasis added).

In March 2009, Duramed filed suit against Paddock under 35 U.S.C. § 271(e)(2), alleging infringement of the '638 patent based on Paddock's Abbreviated New Drug Application ("ANDA") for a generic version of Duramed's hormone replacement therapy product, Cenestin®. Duramed alleged infringement of claims 1, 4, and 6-8 under the doctrine of equivalents, because Paddock's proposed generic product uses a polyvinyl alcohol ("PVA") MBC, marketed as Opadry AMB. Paddock moved for summary judgment of noninfringement, arguing that Duramed was barred by amendment-based prosecution history estoppel from alleging that PVA met the "moisture barrier coating comprising ethylcellulose" limitation of the asserted claims.

In its motion for summary judgment, Paddock relied on several pre-amendment references, including an international patent application filed by Colorcon pursuant to the Patent Cooperation Treaty ("the Colorcon PCT"). The Colorcon PCT, published on January 25, 1996, discloses formulations of PVA-based MBCs, including Opadry AMB, but also, in a section entitled "Description of the Prior Art," notes several technical drawbacks of using PVA as an MBC. Paddock also relied on (1) U.S. Patent 3,935,326 ("the Groppenbächer patent"), which issued in 1976 and discloses the use of PVA in moisture-tight tablets; (2) an article in the December 1995 issue of "Manufacturing Chemist" that tests PVA MBCs and concludes that Opadry AMB is a highly effective moisture barrier formulation; (3) three scientific articles on PVA MBCs authored for distribution at scientific conferences in May 1995, May 1998, and November 1998; and (4) invoices indicating sales of Opadry AMB by Colorcon before September 1996.

The district court granted Paddock's motion for summary judgment of noninfringement, holding that prosecution history estoppel barred Duramed's infringement allegations. *Duramed*, 715 F. Supp. 2d at 555-56. The district court first held that Duramed's amendment adding the ethylcellulose limitation was substantially related to patentability and narrowed the scope of the asserted claims, thus triggering the presumption under *Festo Corp. v. Shoketsu Kinzoku Kogyo Kabushiki Co.*, 344 F.3d 1359, 1366-67 (Fed. Cir. 2003) (*en banc*) ("*Festo IX*"), that Duramed had surrendered all territory between the original and amended claim scope. *Duramed*, 715 F. Supp. 2d at 559-60.

The district court then held that Duramed had failed to rebut the *Festo* presumption based on an argument of, *inter alia*, the unforeseeability of the use of PVA as an MBC in a pharmaceutical formulation. *Id.* at 560. Rather, the court held that PVA MBCs were foreseeable at the time of Duramed's narrowing amendment based on the Colorcon PCT's description of PVA as "a moisture barrier coating for pharmaceutical tablets and the like" and its disclosure of the Opadry AMB formulation used in Paddock's proposed generic product. *Id.* at 560-61. The court noted that several other facts reinforced this decision: (1) the pre-September 1996 invoices for the sale of Opadry AMB; and (2) the Groppenbächer patent, which teaches coating tablets with PVA to ensure "'moisture tight[ness]' and 'insolub[ility] in the gastrointestinal tract.'"[1]   *Id.* at 561-62. Finally, the court rejected Duramed's argument that the Colorcon PCT's disclosure of PVA MBCs' technical drawbacks raised serious questions about PVA's effectiveness as an MBC, concluding that "even if the effectiveness of PVA was unknown in 1998, that would not mean that PVA MBCs were unforeseeable." *Id.* at 563.

Duramed timely appealed to this court. We have jurisdiction pursuant to 28 U.S.C. § 1295(a)(1).

DISCUSSION

We review a district court's grant of summary judgment *de novo*, reapplying the same standard applied by

---

[1]   The district court did not consider Paddock's remaining pre-1998 articles based on Duramed's claim that a bench trial would be necessary to determine if the 1995 "Manufacturing Chemist" article was publicly available in a university library and if the conference articles were actually distributed to the attendees. *Id.* at 561 n.8. The court concluded that these articles were not necessary to establish foreseeability. *Id.*

the district court. *Iovate Health Scis., Inc. v. Bio-Engineered Supplements & Nutrition, Inc.*, 586 F.3d 1376, 1380 (Fed. Cir. 2009). Summary judgment is appropriate if there are no genuine issues of material fact and the moving party is entitled to judgment as a matter of law. Fed. R. Civ. P. 56(c).

Under the doctrine of the equivalents, "a product or process that does not literally infringe . . . the express terms of a patent claim may nonetheless be found to infringe if there is 'equivalence' between the elements of the accused product or process and the claimed elements of the patented invention." *Warner-Jenkinson Co. v. Hilton Davis Chem. Co.*, 520 U.S. 17, 21 (1997) (citing *Graver Tank & Mfg. Co. v. Linde Air Prods. Co.*, 339 U.S. 605, 609 (1950)). However, the doctrine of prosecution history estoppel prevents a patent owner from recapturing through the doctrine of equivalents subject matter surrendered to acquire the patent. *See Festo Corp. v. Shoketsu Kinzoku Kogyo Kabushiki Co.*, 535 U.S. 722, 734 (2002) (*"Festo VIII"*).

Because during prosecution Duramed narrowed the scope of the '638 patent's claims in response to a prior art rejection, a presumption of prosecution history estoppel applies. *See Festo IX*, 344 F.3d at 1366-67. Nonetheless, Duramed may rebut that presumption by showing, *inter alia*, the "alleged equivalent would have been 'unforeseeable at the time of the amendment and thus beyond a fair interpretation of what was surrendered.'" *Id.* at 1369 (quoting *Festo VIII*, 535 U.S. at 738). "[A]n alternative is foreseeable if it is disclosed in the pertinent prior art in the field of the invention. In other words, an alternative is foreseeable if it is known in the field of the invention as reflected in the claim scope before amendment." *Festo Corp. v. Shoketsu Kinzoku Kogyo Kabushiki Co.*, 493 F.3d 1368, 1379 (Fed. Cir. 2007) (*"Festo X"*). Foreseeability is a question of law based on underlying issues of fact. *Id.* at 1375.

On appeal, Duramed argues that the district court applied the wrong legal test for foreseeability and thus held that any mention of an alleged equivalent in the prior art makes that equivalent foreseeable as a matter of law. But, according to Duramed, an equivalent is not foreseeable if it was not understood by one of ordinary skill in the art to be suitable for use in the invention as originally claimed. And, in this case, Duramed asserts, the relevant art did not disclose either PVA or Opadry AMB as suitable MBCs for moisture-sensitive pharmaceutical compounds, like conjugated estrogens.

Paddock responds that the district court applied the correct foreseeability standard, which requires only that PVA be foreseeable as an MBC for pharmaceutical applications at the time of Duramed's narrowing amendment. In this case, according to Paddock, the Colorcon PCT alone renders PVA MBCs foreseeable, but this conclusion is bolstered by Colorcon's commercialization of Opadry AMB, the Groppenbächer patent, and the other references not considered by the district court.

We agree with Paddock that Duramed failed to rebut the presumption of prosecution history estoppel based on unforeseeability. We first note that, to the extent that Duramed argues that foreseeability requires that PVA must have been known as an MBC for use *with conjugated estrogens*, we have previously rejected such a restrictive definition of the field of invention. *See Schwarz Pharma, Inc. v. Paddock Labs., Inc.*, 504 F.3d 1371, 1377 (Fed. Cir. 2007). As we spelled out in *Schwarz*, when the language of both original and issued claims begins with the words "[a] pharmaceutical composition," that language defines the field of the invention for purposes of determining foreseeability. *Id.* Accordingly, PVA MBCs need only to have been known in the field of pharmaceutical compositions as of the time of Duramed's narrowing amendment, *see Festo X*, 493 F.3d at 1379, which we hold that the Colorcon PCT establishes as a matter of law.

The Colorcon PCT discloses PVA MBCs for use with pharmaceutical compositions: "A dry powder moisture barrier coating composition is made to form a moisture barrier film coating for pharmaceutical tablets and the like, which comprises polyvinyl alcohol . . . ." J.A. 4466. In the "Description of the Prior Art" the PCT states that "[t]he use of the polymer polyvinyl alcohol, PVA, as a moisture barrier coating has been previously suggested," but it also notes two drawbacks of PVA MBCs: stickiness and plasticizer compatibility. *Id.* Specifically, the Colorcon PCT states:

> [P]ractical usage [of PVA] has been inhibited by the stickiness of grades of the polymer which have a fast enough rate of going into solution in water to make a dispersion to render them economical to use in making the coating. A further problem with the use of PVA is in identifying or selecting a plasticizer which does not compromise the moisture barrier properties of the final coating.

Id.

The Colorcon PCT then, in the "Summary of the Invention," discloses preferred PVA grades and identifies a plasticizer that does not compromise PVA's properties as a moisture barrier. The application states that "[e]xcellent moisture barrier properties are obtained when hot water soluble grades of PVA are used in the inventive coating," and that "[a] preferred grade of PVA for use in the inventive coating is a grade in the medium range . . . because the step of heating the water of the liquid coating dispersion may not be necessary, while still maintaining excellent moisture barrier properties in the inventive coating." J.A. 4468-69. The Colorcon PCT next discloses that soya lecithin "surprisingly, and unexpectedly, acts as a plasticizer by locking moisture in the coating so the coating stays flexible and not brittle," and thus soya lecithin as a plasticizer "does not compromise the moisture barrier properties of the overall coating." J.A. 4469. Finally, the Colorcon PCT lists a number of PVA MBC formulations, including Opadry AMB. Accordingly, the Colorcon PCT discloses PVA MBCs, including Opadry AMB, in the field of pharmaceutical compositions, rendering such PVA MBCs "known in the field of the invention," and thus foreseeable. *Festo X*, 493 F.3d at 1379.

Duramed argues that the Colorcon PCT's disclosure fails to establish that PVA-based Opadry AMB was suitable as an MBC because it provides only conclusory statements that the inventors had solved the technical drawbacks of PVA MBCs and lacks any data on the stability of the pharmaceutical compounds coated with Opadry AMB. We disagree; foreseeability does not require such precise evidence of suitability. *See Honeywell Int'l, Inc. v. Hamilton Sundstrand Corp.*, 523 F.3d 1304, 1312-13 (Fed. Cir. 2008). And even if the PCT disclosure indicates that PVA is less than ideal in some pharmaceutical uses as an MBC, it is still disclosed to be useful as such, and that renders it foreseeable for purposes of prosecution history estoppel. Foreseeability does not require flawless perfection to create an estoppel.

In rejecting a foreseeability rebuttal in *Glaxo Wellcome, Inc. v. Impax Laboratories, Inc.*, 356 F.3d 1348 (Fed. Cir. 2004), we held that "the record abundantly disclosed [the alleged equivalent's] use as a release agent at the relevant time," *SmithKline Beecham Corp. v. Excel Pharms., Inc.*, 356 F.3d 1357, 1365 (Fed. Cir. 2004) (describing *Glaxo*, 356 F.3d at 1355). Our holding relied on statements from several references disclosing the alleged equivalent's use as an extended-release agent in drug formulations; it did not rely on test data showing the alleged equivalent's precise characteristics or suitability as an extended-release agent, and thus did not rely on the type of evidence Duramed demands in this case. *See Glaxo* 356 F.3d at 1355. Rather, the Colorcon PCT discloses the use of PVA as MBCs in the field of pharmaceutical compounds prior to December 3, 1998, rendering such PVA MBCs foreseeable at the time of Duramed's narrowing amendment.[2]

---

[2]   Although not necessary to our decision, we note that the 1995 "Manufacturing Chemist" article also supports a finding of foreseeability in the case. Like the Colorcon PCT, the "Manufacturing Chemist" article discloses PVA MBCs for use in pharmaceutical applications, and it discloses tests on the performance of PVA-based coatings with moisture-sensitive drugs. The tests compared PVA MBCs with hydroxypropyl-methylcellulose MBCs coating tablets of aspirin or erythromycin ethylsuccinate stored for twelve weeks under high relative humidity. The data reveal that "the PVA formulation gives much superior moisture protection under humid storage conditions." J.A. 4497. The article concludes that "[t]he results presented here have shown a highly effective moisture barrier formulation [based on the water soluble polymer PVA, designated Opadry AMB] has been developed." J.A. 4498. The district court did not rely on this article based on Duramed's claim that a bench trial would be necessary to determine if the article was publicly available. *Duramed*, 715 F. Supp. 2d at 561 n.8. We disagree that there is a genuine issue of material fact on the public availability of an article published in a scientific journal three years before Duramed's amendment. *See, e.g., In re Lister*, 583 F.3d 1307, 1312 (Fed. Cir. 2009).

CONCLUSION

For the foregoing reasons, we affirm the district court's grant of summary judgment of noninfringement.

AFFIRMED

ANNEXURE 8

JUDGEMENT RELATING FIRST INDIAN COMPULSORY LICENSING

BEFORE THE CONTROLLER OF PATENTS
MUMBAI

Present: Mr. P. H. Kurian

Compulsory License Application No. 1 of 2011

IN THE MATTER OF:

NATCO PHARMA LIMITED: ....APPLICANT

Represented by: Ms. Rajeshwari H., Advocate &
                                                Patent Agent

AND

BAYER CORPORATION   ...... PATENTEE/OPPONENT

Represented by: Sh. Sudhir Chandra Aggarwal,
                                                Senior Advocate.
                                                Sh. Sanjay Kumar, Advocate &
                                                Patent Agent
                                                Ms. Arpita Sawhney, Advocate
                                                Sh. Rahul Kumar, Advocate

APPLICATION FOR COMPULSORY LICENCE UNDER SECTION 84(1) OF THE PATENTS ACT, 1970 IN RESPECT OF PATENT NO.215758.

1.   **Overview**

The patent system is a carefully crafted bargain that rewards an inventor in lieu of his contribution towards the society. The inventor is granted an exclusive right for a limited period: a) where the subject matter of the patent is a product, the exclusive right to prevent third parties, who do not have his consent, from the act of making, using, offering for sale, selling or importing for those purposes that product; and b) where the subject matter of the patent is a process, the exclusive right to prevent third parties, who do not have his consent, from the act of using that process, and from the act of using, offering for sale, selling or importing for those purposes the product obtained directly by that process. The benefit derived by the society, *inter alia*, in granting such a comprehensive right to the inventor for twenty years, is the enrichment of knowledge in public domain, which can be utilized to invent further. This cycle goes on and on to take the nation towards socio-economic prosperity. Without the presence of a Patent system, the inventor will not be encouraged to disclose his invention to public and may prefer to keep it as a trade secret, which may result in innovative sluggishness, thereby adversely affecting the prosperity of a nation.

From its very nature, a right cannot be absolute. Whenever conferred upon a patentee, the right also carries accompanying obligations towards the public at large. These rights and obligations, if religiously enjoyed and discharged, will balance out each other. A slight imbalance may fetch highly undesirable results. It is this fine balance of rights and obligations that is in question in this case.

2.   **History of compulsory licenses**

When TRIPS (Trade-Related Aspects of Intellectual Property Rights) Agreement was introduced in 1994, it reduced the discretionary powers of WTO Members to customize key elements of their national intellectual property regimes. In January 1995, when WTO came into existence, the TRIPS Agreement, building on the existing multilateral treaties administered by the World Intellectual Property Organization (WIPO), introduced minimum standards for protecting and enforcing intellectual property rights to an extent previously unseen at the global level, including new monitoring and dispute settlement mechanisms. Article 27.1 of the TRIPS Agreement requires WTO Members to make patents "available for any inventions, whether products or processes, in all fields of technology", which includes patents for pharmaceutical processes and products. At the same time, TRIPS also provides a reasonable fetter on the rights of the Patentee in the form of Article 30 and 31, in line with Paris Convention, thereby allowing member countries to enact provisions, *inter alia*, for granting compulsory license to prevent the abuse of patent right.

Compulsory License (CL) under the Patents system is an involuntary contract between a willing buyer and an unwilling seller imposed and enforced by the State. The WTO states compulsory licensing is when a government allows someone else to produce the patented product or process without the consent of the patent owner. It has been in existence since the 1830s. CL has been reported to be popular in Britain as early as 1850s. Later, this system was recognized by the international community through the Paris Convention of 1883. It is also one of the flexibilities on patent protection included in the TRIPS Agreement.

Provisions for granting a compulsory license exists in the Patent Laws of various countries such as Canada, France, UK, USA, Australia (developed countries), and Zimbabwe, Ghana, Brazil, Equador, Malaysia, Thailand and India (developing countries). In fact, compulsory licenses are being issued by developed as well as developing countries even in recent times.

India joined TRIPS and the deadline for complying with TRIPS obligations was January 1, 2005. The Patents Act, 1970 was amended thrice to make it fully TRIPS compliant i.e. in 1999, 2002 and finally in 2005. The Patents Act, 1970, as enacted originally, contained a provision for grant of a compulsory license, in case the aforementioned balance is disturbed. However, vide the Patents (Amendment) Act, 2002, the provisions relating to compulsory license, i.e. Chapter XVI of the Patents Act, 1970 was substituted with a completely new one. The Patents (Amendment) Act, 2005 allowed product patents to be granted for drugs, which was not allowed under the 1970 Act.

Present case is the first of its kind in the history of Patents Act, 1970, wherein the provisions of Section 84 have been invoked by the Applicant herein for seeking the grant of a compulsory license. As such, there is no precedent to guide this tribunal. Relevant persuasive material has been submitted by both parties. In order to appreciate all the issue involved in the present litigation, the hearings went on for three days for a total of eighteen hours. Reasonable research has also been conducted by this tribunal to study, *inter alia*, the provisions of the International Agreements and Conventions on Intellectual Property Rights as well as laws of other TRIPS member countries to arrive at this order. This includes the articles published by WHO, UNDP, Mr.Carlos M. Correa, University of Buenos Aires, & Professor Shamnad Basheer, The West Bengal National University of Juridical Sciences, Kolkata.

3.   **The Patentee**

M/s. Bayer Corporation, 100 Bayer Road, Pittsburg, PA 15205-9741, USA (hereinafter referred to as 'patentee'), an internationally renowned manufacturer of innovative drugs, invented a drug called 'Sorafenib' (Carboxy Substituted Diphenyl Ureas) useful in the treatment of advanced stage liver and kidney cancer in the 1990s. The patentee first applied for a patent in the United States Patent and Trade

Mark Office on 13.01.1999 and subsequently filed a PCT International Application on PCT/US00/000648 in the 12.01.2000. The Patentee entered the national phase in India on 05.07.2001. After examination under the provisions of the Patents Act, 1970, a patent was granted on 03.03.2008. The Patentee has also obtained patents in many other countries for the same drug including members of the European Patent Office.

In the meanwhile, the Patentee developed the drug and launched it in 2005 under the trade name Nexavar (hereinafter referred to as the 'drug') for treatment of Renal Cell Carcinoma-RCC (kidney cancer) and subsequently got additional approval for treatment of Hepatocellular Carcinoma-HCC (liver cancer) in 2007. The Patentee received the regulatory approval for importing and marketing the drug in India and launched it in India in the year 2008.

4.   **The Applicant**

The Applicant herein M/s. Natco Pharma Ltd, Natco House, Road No. 2, Banjara Hills, Hyderabad-500033, Andhra Pradesh, India (hereinafter referred to as 'Applicant') is a reputed Indian generic drug manufacturer. The Applicant has developed the process to manufacture this drug and received a license from the Drug Controller General of India for manufacturing the drug in bulk and for marketing it in the form of tablets in April 2011.

5.   **The drug**

'Sorafenib tosylate', which is a compound covered by Patent No.215758 and sold under the brand name NEXAVAR by the Patentee is used for the treatment at the advanced stages of kidney and liver cancer. The drug stops the growth of new blood vessels and targets other important cellular growth factors. It is pertinent to mention that the drug is not a life-saving drug, but a life extending drug i.e. in case of kidney cancer, the life of a patient can be extended by 4-5 years, while in case of liver cancer the life of a patient can be extended by about 6-8 months. The drug has to be taken by the patient throughout his lifetime and the cost of therapy is Rs.2,80,428/- per month and Rs.33,65,136/- per year.

6. **The Application and initial developments**

The Applicant filed an Application for Compulsory License (hereinafter referred to as the "Application") on 29.07.2011 under Section 84(1) of The Patents Act 1970 (hereinafter referred to as the Act) r/w Rule 96 of the Patent Rules 2003 (hereinafter referred to as the "Rules") in respect of the Patent No. 215758. The Applicant being a leading manufacturer and distributor of various drugs in India approached the Patentee with a request for a voluntary license to *manufacture and sell the drug, which did not materialize*. The Applicant proposed to sell the drug at a price of Rs.8800/- for one month therapy as compared to the price of about Rs.2,80,428/-, which was being charged by the Patentee at the time of making the Application. Three years had lapsed since the date of grant of patent when the Application was filed. The Applicant is also a *person interested* within the meaning of the Act. Upon arriving at a conclusion that a *prima facie* case under Section 87(1) of the Act has been established, vide order dated 9.8.2011, the Applicant was directed to serve a copy of the Application upon Patentee and the Application was published in the official journal published on 12th August, 2011. On 23.08.2011, the Patentee filed a request seeking an extension of time by one month to file the notice of opposition and the same was allowed in the interest of justice. The Patentee then filed an 'interlocutory petition' dated 07.10.2011 seeking stay in this matter on the ground that an infringement suit was pending before the Hon'ble High Court of Delhi against the Applicant w.r.t. the same Patent. The request of the Patentee was refused vide order dated 27.10.2011. The Patentee filed a petition seeking extension of time to file a review petition and another petition for staying the proceedings on the ground of pendency of a contempt petition against the Patentee in the Hon'ble High Court of Delhi. Both the petitions were refused vide my order dated 21.12.2011.

Meanwhile, the Patentee preferred Writ Petition No. 2194/2011 in the Hon'ble High Court of Judicature at Bombay challenging the said Order dated 9.8.2011. The Writ Petition was disposed of by the Hon'ble High Court of Bombay with the following order dated 11.11.2011:

"Considering the said aspect of the matter, the above petition is not entertained by this Court, with a liberty to the petitioner to file appropriate petition before the Delhi High Court, especially when it has been observed by the Delhi High Court in Injunction Application No. 7343 of 2011 that in view of the pendency of the application before the Controller of Patent, both the parties agree not to proceed further with the present proceedings. Considering the said aspects, the above petition is disposed of with a liberty to the petitioner to move the Delhi High Court regarding the subject matter. Time to file reply before the Controller of Patent is extended till 18.11.2011. Such extension is given without prejudice to the rights and contentions of the parties and with a view to see that the petitioner in the meanwhile, can approach the Delhi High Court by way of appropriate proceedings. It is clarified that we have not expressed any opinion on the merits of the case and the points raised by both the sides in this petition are explicitly kept open."

The Patentee thereafter exercised his constitutional right by approaching the Hon'ble High Court of Delhi by way of Writ Petition

No. 8062/2011, thereby challenging the aforementioned order dated 9.8.2011. The Hon'ble High Court of Delhi disposed of the said Writ Petition with the following order dated 16.11.2011:

"The petitioner impugns the order dated 11.08.2011 passed by the Controller of Patents, Patent Office, Mumbai in C.L.A. No.1 of 2011. It has been pointed out to learned senior counsel for the petitioner that the impugned order merely records a prima facie view that a case under Section 84(1) of the Patents Act has been established. The petitioner is still entitled to contest the said proceedings before the Controller of Patents.

Learned senior counsel for the petitioner submits that before arriving at the said prima facie view, the Controller of Customs has not conducted any enquiry and not recorded any evidence. It shall be open to the petitioner to raise all such pleas before the Controller of Patents in answer to the notice. In view of the aforesaid, the petitioner wishes to withdraw this petition. The petition is accordingly dismissed as withdrawn."

Subsequently, the Patentee filed a notice of opposition on Form-14, along with evidences and the conditions for license, under Section 87(2) of the Act read with Rule 98(1) of the Rules on 18.11.2011, within the timeline as extended by the Hon'ble High Court of Bombay.

7.   **Hearings**

The parties were heard on 13.01.2012. During the course of hearing, counter allegations were raised by both the parties that evidence has not been filed on affidavits. The parties were also informed by me during hearing that the evidence filed by both the sides are not conclusive and that there is a need to lead further evidence on crucial aspects to assist the tribunal in arriving at a conclusive finding. Parties agreed to the same. Accordingly, in the interest of justice, leave was granted for filing further evidence to both the parties and the matter was adjourned to 27th February 2012. Both the parties were given full opportunity to present their side of the case. As the hearing could not be concluded on 27th February, 2012, the same was continued on 28th February 2012, on which day the hearings were concluded.

8. **Preliminary issues raised by the Patentee and decision thereof**

   a. On the first day of hearing, the Patentee submitted that the Applicant has specifically raised only the ground mentioned in S.84(1)(a) of the Act and has failed to mention the grounds enumerated under S.84(1)[(b) and (c)] of the Act. This objection appears to be of a hyper-technical nature as it is found that in the Application all the grounds mentioned in S.84 of the Act have constructively been raised by the Applicant and must accordingly be adjudicated.

   b. The Patentee also contended that the provisions of Section 84(6)(iv) have not been satisfied and that the Application is required to be rejected on this ground alone. The Patentee's contention is that from the tenor of the letter dated December 6, 2010 sent by Applicant seeking voluntary license, it appeared that the Applicant was fulfilling the requirements for filing an Application for compulsory license. Accordingly, this letter cannot be termed as an effort on reasonable terms and conditions. The Patentee further contended that the Applicant failed to mention any terms and conditions that he was willing to accept. Furthermore, the Patentee states that the Applicant was given a time of 14 days to return if he had anything to say.

   I am of the view that the Applicant could have been more humble in writing the said letter dated December 6, 2010 so as not to hurt the sensitivities of the Patentee. Patentee, vide Para 9 of the reply stated as follows:

'In view of what has been stated above, our client does not consider it appropriate to grant voluntary license to manufacture and market the product, Nexavar to NATCO.'

As the Patentee categorically refused to grant a voluntary license, I don't think that the Applicant could have taken further efforts for grant of a voluntary license. Hence, I am of the view that the requirements of Section 86(4)(iv) have been satisfied.

c. The Patentee raised a further objection that the Controller's order dated 09.08.2011 was erroneous as the Applicant did not make out a *prima facie* case and the Controller ought not to have passed an order under Section 87(1) of the Act, without first giving an opportunity to the Patentee to be heard in the matter. It was also argued that this violates the basic principle of natural justice as no *prima facie* case was made out (without there being any evidence) and the Patentee ought to have been given an opportunity to point that out and show the Law on the point of natural justice.

In this regard, while considering the Application, the Form-27 filed by the Patentee was also considered by me. As per the Form-27 submitted by the Patentee, I found that in 2008 the Patentee did not import the drug at all, while in 2009 and 2010 the Patentee imported in small quantities. The quantities imported by the Patentee *prima facie* appeared to be grossly inadequate. In view of this and the submissions made by the Applicant in his Application, and on satisfaction that a *prima facie* case has been made out, an order under Section 87(1) of the Act was passed. The Act does not envisage a hearing for the Patentee while issuing an order Section 87(1), particularly in view of the fact that no right, title or interest of the Patentee is affected by the said order and also because unnecessary delay is not in the interests of public. However, that does not in any way mean that the patentee is prejudiced. The Act affords full opportunity to the Patentee to present his case in the best possible manner, before any order affecting his right, title or interest is passed. Accordingly, I find no force or substance in the submissions of the Patentee that before passing the said order, which merely records a *prima facie* satisfaction of the Controller, an opportunity of hearing should have been granted to the Patentee and this issue is decided accordingly.

d. The Patentee raised a contention that the Applicant has suppressed the fact that M/s. Cipla, another generic drugs manufacturer in India, has been selling the generic version of the drug Sorafenib in India since April-May 2010. This suppression of fact by the Applicant shall entail rejection of the Application on this ground itself. The Applicant replied to this contention and submitted that they were aware of the alleged infringing sale by M/s. Cipa and that the Patentee has filed a infringement suit against M/s. Cipla, which is pending. The Applicant further argued that the failure of the Patentee to discharge his obligations under the Act has led to this Application. The presence of Cipla is not a material consideration so far as this Application is concerned as the alleged infringing sale by Cipla cannot rescue the Patentee and hence there has been no material suppression of any relevant fact. I find merit in the Applicant's pleadings and hence there is no ground for rejecting the Application on this ground. However, the other arguments made by the Patentee relating to sales of M/s. Cipla will be discussed later in the relevant paragraphs below.

9. **Main issues to be decided in the case**

Now I proceed to dwell upon the pleadings by the Applicant and Patentee on the three substantial issues in this Application [Section 84(1)(a, b and c)], i.e. whether,

a. the reasonable requirements of the public with respect to the patented invention have not been satisfied.

b. the patented invention is not available to the public at a reasonably affordable price.

c. the patented invention is not worked in the territory of India.

I will take up the afore-mentioned grounds one by one through consideration of the pleadings by parties, appreciation of evidence on record and my decisions thereof.

10. **Reasonable requirements of the public.**

Section 84 of the Act states as follows:

"84. Compulsory licenses. –

(1) At any time after the expiration of three years from the date of the grant of a patent, any person interested may make an application to the Controller for grant of compulsory license on patent on any of the following grounds, namely –

(a) that the reasonable requirements of the public with respect to the patented invention have not been satisfied.....'

Applicant's submissions

The Applicant has made the following submissions through pleadings and by way of written arguments along with evidence on affidavits. Applicant's submissions in brief are as follows:

a. The reasonable requirements of public have not been fulfilled with respect to Patent No. 215758. As per the data gathered and published in GLOBOCAN 2008 (a publication by GLOBOCAN project of the World Health Organization), the approximate patient base in India, in case of liver cancer is about 20000 (14516 men, 5628 women), while in case of kidney cancer the patient base in India is about 8900. In India, in 90% of the patients, the disease of liver cancer is detected at a late/advance stage. Hence, assuming that 80% of the patients in liver cancer alone require Sorafenib, 16,000 patients having liver cancer are eligible for Sorafenib. Similar is the case with kidney cancer. When one compares the demand with the working statement (Form-27) filed by the Patentee a clear picture of the demand not being met clearly emerges:

	Total Patients	Demand for 80% of patients	Bottles per month (required)	Bottles Imported in 2008	Bottles Imported in 2009	Bottles Imported in 2010
Liver Cancer	~ 20,000	~ 16,000	~ 16,000	-Nil-	~ 200 bottles	Unknown
Kidney Cancer	~ 8,900	~ 7,120	~ 7,120			

b. Patentee imports and sells the drug in India and has not taken adequate steps to manufacture the product in India to make full use of the invention. The drug is exorbitantly priced and out of reach of most of the people. The product is available only in limited quantities. It is available in pharmacies attached to certain hospitals and that too only in metro cities such as Mumbai, Chennai, Kolkata and Delhi. The product is often out of stock or not available in common pharmacies even in metro cities. The product in question is not a luxury item but a life saving drug and it is highly important that substantial part of the demand be met strictly. In the present case, even 1% of the public does not derive benefit of the patented drug.

c. The Patentee received FDA approval for the product in 2005 and launched the same in the world market around 2006. The sales figures for the years 2006-2011 obtained from public records show that the Patentee not only launched the product all over the world in 2006 but made thumping sales which has grown by leaps and bounds every year.

Sales figures of the drug:

	2006	2007	2008	2009	2010
Sales per year (Worldwide)	$165m	$371.7m	$677.8m	$843.5m	$934m
Sales in India	Nil	nil	Nil	16 crores	unknown

These figures clearly demonstrate the neglectful conduct of the Patentee as far as India in concerned. It shows that although the Patentee has fully developed and launched the product in various parts of the world and reported sales atleast since 2006, and despite the fact that the Patentee had filed its application in India in 2000, the Patentee clearly neglected India and did not launch until 2009. The Patent was granted in 2008 and from then till 2011 the Patentee did not bother to fulfill the demand to comply with the duty imposed by the Act.

d. The Patentee only imports the drug into the Indian market and does not manufacture the drug by itself in India, though it does manufacture and sell other products in India. The worldwide sales in various countries over the last three years has exceeded USD

2454 million whereas in India the sales did not exceed USD 32-40 million.

e. On the Patentee's submission that CIPLA entered the market with an infringing product, which was priced at about Rs.30000 against the Patentee's price of Rs.2,80,000, and this has undercut his market share thereby preventing him from selling in sufficient numbers. The Applicant submitted that the presence of Cipla in the market is irrelevant since:

  i. The demand in the market for the drug Sorafenib has to be fulfilled by the Patentee and not by the third parties; the sales by Cipla are not reflected in the working statement filed by the Patentee nor in the annual returns filed by the Patentee which clearly reflects the fact that Cipla's sales are of no relevance;

  ii. Cipla faces a suit for injunction and its sales are that of an infringer which cannot be taken into account;

  iii. Cipla could be injuncted anytime and the supply by Cipla may stop totally. Public cannot be held to ransom or left at the mercy of such uncertain supply.

Further, the mandate of law is not just to supply the drug in the market but to make it available in a manner such that substantial portion of the public is able to reap the benefits of the invention. If the terms are unreasonable such as high cost of Rs 2,80,000/-, availability is meaningless.

f. Availability of the drug is not to be measured in terms of mere Field Force or field strength of the Patentee. If the drug is so highly priced that the ordinary public cannot afford it, then it is a fact that the product is not available to the public on reasonable terms and presence of an army in the field is of no consequence and such high price becomes a barrier to availability of the drug, which is precise evil that the legislation is designed to curb.

The number of patients and the actual demand for the drug far exceeds the supply thereof by the patentee. Furthermore, price of the patented product is too high and simply unaffordable by the common man making the product inaccessible and out of reach. Hence, the demand for the patented product has not been met on reasonable terms.

In view of the above, the reasonable requirements of the public with respect to the patented invention have not been satisfied and this makes out a fit case for the grant of Compulsory License.

Patentee's submissions

The Patentee has made the following submissions through pleadings and by way of written arguments along with evidence on affidavits. Patentee's submissions in brief are as follows:

a. Estimated incidence for kidney cancer in India as per GLOBOCAN 2008 is 8900 patients and mortality is 5733 patients, which accounts 64.4% of total patients. Of the 8900 patients of kidney cancer around 90% account for RCC, which equals to approximately 8010 patients.

Around one third (33.33%) of the initially diagnosed RCC patients are affected with the stage IV disease (33.33% of 8010= 2669). This means there are approximately 5341 stage I, II, III patients, and about **2669** stage IV patients. In 25% of patients having surgical resection for localized disease (stage I, II and III) with a curative intent, recurrence occurs (25% of 5341= 1335). These **1335** patients (from stage I, II and III) eventually may progress to stage IV RCC. Therefore, the total number of patients falling under stage IV of RCC is approximately 2669 + 1335 = 4004 patients. Therefore, the total number of patients with RCC, entitled for treatment with the drug is approximately **4004**.

Hepatocellular Carcinoma (HCC) is classified into early, intermediate, advanced and terminal stage. As per the HCC trials conducted globally, the drug is used in advanced cases of HCC. Therefore, in practice it is being used in advanced HCC based on the available global clinical trial data.

Estimated incidence of HCC in India as per GLOBOCAN is 20,144 patients and mortality is 18043 patients which accounts 89.5% of total patients. Approximately 24% of the patients are in advanced stage of HCC, which require systemic treatment like sorafenib. (This accounts to approximately 4,838 patients out of 20144 total HCC patients.) Therefore, the total number of patients of HCC entitled for treatment with the drug is approximately **4838**. The total number of patients eligible for the drug are 4004 (RCC) and 4838 (HCC) i.e. a total of **8842**. Alternative treatments are also available to the patients and the Applicant has not agitated this fact.

b. The Applicant has provided misleading statistics and a list of cities that are covered by Field Force and Distributors and the list of cancer treatment centers in India has been provided as Annexure-4 to the Notice of Opposition. On perusal of the said annexure, it is evident that the Patentee's Field Force and Distributors do cater to all the cancer treatment centers in India. In addition, the following procedure is followed by the Patentee to ensure that the drug is available wherever it is required:

i. Distributors supply to hospitals, pharmacies, retailers and patients.

    ii. Distributors supply to outstation towns, cities where the drug is required.

    iii. For outstation patients, supply is done through courier.

c. Further, the treatment with the drug should be supervised by Doctors who have experience of anticancer treatments (Oncologists). Hence, the allegation of the Applicant that it is not available in villages is of no consequence as it has to be made available in cancer hospitals and institutes, which duty the Patentee has duly performed. Further, it is available at 50 places in 278 hospitals and institutes. Hence, the drug is accessible to the public at large.

In view of the above, the issue of requirement vs. availability is being appropriately taken care of by the Patentee.

d. The Applicant has erroneously and impermissibly linked the issue of price of the drug to this ground i.e reasonable requirements of the public have not been satisfied. Section 84(7) of the Act clearly lays down as to when the reasonable requirements of public shall be deemed not to have been satisfied. It was further submitted that none of the deeming provision under Section 84(7) relates to the price of the drug or availability to the public at a reasonably affordable price, which is a ground under Section 84(1)(b) of the Act.

e. The purpose behind Section 84(1)(a) is to enhance access to patented inventions. However, access to a patented invention is not identical to affordability thereof and cannot be on the identical footing. For example, for access to medicine, existence of trained healthcare staff and infrastructure, cultural acceptability of treatment, accessibility of healthcare facilities, quality of care and insurance facility all play a role in access. In other words, the parameters/criteria of establishing accessibility or lack thereof and affordability or lack thereof are different. The aforesaid submission is further strengthened by the fact that the Patents Act provides two different/specific grounds Section 84(1)(a) [lack of accessibility] and Section 84(1)(b) [lack of affordability] for the grant of Compulsory License. As such, the aforementioned two grounds cannot be mixed as has been done by the Applicant in the present case. It has to be appreciated that the grounds are distinct and separate.

f. The Patentee in their affidavit submitted through Dr. Manish Ram Mohan Garg, Country Medical Director, that the availability of the drug in India has been considerably enhanced due to its sale by M/s. Cipla. The affidavit reveals the following table of sale by M/s. Cipla and the Patentee during the year 2011:

	Q1A	Q2A	Q3A	Q4 E*	Total
Cipla No. of boxes	532	1071	1358	1725	4686
Growth %		101	27%	27%	
Bayer boxes	119	179	138.5	157	593

*projected for Q4 based on growth trend of last quarter.

The Patentee submitted further data in the form of table through the affidavit giving projections of sales by them and M/s. Cipla upto the year 2015.

	2011	2012	2013	2014	2015
Total No. of Patients (Cipla + Bayer)	3908	4844	6034	7544	9463
Total No. of HCC + RCC patients eligible for Sorafenib	8842	8842	8842	8842	8842
	44%	55%	68%	85%	107%

Based on the above figures, the Patentee argued that the reasonable requirements of the public is being fulfilled by Patentee and M/s.Cipla cumulatively currently and will be fulfilled in future as well. Hence, there exists no case for grant of compulsory license under Section 84(1)(a).

Decision

I have carefully gone through the pleadings of the parties, the affidavits, oral as well as written submissions, and the relevant provisions of the Act. The Applicant has relied upon the GLOBOCAN 2008 for the incidence of Liver and Kidney Cancer in India. The Patentee too has extensively referred to the same statistics. In the absence of any other evidence on record as to the incidence of the two types of cancer, I am constrained to accept the statistics available in the GLOBOCAN 2008 and the projections of incidence given therein.

Patentee by his own logic has derived a figure of number of patients who are eligible for this drug to be around **8842.** The Applicant submitted that both these cancers are generally diagnosed in India at an advanced stage. Given the state of healthcare infrastructure in the country and the income level of its people, I find merit in the argument of the Applicant. I am accordingly of the view that the number of patients requiring treatment by this drug will be much higher than the figure derived by the Patentee.

I am not inclined to accept the argument of the Patentee that the sales of Patentee combined with that of M/s. Cipla satisfy the reasonable requirements of the public. The Application for a compulsory license is filed against the Patentee or his licensee, if any, and it is their conduct that is relevant in this case. The conduct of any other person, especially an alleged infringer, cannot by any stretch of imagination be considered in this case. This view flows from Section 86(6)(i), which states as follows:

"In considering the application filed under this section, the Controller shall take into account, -

(i)............the measures already taken by the patentee or any licensee to make full use of the invention;"

If the conduct of the Patentee is considered with reference to this provision, it follows that the Patentee tried his best to prevent M/s.Cipla by preferring an infringement suit against them, which is at an advanced stage. In such circumstances, the Patentee appears to be indulging in two-facedness by adopting one stand before this tribunal and another stance before the Hon'ble High Court of Delhi, in order to defend the indefensible.

M/s.Cipla is an alleged infringer, as per patentee's own submissions, and accordingly cannot discharge the obligations of Patentee under the Act. The Patentee appears to have treated M/s.Cipla, in this case, as if they are their licensee. M/s. Cipla may be injuncted at any time by the Hon'ble Court. Such an uncertain supply by an alleged infringer cannot be considered while deciding this matter, as it involves the lives of cancer patients, which in my opinion cannot be left to the uncertainties of legal proceedings.

The Patentee has submitted an affidavit of Dr. Garg and has submitted a patient coverage during 2011. It is pertinent to mention that the Patentee refrained from giving the patients covered by his drug and simply submitted a patient coverage by him and M/s.Cipla together. It is noted that the Form-27 for 2009 filed by the Patentee does not provide any logical information about the sales. Form-27 for the year 2010 discloses that the Patentee did not import any 'sale pack' but imported only 340 units [60 tablets pack] of 'support pack' and 340 units [60 tablets pack] of 'sample pack', both having an 'invoice value' of Rs.10,045,692. It appears to me, from the Form-27 filed by the Patentee for the year 2009 and 2010, that only an insignificant quantum of the drug was made available by the Patentee to the public during these two years. As discussed above, I am not inclined to buy the argument of the Patentee by taking shelter of M/s. Cipla's supply.

The Patentee has arrived at a figure of 8842 cancer patients according to his logic and has compared this figure with the combined sales achieved by him and M/s.Cipla. The Patentee has submitted that they have sold about 593 boxes during the year 2011. It is an admitted fact that a liver patient's life is extended by 6-8 months and a kidney cancer patient's life is extended by 4-5 years upon treatment with the drug. Even if I consider that on an average a patient requires three packets (3 months), the patentee would not have supplied the drug to more than 200 patients in 2011. By his own admission, the Patentee has submitted the number of patients eligible for Sorafenib is 8842 per year. Hence, the Patentee has made available the drug only to a little above 2% of the eligible patients. The Applicant submits that the annual requirement of the drug is about 70000 boxes.

From the conclusions drawn about the probable number of patients requiring the drug, the annual requirement could lie between 9000*3=27000, which is the Patentee's figure, and 70000 boxes per annum, which is the Applicant's figure.

For argument sake, even if I consider the sale 4686 packets during 2011 by M/s.Cipla, the supply in India was not anywhere near the requirement.

In the aforementioned circumstances, the Patentee's conduct of not making the drug available as per the requirements of public in

India during four years, since the grant of Patent, is not at all justifiable. This is inspite of the fact that the Patentee was already marketing the drug in other parts of the world from 2006 onwards. It is not the case of the Patentee that he had to develop the drug before launching the same in the Indian market or had no means to market the drug. The Patentee has a considerable Field Force and Distributors, being an old and established force in the Indian market. In the year 2009, the sales of Patentee in India were only Rs.16 Crores, as per the Applicant, which appears to be incorrect as the Form-27 filed by the Patentee for the year 2009 discloses a possible sale of Rs.2 Crores only. It is also not the case of the Patentee that there is no demand for the drug because as per their own submission, there is a requirement for at least 8842 patients. Even after the lapse of three years, the Patentee has imported and made available only an insignificant proportion of the reasonable requirement of the patented product in India.

It is also pertinent to refer to Section 84(7) of the Act, which states as follows:

"(7) For the purposes of this Chapter, the reasonable requirements of the public shall be deemed not to have been satisfied—

(a) if, by reason of the refusal of the patentee to grant a license or licenses on reasonable terms,—

... ...

(ii) the demand for the patented article has not been met to an adequate extent or on reasonable terms; or... ... ."

In the circumstances of this case, it is also clear that Section 84(7)(a)(ii) in invoked beyond doubt. Accordingly, I hold that the reasonable requirements of the public with respect to the patented invention have not been satisfied in this case and consequently a compulsory license be issued to the Applicant under Section 84 of the Act.

11.   **Reasonably affordable price**

Section 84 of the Act states as follows:

"84. Compulsory licenses. --

(1) At any time after the expiration of three years from the date of the grant of a patent, any person interested may make an application to the Controller for grant of compulsory license on patent on any of the following grounds, namely –

… … ….

(b) that the patented invention is not available to the public at a reasonably affordable price …..'

<u>Applicant's submissions</u>

Price of the patented product is too high and simply unaffordable by the common man making the product inaccessible and out of reach – hence the demand for the patented product has not been met on reasonable terms.

The Applicant submitted through the affidavit of Sh. C. Rammanohar Reddy, the Editor of Economic and Political Weekly that there are a number of ways for determining the affordability of a drug. These include the following two methods, as described in following published papers:

i. Shanti Mendis et al, "The availability and affordability of selected essential medicines for chronic diseases in six-low and middle income countries", [Bulletin of the World Health Organization, April 2007, 85(4)]:

As per this approach, the number of days a lowest paid government worker would be required to work to purchase from the public sector, a month's course of medicine at the standard or common dose, has to be considered. It has been argued that in the case of the present drug such a Government Worker would have to work for three and a half years to be able to purchase the drug at a price of Rs.2,80,000. By this time, going by that fact that the life-expectancy is not more than four months, such a government worker would not be able to afford it.

ii. Laurens M. Niens et al, "Quantifying the Improvershing Effects of Purchasing Medicines: A Cross-Country Comparison of the Affordability of Medicines in the Developing World", PLOS Medicine, August 2010, Volume 7, Issue8:

As per this approach, the author has opined that the impoverishment effect of the medicine should be considered i.e. the percentage that would be pushed below a certain income level when having to purchase the medicine. According to the official Government of India norms, a family of five with an income of more than Rs. 4805 (Rs.57,660 a year) in urban areas and more than Rs. 3924 (Rs.47,088 a year) in rural areas, is deemed to be above poverty line. At present an estimated 72% of the population is above this very low poverty line. Hence, a medicine that costs Rs.2,80,000 a month will push a large proportion of the population into poverty. It is also suggested that the price should be arrived at after taking into account the manufacturing costs, administrative expenses, taxes etc. and should provide for a certain minimum profit which would incentivize a company to sustain manufacture and sale of the drug in the market.

Applicant has also submitted an affidavit by Mr. James Packard Love, Director, Knoweldge Ecology International, a non-profit organization located in Washington DC, USA, and co-chair of the Trans-Atlantic Consumer Dialogue (TACD) Policy Committee on Intellectual Property Rights. It was submitted that Mr. James Love is an invited expert on intellectual property issues in meetings and consultations organized by the World Intellectual Property Organization (WIPO), World Health Organization (WHO), the World Trade Organization (WTO), the United National Program on Development (UNDP), the United Nations Conference on Trade and Development (UNCTAD), the UN Human Rights Council, the Hague Conference on Private International Law, the UNITAID, the World Bank and other multilateral and regional bodies. Mr. James Love has also served as an advisor to several national governments on Intellectual Property issues, including the Competition Commission in South Africa where he was the principal consultant to evaluate a complaint that the prices for AIDS medicines were excessive. It has been deposed that the World Bank estimates of Indian Gross National Income per capita for 2010 is $1330, which is approximately Rs.60,455. The present pricing of the drug shatters the notions of cost-effectiveness.

Bayer had received an FDA designation under the US Orphan Drug Act in 2004. The clinical trials that were related to the orphan drug indication, "treatment of renal cell carcinoma", were eligible for a 50 percent orphan drug tax credit, lowering the net cost of the investments to Bayer. There is no publicly available information on the amount of tax credit received by Bayer. The credit was available during the period of the most extensive spending on clinical trials, and for the largest and most expensive trials that were undertaken. The issue of lack of transparency in the reported expenditures on R and D was also raised by Mr. James Packard Love. It has been submitted that while the outlays on research and development related to the drug were not trivial, the revenue from the sales were much larger. In 2006, its first year on the market, Onyx, with whom the Patentee entered into a drug development agreement, reported that in the year 2006, its first year on the market, the drug generated $165 million in sales, an amount nearly equal to all joint outlays on R and D from 1994 to 2004. In 2007, Bayer reported the sales of the drug as $371.7 million. By 2008, the sales were reported at $ 678 million, i.e. a total of $1.2 billion within three years of approval as an 'orphan drug'. It has been submitted that if the Patentee has raised the issue of R and D, then it must also open the doors to look at the revenues and profits from the drug. The deponent has also demonstrated as to how various methods can be utilized for calculating royalty.

In conclusion, the Applicant has submitted that the pricing adopted by the Patentee is exorbitant for its patented life-saving product and is an abuse of its monopolistic rights and such practice is unfair and anti-competitive and has requested for grant of a compulsory license on this ground.

Patentee's submissions

It was submitted that innovation based products cost a price over generics, but this price pays for the pipeline (i.e. the future innovation) and competition. The higher price of the drug covered by the subject patent as compared to generic version thereof is justified inasmuch as for the Patentee, it also involves the Research and Development (R&D) cost of innovators as against the Applicant who merely copies the drug discovered by the Patentee thereby taking advantage of the R & D carried out by the Patentee.

The affidavit filed by Mr. Herald Dinter elaborately explains the complete process to discover and develop a drug. It has been explained that quite a large amount of money is spent in failed projects, which is about 75% of the total R & D cost. The marketed product must pay not only for its own R & D cost but also for the cost of the underlying failed R & D, and further must underwrite the additional R & D for the next generation of innovations. The Patentee and its collaborator continue to invest major sums into further development of Sorafenib. Its potential for treatment of cancers, other than renal and kidney cancer is under investigation in large Phase III trials (e.g. breast cancer, thyroid cancer and non-small-cell-lung cancer). It is therefore important to understand that R & D on a new drug does not at all stop when the drug is launched in the market but actually continues with considerable investments. In conclusion, it is neither possible nor – if it were somehow possible – would it be reasonable to look at past R & D expenditure for a launched product to decide whether its current price is reasonable. Rather one has to take into account the total R & D spending of a company and the need and desire to finance such R & D sustainably to ensure ongoing innovation in healthcare. In 2010, the pharmaceutical division of Bayer invested almost € 1.8 bn or 16% of its net sales into R & D for pharmaceuticals, and 6200 employees worked in the R & D divisions of Patentee globally. Since, the year 2007, the cumulative R & D spending of Patentee was € 8 bn. In this period, 2 NMEs and one new combination product were brought to the market. It thus takes investments of more than €2 bn to bring an NME to the market.

It was submitted that Nexavar has been granted an 'orphan drug' status in the US and Europe. The exact criteria to meet the orphan drug status vary between jurisdictions. In the US, for example, Nexavar was granted 'orphan drug' status on the basis of having fewer than 200,000 patients for each of its indications. In Europe, one of the criteria for a drug to qualify for an orphan designation is that it must be intended for the diagnosis, prevention or treatment of a life-threatening or chronically debilitating condition affecting no more than 5 in 10,000 people in the EU. Therefore, the number of patients for cancer drugs (especially for orphan cancer indications as in the present case of Nexavar) is small when compared to the overall R & D investment of the originator. Further, if one compares this drug vis-à-vis other Oncology brands of innovation based companied, it will be found that the pricing is similar to other comparable drugs.

The Patentee desires to sustainably fund further research in areas of unmet medical needs, which research is in public interest. Replacing the innovation based product with a generic will damage India and Indian patients in the long run as the Patentee as an originator provides more than just the drug product, e.g., education of practitioners on use of the product, pharmacovigilance (observing/evaluating/improving the safety of medicines) etc.

It is the Patentee, being the innovator and having invested resources in developing/marketing the innovation based product, who would decide as to what would constitute a "reasonably affordable price" for such product. It needs to be appreciated that if a higher price of the patented drug with huge investment in R & D by an originator is a good enough argument for the Applicant to request for the grant of

Compulsory License, it will always be applicable and will always circumvent the objective of the Patents Act, which cannot be the intention of the Legislature.

Patents Act provides that the patented invention should be available to "public" at a "reasonably affordable price". "Reasonable" must mean "reasonable" to the public i.e., patients and the patentee as well. If it is not read in this manner, the word "reasonable" would not have been present there. Balance needs to be created. Therefore, the cost of R&D and the cost of manufacture, both have to be taken into account while determining "reasonable affordable price".

There can be no "reasonably affordable price" below the expense incurred in the development of the product and the cost of manufacture is a reasonable element of commercial gain. "Reasonably affordable price" has to be used to balance the interest of the consumer/public without compromising on the interest of the innovator. "Reasonably affordable price" does not relate to the lowest price relative to the cost of manufacturing alone. "Reasonably affordable price" must necessarily take into account the cost of R&D and reasonable gain.

"Public" denotes different sections of public. "The Rich class", "the middle class" and "the poor class". A blanket CL cannot be granted thereby giving the opponents patented drug to <u>all sections</u> of "public" <u>at the same price</u>. Therefore, a method will have to be devised in order to make it "reasonable" for the patentee and to make it "reasonably affordable" for the different sections of "public".

"Treating unequal as equal" is discriminatory and is not permissible under law. Placing "the rich class" and "the lower class" in one category at the expense of the patentee is unreasonable and cannot be the intention of the legislature. In case of a drug, if R&D is not to be killed, this device has to be implemented.

The word "reasonable" necessarily mean affordable to patients, which necessarily is relative *vis-à-vis* to the paying capacity of the patient. "Reasonably" means "reasonable" to the patients and patentee as well. The Patents Act does not envisage the grant of CL unless the product is not reasonably affordable. It will be within the jurisdiction of the Controller (implied power) to reject, resurrect or keep in abeyance an application for the grant of CL if the patentee is willing to meet the "reasonable requirement" and provide the patented product at "reasonable affordable price to the public". It cannot be the intention of the legislature to lower the price for those patients who can afford the opponent's drug. "Reasonableness" is a relative term which has to be interpreted in the circumstances of each case.

The term "affordability" is the capacity to pay. Different classes/sections of the public have vastly different capacity to pay. What may be "affordable" for one class/section may not be "affordable" to another class/section. The phrase "available to the public at a reasonable affordable price", therefore, must be interpreted to mean as to whether the treatment is "affordable" to a particular class/section of public. Therefore, in modern times, one of the means whereby the treatment can become "affordable" is by way of insurance cover. In other words, treatment as a whole is "affordable" including the drug (being one of the factors of treatment) by an insurance cover. Therefore, "affordability" has to be judged from the cost to be incurred on the insurance cover. Question now that arises for consideration is not whether the patient can afford the drug at a given cost but whether the patient can afford the insurance cover. "Affordability" is also required to be judged as to whether the patient can afford insurance cover.

In India, insurance cover is accessible to any person by the following modes:

(1) Voluntary health insurance schemes or private-for-profit schemes;

(2) Employer-based schemes;

(3) Insurance offered by NGOs / community based health insurance, and

(4) Mandatory health insurance schemes or government run schemes (namely ESIS, CGHS).

In the affidavit of Mr. Pradeep Kumar Sharma, Business Unit Head, Specialty Medicine, it has been stated that the New India Assurance Company Limited (NIA) offers an insurance policy which is extremely cheap as compared to general health insurance policies. Two such policies are currently offered by NIA and the maximum sum insured is of Rs. 75000 for the first policy and Rs. 3,00,000 for the second policy. A policy offered by ICICI Prudential secures coverage of Rs. 10 lakhs.

It was submitted that "reasonably affordable price" is the notional price, which has to be determined, and it cannot be obviously lesser than the royalty if fixed under Section 90 (1) (i) and (ii) of the Patents Act.

a. The application for Compulsory License must establish that the drug is not available at "reasonably affordable price". If it is available at "reasonably affordable price", a CL cannot be granted. It is a condition precedent, sine qua non for an application for grant of CL to be adjudicated upon. The applicant has chosen to show that the opponent's drug at Rs. 280,000 per month is not "reasonably affordable price" and has suppressed the fact that

Cipla's same drug is available to public approximately Rs. 30,000 per month.

b. The very bulk of sales of Cipla's drug at approximately Rs.30,000 itself is an evidence to show that it is at least "reasonably affordable price" for those patients who cannot afford the opponents' drug at its original price. The application is laible to be dismissed on this ground alone.

c. The CL ought to be dismissed at as threshold as the Applicant has been guilty of suppressing the fact that Cipla's product was available in the market which is a material fact to adjudicate upon the core issue involved vis-à-vis "reasonable affordable price". The suppression of material fact is a fundamental flaw and is certainly not an innocent one. The Applicant ought to have compared its price with Cipla's price and determined as to how Cipla's price is not "reasonably affordable price". The core issue before the Learned Controller is that Cipla's drug at its quoted price is not a "reasonable affordable price". The pleading of the Applicant is completely silent on this issue. Accordingly, the Applicant has failed to discharge the burden and therefore, the Learned Controller should use the discretion in favour of the patentee/ opponent in rejecting CL application. This fact was well within the knowledge of the applicant and inspite it chose not to disclose the said material fact thereby approaching the Learned Controller with unclean hands. It is further submitted that the motivation for the applicant appears to make a quick profit at the expense of the opponent's R&D.

d. It is submitted that in the absence of an injunction from Hon'ble Delhi High Court in CS (OS) No. 523 of 2010, Cipla is another entity apart from the opponent in the market selling the product covered by the Subject Patent for Rs 27,960. It is further submitted that it is the case of the applicant that the demand of Nexavar is not being met as it is not available to public at "reasonably affordable price". The provisions regarding CL no-where mention that demand is required to be met by only the patentee.

Patentee has further submitted that the intention behind Chapter XVI of the Patents Act is that the patentee should not be allowed to charge exorbitant price so long as it is making a reasonable profit. There is no *suo motu* power upon the Learned Controller to grant CL. It is only upon an application made by "any person interested", that the Learned Controller may grant CL. Emphasis in this regard is laid on the word "may" appearing in Section 84 (4) of the Patents Act, the Learned Controller has a discretion as evident from the said provision. Further, it is submitted that Section 90 (1) (i) of the Patents Act is important in construing "reasonable affordable price". It is submitted that law does not envisage the grant of CL unless the hurdle/condition under the said clause is crossed. The cost of R&D that the patentee has incurred has to be taken into account while fixing royalty. It has no relationship whatsoever with the fact that patentee has already earned/profited so much on Nexavar as has been the case of the applicant. The "reasonable affordable price" cannot be less than the royalty to be fixed by the Learned Controller. "Reasonable affordable price" does not merely depend upon the purchasing power of the public. It will have to be determined on the basis of cost incurred by the patentee on the R&D with some reasonable gain/profit to it. It is submitted that the affidavit of Mr. James Love does not further the case of the applicant as if his deposition is accepted, every time an application for CL will be filed, the Learned Controller shall call for the balance sheets of the patentee. That can certainly not be the intention of the legislature. In any event, it is admitted case of the applicant that even its quoted price is too high.

Decision

I have carefully gone through the pleadings of the parties, the affidavits, oral as well as written submissions, and the relevant provisions of the Act to decide on the issue as to whether the patented invention is not available to the public at a reasonably affordable price in this case.

The Patentee has vehemently argued on 'reasonably affordable price' and has suggested that reasonableness has to be judged with respect to public as well as to patentee. The Applicant has argued that the 'reasonably affordable price' has to be interpreted as reasonable to public. Both the parties have also submitted that 'reasonably affordable price' is a notional price and has to be arrived at from the facts and circumstances on a case by case basis. Patentee has also argued that the sales made by M/s.Cipla at a price of about Rs.30000/- is a relevant factor to be considered in this case. Patentee also submitted that affordable to public is required to be considered as affordable to different classes/sections of public. On this point, I fully agree with the Patentee. I only wonder why the Patentee did not execute this concept by offering differential pricing for different classes/sections of public in India. Further, the Patentee in their affidavit submitted that they offer this drug at a similar price (subject to variation in exchange rate etc.) to patients all over the world.

As I have already decided that the sales by M/s. Cipla cannot be considered in these proceedings, I need not further dwell upon this issue. While deciding this case, I need to only decide as to whether the drug was available to the public at a reasonably affordable price or not.

I do not fully agree with the submission of Patentee that reasonably affordable price has to be construed with reference to the public as well as patentee. I am of the view that reasonably affordable price has to be construed predominantly with reference to public. Given the 'admitted facts' in this case, I need not go into these issues in detail as the admitted facts fully enable me to decide this issue.

As concluded in 10 above, during the last four years the sales of the drug by the Patentee at a price of about Rs.2,80,000/- (for a therapy of one month) constitute a fraction of the requirement of the public. It stands to common logic that a patented article like the drug in this case was not bought by the public due to only one reason, i.e. its price was not reasonably affordable to them. Hence, I conclude beyond doubt that the patented invention was not available to the public at a reasonably affordably price and that Section 84(1)(b) of the Patents Act, 1970 is invoked in this case. Consequently, a compulsory license be issued to the Applicant under Section 84 of the Act.

12.   **Patented invention not worked in the territory of India**

Section 84 of the Act states as follows:

"84. Compulsory licenses. –

(1) At any time after the expiration of three years from the date of the grant of a patent, any person interested may make an application to the Controller for grant of compulsory license on patent on any of the following grounds, namely –

....

(c) that the patented invention is not worked in the territory of India. '

<u>Applicant's submissions</u>

The patented product is being imported into India and hence the product is not worked in the territory of India to the fullest extent that is reasonably practicable. As per the Act, the law expects the Patentee to work the invention in the country to the fullest extent possible. The provision of 'working' is to be read in the context of principles stipulated under Section 83[(a) and (b)] of the Act and with reference to the debates in the Lok Sabha.

It is pertinent to note that Patentee has been working the Patent in other countries since 2006; however, the Patent has not been exploited in India and no reason has been ascribed for such neglect. This is especially in view of the fact that the Patentee claims to have manufacturing facilities in India for several products, including Oncology products. As such there is no hurdle preventing the Patentee from working the Patent in India. A comparison of the working statement with the Patient base would clearly show that the Patent has not been worked in India.

Patentee's argument that even minimal working would satisfy the requirements of Section 84(1)(c) is flawed and fallacious for the reason that the expression "working" in Section 84 has to take color from Section 83(a). If the argument of Patentee were to be accepted then it would render Section 84(1)(c) otiose. As per Heydon's Rule, where two different interpretations are advanced, the one that suppresses mischief and advances the cause of the Act should be taken. Accordingly, the correct interpretation of Section 84(1)(c) would be that minimal working is no working at all and the invention must be worked to the fullest extent to escape from the rigours of Section 84(1)(c).

<u>Patentee's submissions</u>

The local working requirements in the Patents Act are directed towards ensuring that inventions are domestically "worked" i.e. supplied to the Indian market. An attempt to impose local working requirements – in the sense of local manufacturing – on patents granted in India would be beyond the scope of the Patents Act and against the intent of the legislature. The intent of the legislature is clear from the fact that the phrase "manufactured in India" was deleted from Section 84(7)(a)(ii) of the Patents Act during the amendment to the Patents Act in 2002, thus negating the requirement of local manufacture in order to make it consistent with Article 27(1) of TRIPS Agreement. This is also relevant to Section 84(7)(e) of the Patents Act, which states that a compulsory license should be available "if the working of the patented invention in the territory of India on a commercial scale is being prevented or hindered by the importation from abroad of the patented article." Section 84(7)(e) should be interpreted, consistently with settled proposition of law, to apply where the patentee, or other entity claiming under the same right holder, was not supplying the patented product to the market.

The economies of scale ought to be appreciated which provides valid reason for not locally manufacturing the drug. Manufacturing of the drug requires huge investment in terms of infrastructure and logistics. Nexavar is a product of small global demand and hence is required to be produced in small volumes. With a view to achieving economies-of-scale with such a small-volume product and keeping manufacturing costs at a reasonable level, the Patentee made a strategic decision to consolidate both chemical API synthesis and pharmaceutical bulk production of the product covered by the Subject Patent within its manufacturing facilities in Germany. Further, manufacturing bundled in Germany allows for maintaining a harmonized high quality production at reasonable manufacturing costs due to volume scale. In addition, production in Germany allows for taking advantage of good infrastructure for supplying global markets as good downstream and upstream industries ensure a smooth supply chain process. The quantities required in India do not economically justify setting up a manufacturing facility by Bayer in India. However, these can, due to the local nature of their sales, be manufactured on contract manufacturing basis with other manufactures who are expert *in manufacturing those specific dosage forms.*

The Patentee also submitted a detailed list of contract manufacturers (Annexure-6 of the Notice of Opposition). It is a settled proposition of Law that importation does indeed satisfy the working requirements mandated under the Patents Act.

Decision

I have carefully gone through the pleadings of the parties, the affidavits and oral as well as written submissions to decide the issue as to whether the patented invention is worked in the territory of India or not. The term 'worked in the territory of India' has not been defined in the Act. Hence, one has to seek its meaning from various International Conventions and Agreements on intellectual property, provisions contained in the Patents Act, 1970, the context in which this concept appears, and also the legislative history.

It appears that the arguments of the patentee referring to the deletion of the phrase 'manufactured in India' from Section 84(7)(a)(ii) by the Patents (Amendment) Act, 2002 are misplaced. In fact, the phrase was deleted from Section 90(a) of the unamended Patents Act, 1970 [hereinafter referred to as the 'erstwhile Act']. It may be noted that Section 84 (7) is the corresponding provision under the existing Act [hereinafter referred to as the 'amended Act']. The Patentee argues that the legislature deleted 'default of the patentee to <u>manufacture in India</u> to an adequate extent and supply on reasonable terms the patented article' [hereinafter referred to as the 'concept'] from Section 90(a) of the erstwhile Act, to make the Patents Act, 1970 consistent with Article 27 of the TRIPS Agreement.

It is necessary to address this crucial argument of the patentee in detail. It is pertinent to mention that Section 90 of the erstwhile Act appeared in a different context, i.e. with reference to the issue of 'reasonable requirements of public'. The deletion of this concept was one face of the coin, which is being tossed by the Patentee to suit his convenience. However, there is another face of the coin, which is that this concept was removed from 'a context', i.e. 'reasonable requirements of public', and was made a separate ground for grant of a compulsory license under Section 84(1)(c), with a substantially altered scope.

It must be appreciated that this is not a simple case where a concept is removed from one place of an Act. It is in fact a complicated case where a concept is removed from one place of an Act and is incorporated at a different place, in a different context, and with a substantially altered scope. Accordingly, it cannot be said in such a straightforward manner that the intention of the Legislature, in removing the concept from Section 90(a) of the erstwhile Act, is to totally remove the concept of local manufacturing in India. In fact, this amendment has to be decoded by considering all the International Conventions and Agreements and the Patents Act, 1970 itself.

I have considered the Paris Convention, TRIPS Agreement and The Patents Act, 1970 in detail. Even though the TRIPS Agreement marked a new era of obligations regarding the protection and enforcement of intellectual property, WTO Members retained *important policy options, flexibilities and safeguards, including the* liberty to determine the grounds for issuing compulsory licenses. In addition, certain key terms relating to TRIPS obligations are not defined in the Agreement itself, which leaves considerable discretion to WTO Members as to how to apply the criteria within their national laws. The use of these policy options and other flexibilities can directly or indirectly help the low and middle-income countries to achieve a balance between intellectual property protection and specific developmental priorities, including the attainment of national public health objectives.

It may be noted that Article 2(1) of the TRIPS Agreement states that provisions of the Paris Convention shall be complied with by the member states. This implies that the Paris Convention is to be read as a part and parcel of the TRIPS Agreement. Article 5(A)(1) of the Paris Convention provides that importation of patented articles by the patentee shall not entail forfeiture of the patent. This would seem to suggest that importation could entail something less than forfeiture, such as a compulsory license. Such a conclusion is further fortified by the fact that Article 5(A)(2) of the Convention goes on to state that each member shall have the right to take legislative measures providing for the grant of compulsory licenses in order to prevent any abuse of patent rights, for example, failure to work. It is pertinent to note that the Paris Convention did not define the term 'working' and left it to the wisdom of Legislatures of member countries in a manner conducive to their socio-economic requirements.

Article 27(1) of the TRIPS Agreement, *inter alia*, states that "patents shall be available and patent rights enjoyable without discrimination as to the place of invention, the field of technology and whether products are imported or locally produced." When the Article 27(1) of TRIPS Agreement is read with the afore-mentioned provisions of TRIPS Agreement and the Paris Convention, it follows that importation of a patented invention shall not result in forfeiture of a patent. However, a reasonable fetter on the patent rights in the form of a compulsory license is very well within the purview of the Paris Convention and TRIPS Agreement, when there is an abuse of patent rights. It is this flexibility that the Parliament have invoked in Chapter XVI of the Patents Act, 1970 by incorporating a provision for grant of compulsory license upon failure to work the invention within the territory of India.

I now turn to the indications that the Patents Act, 1970 provides with reference to working of the patented invention. The Patentee contended that working means working on a commercial scale as is evident from Section 84(7)(e). It may be noted that while deciding 'the reasonable requirements of public', one relevant consideration, as provided under Section 84(7)(e), is that the 'working of patented invention in the territory of India on <u>a commercial scale</u> is being prevented by importation by the Patentee'. However, it must be appreciated that Section 84(7)(e) relates to Section 84(1)(a) and not Section 84(1)(c). Accordingly, it does not appear logical to me to accept the Patentee's contention that working means working on a commercial scale only as I find no such limitation in Section 84(1)(c). If such was the case, then there was no need to incorporate Section 84(1)(c) as a separate ground for grant of a compulsory license, as it would be an absurdity (emphasis added). Due to this, I am of the view that the term 'worked in the territory of India' cannot be restricted to mean as 'worked in India on a commercial scale' only as submitted by the Patentee. To my mind, it is something more than that.

I now turn to Section 83, which is the over-riding legislative policy and the key to decoding the various provisions contained in Chapter XVI of the Act.

Section 83(b) states that Patents are not granted merely to enable patentees to enjoy a monopoly for importation of the patented article. Upon a reading of this provision, it becomes amply clear to me that mere importation cannot amount to working of a patented invention.

Section 83(c) buttresses this interpretation by stating that the grant of a patent right must contribute to the promotion of technological innovation and to the transfer and dissemination of technology. Section 83(f), clears all ambiguity that the patent right should not be abused and the patentee should not resort to practices that unreasonably restrain trade or adversely affect the international transfer of technology. Upon a combined reading of Section 83(c) and (f), it is clear to me that a patentee is obliged to contribute towards the transfer and dissemination of technology, nationally and internationally so as to balance the rights with the obligations. A patentee can achieve this by either manufacturing the product in India or by granting a license to any other person for manufacturing in India. Unless such an opportunity for technological capacity building domestically is provided to the Indian public, they will be at a loss as they will not be empowered to utilise the patented invention, after the patent right expires, which certainly cannot be the intention of the Parliament. Hence it follows that 'worked in the territory of India' implies manufactured in India to a reasonable extent so that the principles enumerated in Section 83 can be brought into effect. In the absence of manufacturing in India, Section 83 will be a dead letter.

Another indication is provided by Section 84(6) and Section 90(2) of the Act, which state as follows:

Section 84(6)

"In considering the application filed under this section, the Controller shall take into account,—

... ...

(ii) the ability of the applicant to <u>work the invention</u> to the public advantage;

(iii) the capacity of the applicant to undertake the risk in providing capital and working the invention, if the application were granted;"

Section 90(2)

'......no license granted by the Controller shall authorise the licensee to import the patented article or an article or substance made by a patented process from abroad.....'.

The term 'work the invention' does not include imports as a compulsory license holder has to necessarily work the patent by manufacturing the patented invention in India. If, the licensee cannot import the product into India, for working the invention under the terms of License, barring exceptional circumstances mentioned in Section 90(3) of the Act, then is implies that importing cannot amount to working for a licensee. A combined reading of these provisions implies that the same logic must apply with respect to the Patentee as well.

From all the aforementioned indications, it is clear to me that the Paris Convention and TRIPS Agreement and Patents Act, 1970 read together do not in any manner imply that working means importation. I am therefore convinced that 'worked in the territory of India' means 'manufactured to a reasonable extent in India'.

In the instant case, the Patent was granted in the year 2008. It is an admitted fact that the Patentee does have manufacturing facilities for manufacturing drugs in India, including Oncology drugs. However, even after the lapse of four years from the date of grant of patent, the Patentee failed to do so. The Patentee has also failed to grant a voluntary license on reasonable terms to anyone including the Applicant herein to work the invention within the territory of India. Accordingly, I hold that Section 84(1)(c) is attracted in this case and consequently a compulsory license be issued to the Applicant under Section 84 of the Act.

13. **Request for adjournment under Section 86**

Patentee's submissions

The allegation against the Opponent/ Patentee is that it is not working the patent to its "fullest extent that is reasonably practicable" as it is highly priced. In order to work the patent to its "fullest extent that is reasonably practicable", the opponent is prepared to modify the current PAP thereby reducing the price of the drug for those patients who cannot afford the original price to a level by which it has been proven by Cipla's sale figures (as mentioned in the affidavit dated February 8, 2012 of Dr. Manish Garg) to cover a very large number of patients.

It was submitted that Cipla being in the market has cut the opponent's market share thereby preventing them to work the invention to the fullest extent that is reasonably practicable.

Section 86 in fact gives preference and the first right option to the patentee to work the patent to the fullest extent that is reasonably practicable before any CL is granted. For this purpose, the present CL proceedings may be adjourned for one year.

It was submitted that Section 86 of the Patents Act obliges the Learned Controller to first consider and give first option right to the inventor/patentee to work the patent to its fullest extent that is reasonably practicable. If the allegation is that the patent is not being fully worked because of the high price, it is in the interest of justice that an opportunity has to be given to the inventor/patentee to reduce the price below the "reasonably affordable price" to those who cannot afford the original price.

In so far as the compliance of conditions imposed by the Learned Controller for the adjournment is concerned, in the event of non-compliance, it is submitted that the Controller can simply grant the CL on the expiry of the adjournment period under Section 86 of the Patents Act.

<u>Applicant's submissions:</u>

The Patentee at the time of hearing made an oral request for adjournment of the hearing under Section 86 (of the Patents Act) by 12 months so as to enable the patentee to work the invention in India to the fullest extent. In addition, the Patentee came up with a proposal that they would provide the product to deserving patients at Rs 30,000 per month and <u>sought adjournment on that basis.</u> Such request being a mere demurrer, cannot be entertained at all even on merits because:

- Section 86 would require the Ld.Controller to first arrive at a finding, the "**time**" that has elapsed after sealing of the patent has been "*insufficient*" to enable the patentee to work the invention in India. Further, the power to adjourn is curtailed by Section 86(2) which clearly stipulates that the adjournment shall **not** be granted for the asking, but only upon a clear satisfaction that the Patentee has taken with promptitude, steps to work the invention in India on a commercial scale to an adequate extent.

- A proper reading of section 86 would require *fulfillment* of following conditions before any adjournment is granted:

  - Application from the Patentee conceding that they have not been able to work the patented invention after its grant, and giving reasons why they could not do so from date of grant till date of CL application and steps that they plan to take to work the patented invention in future

  - On the basis of the above, the Ld. Controller could arrive at a finding and be "satisfied" that the invention though not worked till date, could be worked in future by the Patentee.

- In the case at hand no application from patentee- only oral plea: Patentee has made no serious plea for adjournment; no specific application was filed. Even *in its* oral arguments, the Patentee did not concede that they could not work the invention in a timely manner after its grant and no request for working has been made so far. The argument made is a mere request for adjournment without any assurance that the Patentee shall work the invention nor any details of the mode and manner of working the invention- no change in market price or assurance of greater availability of the drug in the market has been made. In the absence of such reasons, any adjournment is unwarranted and unsustainable.

- Patentee is guilty of absolute neglect and delay: Despite launching the product in the world market in 2006, the Patentee did not launch it in India until 2009- though the patent was granted in 2008 thus the patentee waited for 2 years and no logical reason for such delay has been ascribed till date- neither Patentee has conceded to the delay nor given reasons for the delay ; The key feature of Section 86 is the time factor and the satisfaction that time was insufficient- the satisfaction of the Ld Ld Controller can be gleaned only from reasons if any and ascribed by the Patentee. And, Section 86(2) specifically intends to curb such unexplained delay. In the teeth of such intendment of the legislation, and the unexplained delay and latches by the Patentee in working the patented invention, no adjournment is warranted and not reasonable.

- Bayer as a company with all its supply infrastructure existed as of 2005, as well as 2007 as well as 2011. It is pertinent to note that the demand for the drug always existed whether in 2007 or 2009 or 2011 and the Patentee has not explained why there was delay in working the patent. Thus, the basic requirement of Section 86 remains unfulfilled making out no case for adjournment at all.

- It is pertinent to note that the law makers while framing of Sec 84 of Patents Act had given the Patentee 3 years from the date of grant of Patent as a reasonable period for the Patentee to work the invention. Failure to do so invites consequences outlined in Chapter XVI, Section 84. In this case, even though the Patent was granted in 2008, Patentee not taken any effective steps all these four (4) years to see that the Patent is worked in India as in other countries; which amply demonstrates the neglect on part of the Patentee.

- Further the Patentee, though pleads for adjournment, does not plead that "time" has been insufficient to work the invention in India- rather the Patentee vehemently contests this fact and states that they have worked the patent in India to an adequate extent : hence, even for this reason, the request for adjournment must be dismissed in limini.

- Section 84(6)(iv) precludes consideration of matters after the date of filing of the compulsory license application: Section 84(6)(iv) clearly states that "… *but shall not be required to take into account matters subsequent to the filing of the application*" meaning thereby that the Ld Controller is only required to consider the state of affairs that existed **on the date of filing of the Application for compulsory license** and not beyond; considering any proposal by the Patentee made at the time of hearing would be beyond the scope of Section 84(6)(iv);

- Even with the proposal, product price in Open market price remains unchanged and Section 84 is only concerned with market price: Patentee maintains that it shall continue to sell the patented invention at the rate Rs. 2,80,000/- in the open market (chemist shop) to the affordable patients and the reduced price is only for certain deserving patients- the scope of inquiry under section 84 and the present application centers around whether the product is available in the open market at reasonably affordable price, and not the merits of the patient assistance program of the patentee; hence the proposal is no proposal at all and there is nothing for consideration by the Ld Controller in this respect also;

- No rational classification: No logic or rationale including criteria has been defined by the Patentee as to how the "deserving class" would be carved out from the patient base;

- Ld Controller has no power to arbitrate, mediate or settle: Ld Controller has no power under section 86 or any other provision to settle matters in lieu of grant of Compulsory license– such powers are bestowed on a civil court under Section 151 of the CPC;

- <u>Ld Controller has no power to classify public</u>: Ld Controller has no power under the Act to classify the public into deserving and non-deserving for any reason whatsoever; accepting the proposal would necessarily require the Ld Controller to make such classification which is beyond the jurisdiction of the Ld Controller;

- <u>Ld Controller has no power to grant adjournment on the basis of proposal given by Patentee- such power can be exercised only on a finding of insufficient time:</u> It is important to note that the Ld Controller has no power to take into Account any settlement proposals and grant adjournment on that basis. Ld Controller under the Act especially Section 86 is only empowered to arrive at a finding that *time for working has been insufficient,* and on that basis grant adjournment. Hence Patentee's <u>proposal cannot form basis for adjournment;</u>

- <u>Ld Controller has no power to take into account subsequent events:</u> It is pertinent to note that Sorafenib was launched in the world in 2006; Cipla entered the market around April-May 2010 and till date, the Patentee has not bothered to work the invention. However, now, upon filing of the Application for Compulsory license, the Patentee has expressed a desire to work the invention- the material date for adjudication under Section 84 is "the *"date of the compulsory license Application"*- same can be gleaned from Section 84(6)(iv)-*"..but shall not be required to take into account matters subsequent to the filing of the date of filing of the application" ;* Section 84(a)-*"… have not been satisfied"*;

- <u>Proposal is an attempt to remedy an irrational PAP program:</u> Under the PAP program, the patient was required to pay Rs 2-5 lakhs upfront regardless of whether he lived or not; same has been modified and now same amount is being collected in installments [Rs 2,80,000/9= 30,000].

<u>Decision</u>

Section 86 of the Patents Act, 1970, under which the adjournment has been sought by the Patentee is as follows:

"86. Power of Controller to adjourn applications for compulsory licenses, etc., in certain cases.

(1) Where an application under section 84 or section 85, as the case may be, is made on the grounds that the patented invention has not been worked in the territory of India or on the ground mentioned in clause (d) of sub-section (7) of section 84 and the Controller is satisfied that the time which has elapsed since the sealing of the patent has for any reason been insufficient to enable the invention to be worked on a commercial scale to an adequate extent or to enable the invention to be so worked to the fullest extent that is reasonably practicable, he may, by order, adjourn the further hearing of the application for such period not exceeding twelve months in the aggregate as appears to him to be sufficient for the invention to be so worked:

Provided that in any case where the patentee establishes that the reason why a patented invention could not be worked as aforesaid before the date of the application was due to any State or Central Act or any rule or regulation made thereunder or any order of the Government imposed otherwise than by way of a condition for the working of the invention in the territory of India or for the disposal of the patented articles or of the articles made by the process or by the use of the patented plant, machinery, or apparatus, then, the period of adjournment ordered under this sub-section shall be reckoned from the date on which the period during which the working of the invention was prevented by such Act, rule or regulation or order of Government as computed from the date of the application, expires.

(2) No adjournment under sub-section (1) shall be ordered unless the Controller is satisfied that the patentee has taken with promptitude adequate or reasonable steps to start the working of the invention in the territory of India on a commercial scale and to an adequate extent."

The Applicant's contention that only an oral submission was made is misplaced. The Patentee has given the request in writing supported by an affidavit on the issue of modified Patient Assistance Program (PAP).

The Patentee's main contention is that due to the presence of Cipla in the market, the Patentee could not work the invention to the fullest extent that is reasonably practicable as Cipla undercut them. It is pertinent to mention that the drug was developed and marketed globally right from the year 2006, i.e. two years prior to the grant of patent in India. The present proposal of the patentee is that they are willing to offer the drug at a price of Rs. 30,000 through their PAP program. As per their own submission, the Patentee has two schemes under its PAP program. Under the first scheme termed as 1+6, the patient has to pay for one month stock of the drug and will get the supply for six months free. Under the second scheme termed as 2+10, the patient has to pay for two months stock of the drug and will get the supply for ten months free. The Patentee has proposed that they will supply the drug to needy patients based on the recommendation of the Oncologist that the patients is needy and has no means to pay.

The Patentee launched the product in other countries in 2006, as is evident from their sales provided by the Applicant, which have not been controverted by the Patentee. The Patentee got the License for importing and marketing the drug in India on 01.08.2007. The Patentee got another License from the Directorate General of Health Services to import and market the drug on 22.01.2008. Assuming that the actual permission to import and market the drug was given on 22.01.2008, the Patentee's conduct of not importing the drug till 2008 and importing in small quantities in 2009 and 2010, is beyond explanation. The Patentee *has alleged that Cipla did not allow the sales to flourish. However, it is* pertinent to mention that M/s.Cipla entered the market only in April-May 2010 and the Patentee had approximately 2 years after that to suitably modify its pricing strategy so as to work the invention on a commercial scale to an adequate extent. The Patentee thus took no adequate or reasonable steps to start the working of the invention in the territory of India on a commercial scale and to an adequate extent.

The Patentee argued that "treating unequal as equal" is discriminatory and is not permissible under law. Placing "the rich class" and "the lower class" in one category at the expense of the patentee is unreasonable and cannot be the intention of the legislature. The Patentee was not estopped in any manner from treated equals as equals and unequals as unequals. The Patentee had four years from the date of grant to apply differential pricing for different sections of the public in India.

In my view the two essential conditions for invocation of Section 86 of the Act are as follows:

(1) the **time** which has elapsed since the sealing of the patent has for any reason been insufficient to enable the invention to be worked on a commercial scale to an adequate extent or to enable the

invention to be so worked to the fullest extent that is reasonably practicable; **and**

(2) the patentee has taken with promptitude adequate or reasonable **steps** to start the working of the invention in the territory of India on a commercial scale and to an adequate extent.

As discussed in 9 above, the Patentee did not import the drug at all in 2008, and imported in small quantities in 2009 and 2010. In the facts and circumstances of this case, I do not believe that the time which has elapsed since the grant of the patent has been insufficient to enable the invention to be worked on a commercial scale to an adequate extent or to enable the invention to be so worked to the fullest extent that is reasonably practicable. Further, I do not also see any prompt action on the part of the Patentee to start the working of the invention in the territory of India on a commercial scale and to an adequate extent.

Another reason for non-invocation of this provision is the Section 84(6), which states as follows:

"(6) In considering the application filed under this section, the Controller shall take into account,—

(i) the nature of the invention, the time which has elapsed since the sealing of the patent and the measures already taken by the patentee or any licensee to make full use of the invention;

… … … … …

but shall not be required to take into account matters subsequent to the making of the application."

This provision specifically bars the Controller from considering any measures taken by the Patentee subsequent to the making of the Application. The intention of the Legislature appears to be that subsequent measures by the Patentee to frustrate the proceedings shall not be considered. In my view, the present proposal falls within the four corners of this prohibition.

The proposal of the Patentee appears to be philanthropic in nature, as per the submission of the Patentee. In the present proceedings, we are not concerned with philanthropy, which no doubt is appreciable. Such actions cannot be construed as steps to work the invention on a commercial scale to an adequate extent. The request of the Patentee for adjournment is therefore rejected.

14.   **Terms and conditions**

Having decided to grant the Compulsory License under Section 84 of the Act, I now proceed to settle the terms and conditions of the License in the light of the provisions contained in Section 90 of the Act.

Applicant's submissions

Following terms and conditions are acceptable to the Applicant:

i. Right to manufacture and sell Sorafenib shall be limited to the Territory of India.

ii. The products under license shall be manufactured only to cover the patients who are afflicted by renal and hepatic carcinoma.

iii. Royalty shall be paid to the Patentee at the rate as fixed by the Controller of Patents.

iv. Initially, a price of Rs. 74/- per tablet is proposed, which works out to be Rs.8,800/- per month for therapy.

v. The Applicant also commits to give the product free of cost to atleast 600 needy and deserving patients per year.

The Applicant has also submitted the cost break-up as follows:

Particulars	Amount (Rs.)
M.R.P. (inclusive of sales tax)	8900
Margin to distributor, stockiest and retailer (approximately 30% on M.R.P.)	2670
Cost of manufacture of the product SORAFENAT	4856
Billing price of company to distributors	6105
Margin to the company	1250

The Applicant also submitted that royalty shall be paid from the margin to the Applicant.

<u>Patentee's submissions</u>

The Patentee has submitted the following terms and conditions:

i. Non-exclusive license to make sorafenib tosylate (API of Nexavar), to formulate into tablet form, to sell for the purpose of treating HCC and RCC in humans; all rights non-transferable and limited to the Applicant only (no right to sublicense, assign, or delegate to others) and to India only (no right to import or export);

ii. License does not include any right to represent publicly or privately that the Applicant's product is the same as the Patentee's or that the Patentee is in any way associated with the Applicant's product. The Applicant's product must be visibly distinct from the Patentee's product (e.g. in color and / or shape); the name must be distinct, and the packaging must be distinct. The Patentee expressly does not grant any copyright or trademark rights with he license and will provide no legal, regulatory, medical, technical, manufacturing, sales, marketing, or any other support of any kind.

iii. Raising the prices, failing in market in all states in India, and failing to provide free drug to indigent persons shall each be considered a material breach;

iv. The Applicant is solely and exclusively responsible for its product and for all associated product liability, and will indemnify the Patentee, its Directors, Officers, Employees, Agents, and affiliates against any and all damages arising from or associated with the Applicant's activities. The Applicant will carry insurance in an amount sufficient to cover such damages ($10 million) and upon request will provide certificates evidencing such coverage;

v. Royalty – 15% of net sales, payable in US dollars. There are no milestones or guaranteed minimums but there are also no credits or deductions for any other fees or royalties paid to any third parties;

vi. Term is until first to occur of: a) decision by the relevant government authority that the conditions for granting compulsory license no longer exist, or b) expiration of Indian Patent 215758. This agreement will be terminated upon a) the Applicant's breach of any term, representation, or warranty if such breach is not cured within 30 days; or b) upon bankruptcy of the Applicant.

vii. There are no additional implied licenses to any other patents owned by the Patentee now or in future. There are no representations or warranties of validity or enforceability. The Patentee is not obligated to enforce against infringement by third parties;

viii. The Applicant not to challenge the validity of Indian Patent 215758 in any way, directly or indirectly;

ix. The Patentee is free to do whatever it wishes with its residual patent rights subject to the non-exclusive license to the Applicant, and is free to compete with the Applicant and to grant licenses to third parties to compete with the Applicant; and

x. The license will include such other terms as are normal in the Industry (e.g. record keeping, reporting, mechanisms for conversion from rupees to dollars, details of indemnification etc.)

<u>Decision</u>

Royalty

Article 31 (h) of TRIPS Agreement states as follows:

"(h) the right holder shall be paid adequate remuneration in the circumstances taking into account the economic value of the authorization;...."

The unamended Patents Act, 1970 provided for a ceiling of 4 percent royalty to be paid to the patentee in case of a compulsory license. However, this ceiling was removed by the Patents (Amendment) Act, 2002 and it was left to the Controller to decide on a case to case basis as to quantum of royalty or other remuneration to be paid to the patentee by the compulsory license holder.

Section 90(1) of the Act states as follows:

"90. Terms and conditions of compulsory licences. –

(1) In settling the terms and conditions of a license under section 84, the Controller shall endeavour to secure—

> *(i) that the royalty and other remuneration, if any, reserved to the patentee or other person beneficially entitled to the patent, is reasonable, having regard to the nature of the invention, the expenditure incurred by the patentee in making the invention or in developing it and obtaining a patent and keeping it in force and other relevant factors;… …"*

During the course of hearings, the Patentee submitted that the cost of making the invention and developing a new medical entity (NME), like the drug in this case, works out to be about 1.8bn€. However, the figure arrived was for the cost of R&D for five years preceding 2010. In the absence of any definite figure on the cost of developing and making it available in the market, including the cost of patenting and maintaining the patent made available to me, I am unable to arrive at the actual cost involved in making this particular invention and developing the same. However, I am inclined to believe that the Patentee has spent considerable sum of money for purpose of making and developing this invention.

I am obligated to consider the nature of this particular invention especially with regard to the possible number of consumers, who require the drug in this case in order to arrive at a reasonable royalty to the Patentee. Going by the GLOBOCAN 2008, I find that the number of patients requiring this drug in India is not very high when compared to other recently patented drugs like HIV drugs.

I have also carefully analysed the royalty practices / guidelines generally adopted globally. United Nations Development Program (UNDP) specifically recommended that rates normally be set at 4% and adjusted upwards as much as 2% for products of particular therapeutic value or reduced as much as 2% when the development of the product has been partly supported with public funds, i.e. for a range of 2 to 6%. In the present case, I am satisfied that anything lesser than 6% would not be just and reasonable given the facts and circumstances of this case as discussed above. Hence, I hereby settle that the royalty be paid to the patentee in this compulsory as 6% of the net sales of the drug by the Licensee. I have also considered the other terms and conditions agreed by the Applicant and sought by the Patentee.

15.   **<u>ORDER</u>**

I hereby grant a compulsory license (hereinafter referred to as 'license') under Section 84 of the Patents Act, 1970 to M/s. Natco Pharma Ltd, Natco House, Road No. 2, Banjara Hills, Hyderabad-500033, Andhra Pradesh, India (hereinafter referred to as 'licensee') in patent number 215758 (hereinafter referred to as 'patent') granted to M/s. Bayer Corporation, 100 Bayer Road, Pittsburg, PA 15205-9741, USA (hereinafter referred to as 'licensor') with the following terms and conditions:

a. The price of the drug covered by the Patent, sold by the licensee shall not exceed Rs.8880 for a pack of 120 tablets, required for one month's treatment.

b. The licensee shall maintain accounts of sale etc. in a proper manner and shall report the details of sales to the Controller as well as the

Licensor on a quarterly basis, on or before fifteenth day of the succeeding month.

c. The licensee shall have the right to manufacture the drug covered by the Patent only at his own manufacturing facility and shall not in any whatsoever outsource the production.

d. The license is non-exclusive.

e. The license is non-assignable.

f. The licensee shall pay royalty at the rate of 6% of the net sales of the drug on a quarterly basis and such payment shall be affected on or before fifteenth day of the succeeding month.

g. The license is granted solely for the purpose of making, using, offering to sell and selling the drug covered by the patent for the purpose of treating HCC and RCC in humans within the Territory of India.

h. The licensee shall supply the drug covered by the Patent to atleast 600 needy and deserving patients per year free of cost. The licensee shall annually submit in the form of an affidavit the details of such patients, i.e. name, address and the name of the treating oncologist, to the Office of the Controller of Patents and such report shall be submitted on or before 31st January of the year, in respect of the preceding year.

i. The licensee shall not have the right to import the drug covered by the Patent.

j. The license is for the balance term of the patent.

k. The license does not include any right to represent publicly or privately that the Licensee's product is the same as the Licensor's or that the Licensor is in any way associated with the Licensee's product. The Licensee's product must be visibly distinct from the Licensor's product (e.g. in color and / or shape); the trade name must be distinct, and the packaging must be distinct. The Licensor will provide no legal, regulatory, medical, technical, manufacturing, sales, marketing, or any other support of any kind to the Licensee.

l. The Licensee is solely and exclusively responsible for its product and for all associated product liability. The Licensor, its Directors, Officers, Employees, Agents, and affiliates shall not be held liable in any manner whatsoever for any action of the licensee.

m. The Licensor is free to do whatever it wishes with its residual patent rights subject to the non-exclusive license to the Licensee, and is free to compete with the Licensee and to grant licenses to third parties to compete with the Licensee.

Granted under my hand and seal on this the 9th day of March 2012.

(P. H. Kurian)

Controller of Patents

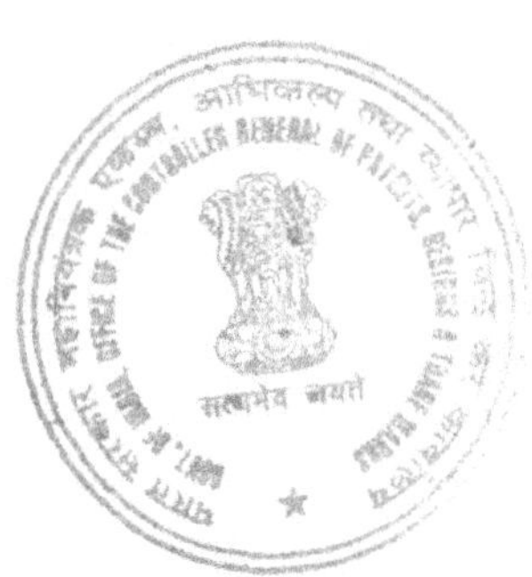

ANNEXURE 9

REJECTION OF COMPULSORY LICENSE APPLICATION
CASE STUDY

THE CONTROLLER OF PATENTS,
PATENT OFFICE,
MUMBAI.

<u>C.L.A. No. 1 of 2013</u>

IN THE MATTER OF:

M/s. BDR Pharmaceuticals International Pvt. Ltd.

.... Applicant

VERSUS

M/s. Bristol Myers Squibb Company

.... Patentee

O R D E R

APPLICATION

1.   An application under Section 84 of the Patents Act, 1970 (hereinafter referred to as the 'Act') was filed by the applicant on 4th March 2013, seeking the grant of a compulsory licence for patent number 203937 titled "A compound 2-amino-thiazole-5-carboxamide" granted to the patentee on 16th November 2006 on the patent application number IN/PCT/2001, 01138/MUM. The active pharmaceutical ingredient DASATINIB (hereinafter referred to as the 'drug', unless the context suggests otherwise), used by patients with Chronic Myeloid Leukemia (hereinafter referred to as 'CML'), was stated to be covered by this patent and was sold by the patentee under the brand name SPRYCEL. It was also submitted that DASATINIB had received Orphan Drug Status in USA, Europe and Switzerland.

DASATINIB

2.   The applicant claims that DASATINIB is a suitable chemotherapeutic option for the treatment of CML and is prescribed when a patient is resistant or develops resistance to the drug IMATINIB, in view of the improved tolerance and efficacy of the drug. DASATINIB is administered as 50 mg tablets with a dosage of 100 mg per day. Thus, two tablets are to be consumed per day until disease progression or until the patient can no longer tolerate the medicine. It has also been submitted that the price of each tablet sold by the patentee is Rs.2761/- which works out to Rs.1,65,680/- for 60 tablets per month per patient and about Rs.19,88,160/- per year per patient.

TERMS AND CONDITIONS

3.   The applicant voluntarily submitted the following terms and conditions:

    a) The drug will be made available to the public at a proposed price of Rs.135/- per tablet working out to Rs.8100/- per month for the treatment of a CML patient. A breakup of the cost was also submitted.

    b) Product under licence shall be manufactured with indication for CML.

    c) Royalty will be paid to the patentee as per the rate fixed by the Controller.

    d) Special care will be taken to make the patented product available to patients who are economically weak and also to the patients residing in remote and rural areas.

    e) The drug will be offered free of cost to a certain percentage of patients suffering from CML as determined by the cancer specialists.

PENDING LITIGATION

4.   The applicant submitted that an infringement suit CS(OS) 2303 of 2009 with respect to the subject patent was filed by the patentee against the applicant before the Hon'ble High Court of Delhi as the applicant had filed an application before the Drug Controller General of India for obtaining approval to market DASATINIB in India. The applicant submitted that the above suit was being adjourned over the last four years and that the patentee was indulging in delaying and blocking tactics. The applicant also informed that another suit CS(OS) 679 of 2013 was filed by the patentee against the applicant. No stay order so as to affect the present proceedings has been placed on record by the applicant. Also, no such order has been received from any Court.

NOTABLE EVENTS

5.   The chronological list of notable events is as follows:

2nd February 2012	Applicant requested the patentee for a voluntary licence.
13th March 2012	Patentee raised certain queries.
4th March 2013	Applicant filed the application for grant of a compulsory licence under section 84 of the Patents Act, 1970.
4th May 2013	Notice was issued by the undersigned to the applicant informing that upon consideration of the application under section 84, a *prima facie* case has not been made out for the making of an order.
10th May 2013	Applicant replied to the letter of the Patentee dated 13th March 2012.
13th May 2013	Applicant submitted a reply to the notice dated 4th May

*Table **Contd**...*

	2013 and requested to be heard.
23rd May 2013	Applicant attended the hearing and defended his case. Applicant sought more time to file written arguments and one month time was given.
23rd May 2013	Applicant filed a petition under rule 137 of the Patents Rules, 2003 (hereinafter referred to as the 'rules') for condonation of delay in complying with procedural irregularities.
24th June 2013	Applicant filed the written arguments.
1st July 2013	Patentee replied to the letter of the applicant dated 10th May 2013.
9th July 2013	Applicant replied to the letter of the patentee dated 1st July 2013.
15th July 2013	Another petition under rule 137 of the Rules was filed by the applicant for condoning the delay in complying with procedural irregularities and requesting that the documents filed on 10th July 2013, namely the Applicant's letter dated 9th July 2013 and the patentee's letter dated 1st July 2013, be taken on record.
15th July 2013	Notice issued fixing a hearing on 31st July 2013.
17th July 2013	The applicant confirmed his presence in the hearing on 31st July 2013.
27th July 2013	The applicant requested for adjournment.
5th August 2013	Notice issued fixing a hearing on 9th August 2013.
7th August 2013	The hearing was adjourned, 9th August 2013 being a holiday.
14th August 2013	Hearing was fixed on 21st August 2013.
19th August 2013	Hearing was adjourned by the undersigned due to unforeseen circumstances.
2nd September 2013	Applicant filed a petition under rule 137 of the Rules for condonation of delay and requested that the reply of the Patentee submitted in the matter of CS(OS) 679/2013, where the applicant had filed an application for rejection of the suit/plaint under Order 7 Rule 11 read with Section 151 of the Code of Civil Procedure Code, be taken on record.
2nd September 2013	Notice issued fixing a hearing on 10th September 2013.
3rd September 2013	Applicant requested for adjournment.
7th September 2013	Notice issued fixing a hearing on 16th September 2013.
16th September 2013	Hearing was held.

An effort was always made during the course of proceedings to fix a date that was convenient to the applicant to afford full opportunity to the applicant to present his case.

PROVISIONS

6.   (I) Section 84(1) of the Patents Act, 1970 states as follows:

"84. Compulsory licences.

(1) At any time after the expiration of three years from the date of the grant of a patent, any person interested may make an application to the Controller for grant of compulsory licence on patent on any of the following grounds, namely:—

> *(a) that the reasonable requirements of the public with respect to the patented invention have not been satisfied, or*
>
> *(b) that the patented invention is not available to the public at a reasonably affordable price, or*
>
> *(c) that the patented invention is not worked in the territory of India."*

In the application, it was claimed that all the aforementioned three grounds are applicable in the case of patent number 203937.

(II) Section 87 of the Act read with Rule 97 of the Rules, lays down the procedure to be followed while dealing with applications under Section 84 of the Act.

i.   Section 87 of the Act states as follows:

> **"87. Procedure for dealing with applications under sections 84 and 85.**
>
> (1)   Where the Controller is satisfied, upon consideration of an application under section 84, or section 85, that a *prima facie* case has been made out for the making of an order, he shall direct the applicant to serve copies of the application upon the patentee and any other person appearing from the register to be interested in the patent in respect of which the application is made, and shall publish the application in the Official Journal.
>
> (2)   The patentee or any other person desiring to oppose the application may, within such time as may be prescribed or within such further time as the Controller may on application (made either before or after the expiration of the prescribed time) allow, give to the Controller notice of opposition.
>
> (3)   Any such notice of opposition shall contain a statement setting out the grounds on which the application is opposed.
>
> (4)   Where any such notice of opposition is duly given, the Controller shall notify the applicant, and shall give to the applicant

and the opponent an opportunity to be heard before deciding the case.

ii.   Rule 97 of the Rules states as follows:

"**97. When a prima facie case is not made out. –**

(1)   If, upon consideration of the evidence, the Controller is satisfied that a prima facie case has not been made out for the making of an order under any of the sections referred to in rule 96, he shall notify the applicant accordingly, and unless the applicant requests to be heard in the matter, within one month from the date of such notification, the Controller shall refuse the application.

(2)   If the applicant requests for a hearing within the time allowed under sub-rule (1), the Controller shall, after giving the applicant an opportunity of being heard, determine whether the application may be proceeded with or whether it shall be refused.

(III) In accordance with the scheme of the Act, the Controller, while considering an application under Section 84 of the Act is also required to take into account the factors mentioned in sub-section (6) of section 84 of the Act. The said provision is as follows:

"*84. Compulsory licences. –*

… … ….

(6) In considering the application filed under this section, the Controller shall take into account, -

(i) the nature of the invention, the time which has elapsed since the sealing of the patent and the measures already taken by the patentee or any licensee to make full use of the invention;

(ii) the ability of the applicant to work the invention to the public advantage;

(iii) the capacity of the applicant to undertake the risk in providing capital and working the invention, if the application were granted;

(iv) as to whether the applicant has made efforts to obtain a licence from the patentee on reasonable terms and conditions and such efforts have not been successful within a reasonable period as the Controller may deem fit.

Provided that this clause shall not be applicable in case of national emergency or other circumstances of extreme urgency or in case of public non-commercial use or on establishment of a ground of anti-competitive practices adopted by the patentee,

but shall not be required to take into account matters subsequent to the making of the application.

Explanation. – For the purpose of clause (iv), "reasonable period" shall be construed as a period not ordinarily exceeding a period of six months."

PERSON INTERESTED AND CAPACITY

7.   The applicant states that more than 6 years have lapsed since the patent was granted and that the patentee primarily imports the drug. The applicant is also a 'person interested' and is into the field of pharmaceuticals, *inter alia*, manufacturing, distributing and exporting pharmaceutical active ingredients and dosage forms. It has been submitted that the applicant is extensively manufacturing anti-cancer products which are being marketed in India to a large extent and the manufacturing facilities of the applicant are approved under WHO's GMP (Good Manufacturing Practice). *Prima facie*, the applicant appears to have the capacity to undertake risk in providing capital to manufacture and make DASATINIB accessible in India as the applicant has his own manufacturing and marketing infrastructure. The applicant also claims to have access to a network of cancer hospitals and specialists.

COMMUNICATIONS PRIOR TO THE MAKING OF APPLICATION

8.   In the present case, the applicant sent a letter dated 2nd February 2012, to the patentee requesting for a voluntary licence for manufacturing Dasatinib. By letter dated 13th March 2012, the patentee raised certain queries such as *"facts which demonstrate an ability to consistently supply high volume of the API, DASATINIB, to the market"*, *"facts showing your litigation history or any other factors which may jeopardize Bristol-Myers Squibb's market position"*, *"quality related facts and in particular compliance with local regulatory standards and basic GMP requirements"*, *"quality assurance systems due diligence"*, *"commercial supply teams"*, *"safety and environmental profile"*, *"risk of local corruption"*. The applicant took this reply of the patentee as *'clearly indicative of the rejection of the application for voluntary licence'* and did not pursue the matter and made no further effort to arrive at a settlement with the patentee. The present application for compulsory licence was filed on 4th March 2013 i.e. after almost one year from the date of receiving reply from the patentee.

NOTICE

9.   By notice dated 4th May 2013, the applicant was informed that a *prima facie* case has not been made out for the making of an order under Section 84 of the Act as 'the applicant has not acquired the ability to work the invention to the public advantage', in the absence of the requisite approval from the DCGI, and 'the applicant has also not made efforts to obtain a licence from the patentee on reasonable terms and conditions' (hereinafter referred to as 'efforts'). The applicant was informed that in accordance with the provisions of Rule 97(1) of the Rules, a request for being heard is required be filed

within one month from the date of this order failing which the application shall be refused.

CLARIFICATIONS

10.   The undersigned clarified to the applicant during the course of proceedings, that in the notice dated 4th May 2013:

   I.   the undersigned had merely quoted the submissions forwarded by the applicant with respect to clause (a), clause (b) and clause (c) of sub-section (1) of section 84 of the Act and that such mention does not by any stretch of imagination amount to a finding of any kind, whatsoever, on these clauses.

   II.   the undersigned had not in any manner suggested that 'a specific rejection of the offer made by the applicant to the patentee' was required in order to demonstrate that 'efforts' have been made by the applicant. In fact, in the notice it was clearly mentioned that *"More than four and a half months remained unutilized out of the 'reasonable period' prescribed by the legislature for the purpose of mutual confabulations but the applicant chose not to take any action during this precious time period that was available with the applicant."*

EFFORTS

11.   The applicant submitted that by not specifically replying to the request for voluntary licence, the patentee can continue to correspond asking for more and more information and keep the request for voluntary licence in abeyance. This clearly leads to unfair exploitation of the provisions of Section 84(6)(iv) of the Act. Moreover, the patentee can also use the information sought from the applicants against the applicants themselves in ongoing suits for patent infringement. If the patentee avoids to specifically reject the request for voluntary licence or does not address the terms for grant thereof, the application for compulsory licence could be indefinitely delayed for want of specific denial from the patentee, unless the Ld. Controller exercises his powers in appreciating the efforts made by the applicant towards fulfilling the requirements of Section 84(6)(iv). It was also submitted that this strategy is presently being adopted by all attorneys representing patentees in voluntary licence applications.

12.   The contentions of the applicant that an application for compulsory licence can be indefinitely delayed for want of specific denial from the patentee are misplaced. The 'explanation' to Section 84(6) of the Patents Act, 1970, clarifies beyond doubt that a patentee cannot indefinitely prevent an applicant

for voluntary licence from making an application for compulsory licence under section 84 of the Act. At the most, if at all, the patentee can prevent a prospective applicant for six months from making an application for compulsory licence.

13. In the notice dated 4th May 2013 it was stated that some of the queries raised by the patentee appeared to be reasonable. In response to the notice, the applicant submitted that the applicant had approached the patentee for a voluntary licence with a clear conscience. The patentee however responded by their letter dated 13th March 2012 with a list of questions which were unreasonable and ambiguous. Under the guise of the questions, the patentee sought to extract information for use against the applicant themselves.

14. It is pertinent to mention that the applicant did not justify the contention that under the guise of the questions, the patentee sought to extract information for use against the applicant themselves. No query raised by the patentee has been specifically highlighted by the applicant that would jeopardize his position either before this forum or before the Courts. In the absence of any kind of reasoning / justification, I am not inclined to accept the 'mere' arguments put forth by the applicant. In fact, it is evident from the proceedings that the applicant realized his mistake and thereafter tried hard to somehow justify his inaction of not replying at all to the letter of the patentee dated 13th March 2012 due to which these submissions can only be termed as an afterthought.

15. It was submitted that to the utter surprise of the applicant, in the April 2012 issue of 'Indian Business Law Journal', the attorney for the patentee publicly declared that the strategy on behalf of the patentee was 'to keep the potential licensee of a compulsory licence engaged without a clear outright rejection' and continue with fresh queries. According to the applicant, this led them to conclude that there would be no purpose in responding to the said letter of the patentee seeking more information, because any response on the part of the applicant would have been treated by the patentee on these lines or in the same manner as publicly stated by their attorney. The applicant submitted that this is further exemplified by a subsequent reply received by the applicant from the same patentee in response to a request for voluntary licence for <u>another drug,</u> that demonstrates and fortifies their stand that simply raising queries without rejecting or accepting their application for grant of voluntary licence is a pre-meditated and well planned strategy to frustrate the efforts of the applicant to obtain a compulsory licence.

16. The applicant ought to have appreciated that a statement / opinion given by the attorney of the patentee in a journal cannot be taken as evidence against the patentee in the present case. Even if the applicant sincerely believed that

the statement / opinion was directly attributable to the present case, the applicant did not have, in light of the scheme of the law, the freedom to bypass the procedure namely sincere mutual deliberations for a reasonable period that have been mandated by the law.

17. The applicant submitted that the timelines accompanied by the word 'ordinarily' need to be distinguished from timelines that are not accompanied by the word 'ordinarily'. It was submitted that the latter timelines are considered **absolute and inflexible, without any exceptions or extensions**, whereas the former ones are considered to be flexible. Section 84(6)(iv) of the Act states that "for the purpose of clause (iv), 'reasonable period' shall be construed as a period not ordinarily exceeding a period of six months". Applicant submitted that this limit is the upper limit and in this case it is unreasonable to assign the time limit of six months as the 'reasonable period' especially due to the on-going litigations between the parties and the attempts by both sides to protect what they deem to be their rights. Precisely, the applicant sought to argue that in this case the reasonable time period should be construed as something less than six months.

18. If the applicant really believed that the 'reasonable period' is something less than 'six month' why did he not take action in accordance with his beliefs. That is, after making an offer on 2nd February 2012 to the patentee and after receiving the patentee's reply dated 13th March 2012, why did the applicant wait till 4th March 2013 to file the present application. On the other hand, it is pertinent to mention that the term 'efforts' is not accompanied by the qualifying term 'reasonable' and the applicant ought to have appreciated that the duty cast upon the applicant to make 'efforts' is **absolute and inflexible and without exceptions.** The conduct of the applicant in sending a letter (dated 4th February 2012) to the applicant and not at all responding to the reply of the patentee (dated 13th March 2012) cannot be termed as an 'effort'. In fact, the applicant did not reply to the patentee's letter (13th March 2012) even till the date of filing of the application for compulsory licence (4th March 2013).

19. Looking at the scheme of the Act, it is clearly apparent that the legislature was fully aware that while a patentee may try to prolong the process of mutual deliberations by raising unnecessary queries, he was also entitled to satisfy himself regarding the credentials and capability of the applicant for a voluntary licence as well as the terms and conditions. The decision to grant a voluntary licence, particularly on a subject matter covered by a patent, is an important decision for a patentee. While, it is possible that some of the queries raised by the patentee may not be strictly reasonable, it is natural that the patentee may seek additional information from the requesting party to satisfy himself about the credentials and capability of the said party.

20. The applicant ought to appreciate that there was intent behind insertion of the 'explanation' to Section 84(6) of the Patents Act, 1970, which explained that the 'reasonable period' available with the parties to engage in a dialogue for the purpose of exploring the possibility of a voluntary licence on reasonable terms and conditions was to be construed as a period not ordinarily exceeding a period of six months. However, if an applicant desirous of getting a voluntary licence were to send a letter to the patentee seeking a licence and upon receipt of a reply were not to take any further step under a preconceived notion that the patentee was engaging in delay tactics, the very purpose of Section 84(6)(iv) of the Patents Act, 1970 would be defeated.

21. In the present case, the applicant made the request for a voluntary licence on 2nd February 2012 to the patentee who, by letter dated 13th March 2012, raised some queries. More than four and a half months remained unutilized out of the 'reasonable period' prescribed by the legislature for the purpose of mutual confabulations but the applicant chose not to take any action during this precious time period that was available with the applicant. In fact, after receiving the reply from the patentee, dated 13th March 2012, the applicant waited for 1 year to file the present application, which demonstrates that the applicant did not intend to engage in any kind of dialogue, whatsoever, after making the initial offer to the patentee.

22. On the face of the record, I am of the view that the applicant's contention that the said letter is *'clearly indicative of the rejection of the application for voluntary licence'* does not hold good, as the aforementioned queries raised by the patentee appear largely to be reasonable. Even if the applicant was under an impression that the patentee was engaging in delaying tactics, the omission of not replying at all to the patentee's said letter dated 2nd February 2012 is unexplainable as it goes against the golden thread apparently visible in section 84(6)(iv). Applicant ought to have appreciated that the provisions relating to compulsory licence are to be invoked as the last resort, i.e. if the mutual deliberations do not lead to a result within six months, in accordance with the scheme of the law.

In my opinion, the applicant did not make efforts to obtain a licence from the patentee on reasonable terms and conditions.

MATTERS SUBSEQUENT TO THE MAKING OF APPLICATION

23. The applicant by letter dated 10th May 2013, i.e. after receiving the notice dated 4th May 2013, replied to the patentee's letter dated 13th March 2012. It is pertinent to mention that this reply was sent after a delay of about 14 months. It was submitted by way of petitions under rule 137 that the

correspondence that took place between the applicant and the patentee subsequent to the filing of the application for compulsory licence, be taken on record.

24.   The applicant raised a contention that in the matter of C.L.A. No. 1 of 2011, the Controller had noted that Section 84(6), where it states that '*but shall not be required to take into account matters subsequent to the making of the application*' (hereinafter referred to as the 'restrictive clause'), specifically bars the Controller from considering any measures taken by the Patentee subsequent to the making of the Application and that the intention of the legislature appears to be that subsequent measures by the Patentee to frustrate the proceedings shall not be considered. It was argued that in view of the above this restrictive clause is applicable only to the patentee.

25.   Section 84(6) mandates certain aspects that are required to be taken into account by the Controller while considering an application under section 84 of the Act. This provision also states what the Controller is not required to take into account as it states that '*but shall not be required to take into account matters subsequent to the making of the application*'. In my view, the restrictive clause is also applicable to the applicant in the present case due to the following reasons:

    I.   In the matter of C.L.A. No. 1 of 2011, the opinion expressed therein was limited to the facts of that case and was not exhaustive. That is, it was not suggested / decided in any manner that the efforts made by the applicant subsequent to the filing of the application for compulsory licence can be considered. In fact, the situation for making an observation on the applicability of the restrictive clause vis-à-vis the applicant did not arise in that case.

    II.   It is clearly evident that mutual deliberations between the applicant and the patentee cannot succeed if they happen under the constant shadow of a pending application for compulsory licence. Even if they succeed, in most of the cases the success would be attributable to the shadow, which would amount to coercion of the patentee which is strictly not allowed under the scheme of the law.

    III.   This is a case where the parties are engulfed in litigation. The restrictive clause will equally be applicable whether there is on-going litigation or not between the parties. It cannot be said that in the present case, the litigation would have affected the mutual deliberations and hence the application of this clause should not be considered. The law has to apply with equal vigor, with the same intent and in the same manner to all situations falling within the purview of a provision.

    IV.   I am convinced that considering such subsequent communication would amount to granting an undue advantage to an applicant seeking a compulsory licence, empowering him to file an application for compulsory licence and simultaneously enter into negotiations with the patentee. In such a case, the applicant would always have an undue advantage and the patentee will always be prejudiced, which is against the underlying intent behind the said restrictive clause.

ANTI-COMPETITIVE PRACTICES

26.   It was submitted that the acts of the patentee, purportedly the filing of court cases and delay tactics, fall within purview of 'anti-competitive practices'. The applicant contended that the infringement suits on products such as Dasatinib, Sunitinib, and Sorafenib have been filed before the Hon'ble High Court of Delhi and Bombay against the applicant and that the protracted litigation in progress against the applicant clearly indicates anti-competitive acts adopted by the Patentee.

27.   In this regard, sub-section (5) of Section 3 of the Competition Act, 2002, so far as relevant, is reproduced below:

"(5) Nothing contained in this section shall restrict—
(i) the right of any person to restrain any infringement of, or to impose reasonable conditions, as may be necessary for protecting any of his rights which have been or may be conferred upon him under—
(a) the Copyright Act, 1957 (14 of 1957);
(b) the Patents Act, 1970 (39 of 1970);
(c) the Trade and Merchandise Marks Act, 1958 (43 of 1958) or the Trade Marks Act, 1999 (47 of 1999);
(d) the Geographical Indications of Goods (Registration and Protection) Act, 1999 (48 of 1999);
(e) the Designs Act, 2000 (16 of 2000);
(f) the Semi-conductor Integrated Circuits Layout-Design Act, 2000 (37 of 2000);"

Section 61 of the Competition Act, 2002 is reproduced below:
"Exclusion of jurisdiction of civil courts
61. No civil court shall have jurisdiction to entertain any suit or proceeding in respect of any matter which the Commission or the Appellate Tribunal is empowered by or under this Act to determine and no injunction shall be granted by any court or other authority in respect of any action taken or to be taken in pursuance of any power conferred by or under this Act."

28.   Prima facie, in view of sub-section (5) of Section 3 of the Competition Act, 2002, the acts of filing of infringement suits cannot not be classified as 'anti-competitive'. Even if the acts are, for the sake of argument, considered to be anti-competitive, by virtue of section 61 of the Competition Act, 2002, the undersigned is not entitled to decide such an issue. I am of therefore of the view that these submissions are of no consequence so far as the present application is concerned.

PRIMA FACIE CASE

29. The applicant sought to argue that the three substantive requirements under clause (a), clause (b) and clause (c) of sub-section (1) of section 84 of the Act have been met singularly and independently satisfied by the applicant due to which any irregularity in procedure / timeline may be either waived or condoned or declared to be not applicable.

30. The stage for making a ruling on the applicability of clause (a), clause (b) and clause (c) of sub-section (1) of section 84 of the Act on merits has not yet arrived. I am of the considered opinion that the deliberate intent on part of the applicant to refrain from entering into any kind of dialogue with the patentee for the purpose of securing the grant of a voluntary licence, and the exercise of a deliberate choice to only invoke the provisions relating to compulsory licences without taking the requisite steps laid down by the law, cannot be classified as an 'irregularity in procedure / timeline', which can be waived or condoned or declared to be not applicable.

The applicant did not follow the scheme of the law as well as the procedure mandated by the law. I am therefore of the considered opinion that the applicant has failed to make out a *prima facie* case for the making of an order under section 87 of the Act. The application for compulsory licence, along with all the petitions for condonation of delay / irregularity, is hereby rejected.

Given under my hand and seal on this 29th day of October 2013.

(Chaitanya Prasad)
Controller General of Patents, Designs and Trade Marks

ANNEXURE 10

PREGRANT OPPOSITION
CASE STUDY

THE PATENTS ACT, 1970
(As amended by Patent Act 2005)
&
The Patent Rules 2003
(As amended by Patent Rules, 2006)

**In the matter of an application for patent
Having no.2485/DEL/1998 made by** Boehringer
Ingelheim Pharmaceuticals, INC.,of 900
Ridgebury Road, P.O. Box 368, Rigefield,
Conn. 06877-0368, United States of America
AND
In the matter of representation of an opposition

thereto by Indian Network for People Living with

HIV/AIDS(INP+) And Positive Womens network

(PWN) India, New Delhi

AND

IN THE MATTER of Opposition u/s 25(1) of the Patents

Act, 1970 and rule 55 of the Patent Rules, 2003

Hearing held on 31st August 2007

Present:

Mr. Deepak Mundra,.................... Agent for the Applicant

Ms. Ranjana Mehta....................... Agent for the Applicant

Sh.Anand Grover......................... Agent for the Opponent

Ms.Shivangi Rai .... **Representative From NPL With HIV/AIDS**

<u>Hearing held on 31st August 2007</u>

DECISION

An application **2485/DEL/1998** titled "Pharmaceutical composition" was
filed on 24th August 1998 by Boehringer Ingelheim Pharmaceuticals
Inc. hereinafter referred as Applicant through M/s Remfry and Sagar,
Attorneys for the Applicant, New Delhi for grant of the Patent. The

invention relates to a pediatric suspension of Nevirapine Hemihydrate used for treating HIV.

The prior art in the application relates to the nevirapine, the active ingredient which is a known agent for the treatment of infection by HIV-1.Its synthesis and use are described in various prior art documents US 5366972, US 5571912, US 556, 9760, EP0429987 and EP0482481.According to the applicants, the stable suspension form of this compound in its hemihydrate form is not disclosed in any prior art documents.

The application was filed with total no. of 6 claims and was published U/S 11A of the Patents Act on 4th March 2005. The application came up for examination and the first examination report was issued on 12/06/06. The examiner raised objections on the grounds of non-patentability u/s 2(1) (j) and definitiveness of the claims. The claims were then amended by the Applicant to comply with the objections.

The present claim 1 reads as follows -

"A pharmaceutical composition consisting essentially of the following constituents in the specified relative range amounts:

Constituent	Range of amount (g/100ml)
Nevirapine hemihydrate	0.1-50
Carbomer934P,NF	0.17-0.22
Polysorbate 80,NF	0.01-0.2
Sorbitol solution,USP	5-30
Sucrose	5-30
Methylparaben,NF	0.15-0.2
Propylparaben,NF	0.02-0.24
Sodium hydroxide,NF	q.s to pH 5.5-6.0
Purified water,USP	q.s ad 100.0 ml

wherein the nevirapine particle size is between about 1 and 150 microns in diameter.

A pre-grant opposition by way of representation was filed by Indian Network for People Living with HIV/AIDS and Positive Women Network hereinafter referred as opponent under section 25(1) of the Patents Act on 9th May 2006 in response to the publication of the application. Consequently, both the parties were heard on 31st August, 2007 as requested under section 25(1) and rule 55(1).

The grounds of opposition relied upon by the opponents are as follows –
 (i) Lack of novelty
(ii) Lack of inventive step
(iii) Non-patentability of Claims under Section 25(1)(f)
(iv) Under Section 3(d)
(v) Under Section 3(e)

At the onset the opponents put forth certain propositions of law and facts.

Patent office should give a strict interpretation of patentability criteria as decision of thereof shall affect the fate of people suffering from HIV/AIDs for want of essential medicine.

The opponents put forth the examples of the Novartis v Union of India and others, which affirmed the principle while examining the validity of section 3(d) of the Act. The Honorable Court in upholding section 3(d) against a Constitutional challenge stated" *We have borne in mind the object which the Amending Act wanted to achieve namely to prevent ever greening: to provide easy access to the citizens of this country to life saving drugs and to discharge their Constitutional obligation of providing good health care to its citizens."*

The opponents talked in length about the TRIPS Agreement and were interrupted by the applicant, as these are not being grounds of opposition.

The opponents referred to below mentioned documents to support their statements.

a) Novartis AG & Anrv.Union of India & ors.,W.P.Nos.24759 & 24760 (hereinafter referred as D1)

b) Paris Convention for the Protection of Industrial Property (hereinafter referred as D2)

c) Guidelines for the Examination of Pharmaceutical Patents: Developing a Public Health Perspective," (hereinafter referred as D3)

The opponent argued that D1 refers to the spirit by which the patentability criteria and section 3(d) was inserted into the Patents Act, 1970, Amendment, 2005. The opponents also put forth the Article 4 bis of the Paris Convention for the Protection of Industrial Property (D2) which states

"Patents applied for in the various countries of the Union by nationals of countries of the Union shall be independent of patents obtained for the same invention in other countries, whether members of the Union or not. Further "the general terms used in Aricle 27.1[of the TRIPS Agreement] have permitted Member countries to keep different criteria to assess patentability.

Continuing with D3, which relates to defining patentability and disclosure standards wherein the definitions of novelty and nonobviousness are discussed. Since the TRIPS agreement does not make it mandatory for the member states to stick to a certain definition, the member states can decide their definitions best suited to their local conditions.

The Applicants did not provide any arguments regarding the above mentioned documents as they agreed to the statements as given above but opined that these documents in no way provided any technical data to establish as to why patents cannot be granted for the said invention.

The Applicant submitted that the section 25(1) of Patents Act, 1970, Amendment 2005 does not have mention this particular criteria as a ground of opposition.

In as such I would not consider the submissions offered in the above paras as a ground of opposition but will consider them facts of law.

I will now consider the grounds relied upon by the opponents in their statement.

Novelty

The following prior art documents were furnished by the Opponents to support the ground of anticipation –

- Angel et al,Electron Microscopy Society of America,1992,132-1327) (hereinafter D1)
- McCrone,W.'"the   Microscope"Vol   45,Third   Quarter,1997 (hereinafter D 2)
- US Patent no. 5620974 (hereinafter D3)

While going through the articles   Angel et al,Electron Microscopy Society of America,1992,132-1327) John A Smoliga- Boehinger Ingelheim-1997 (D1) and McCrone,W.'"the Microscope"Vol 45,Third Quarter,1997(D2) it is well established that it was known that nevirapine hemihydrate exists as both hemihydrate and anhydrous forms.

US5620974 (D3) describes dipyridodiazepines, methods of making these compounds and a method for preventing or treating HIV infection. Example 12 deals with the method of synthesis of nevirapine. This document discloses that pharmaceutical preparations may be prepared in a conventional manner and finished products may include liquid dosage forms like solutions, suspensions, emulsions etc. and may contain conventional adjuvant such as preservatives, stabilizers emulsifiers flavor improvers wetting agents buffers, salts etc. Infact the document mentions the use of the compound being administered in an aqueous or nonaqueous solution in a pharmaceutically acceptable oil or a mixture of liquids which may contain bacteriostatic agents, antioxidants, preservatives, buffers or other solutes to render the solution isotonic with the blood ,thickening agents suspending agents or other pharmaceutically acceptable additives which include tartarate, citrate and acetate buffers, ethanol, polyethylene glycol, polypropylene glycol, EDTA, sodium bisulphate, sodium metabisulphite ascorbic acid, high molecular weight polymers such as liquid polyethylene oxides for viscosity regulation and polyethylene derivatives of sorbitol anhydrides. preservatives like benzoic acid methyl or propyl paraben, benzalkoniumchloride and other qurternary ammonium compounds. The example disclosed for

Parenteral solutions includes :

compound of example 2	5oo mg
tartaric acid	1.5 mg
benzyl alcohol	0.1 by weight
water for injection	q.s.to 1oo ml

for nasal solutions

compound of example 2	100 mg
citric acid	1.92 g
benzalkonium chloride	0.025 percent by weight
EDTA	0.1
polyvinylalcohol	10
water	q.s.to 1oo ml

US5620974(D3) also discusses the use of a parenteral solution with the compound nevirapine for HIV infections. However the cited document does not disclose the said nevirapine hemihydrate 1-150 microns in a suspension form. Also the examples in this document do not show the use of the specific components used in the composition of the alleged invention.

The applicants explained the novel feature of the invention to be the use of suspension of nevirapine hemihydrate maintained between 1 and 150 microns, which has not been cited in any of the documents.

I agree to the contention of the Applicant that all features of claims should be found in single document.

Since no single document cited above do teaches all the features of the claim of the invention; therefore none of the documents challenge the novelty of the invention.
Consequently, the composition claimed is novel.

Inventive step

The opponents provided arguments challenging the inventiveness of the invention. The following documents were relied upon to substantiate the same:

- Angel et al,Electron Microscopy Society of America,1992,132-1327) (hereinafter D1)
- McCrone,W. '"The Microscope" Vol 45,Third Quarter,1997(hereinafter D2)
- US 5620974 (hereinafter D3)
- US 5366972 (hereinafter D4)
- US 5569760 (hereinafter D5)
- Pharmaceutical dosage forms, Lieberman,et al,eds.,vol1(1988),Page 158-Standard textbook on Pharmaceutical dosage forms(hereinafter D6)

Opponent further quoted the :

- Decision of Novartis AG v.Cancer Patients Aid Association in the matter of an application for patent no.1602/Mas/98 filed on July 1998(hereinafter D7)

D1 and D2   discloses that the neviraprine existing in both anhydrous and hemihydrate forms and that during manufacture the hemihydrate is crystallized from solution which may be either be dried at low temperature (35-45^0C) and formulated into an aqueous suspension of neviraprine hemihydrate.

D6 teaches that crystal growth and changes in particle size distribution can be largely controlled by employing one or more of the following procedures and techniques:

a) Selection of particles with narrower range of particle sizes

b) Selection of a more crystalline form of the drug

D3 discloses that nevirapine may be administered as medicaments in the form of pharmaceutical preparations which contain nevirapine in association with a compatible pharmaceutical carrier material.

Example 12 deals with the method of synthesis of nevirapine which yields only the anhydrous form. Even though the document says that pharmaceutical preparations may be prepared in a conventional manner and finished products may include liquid dosage forms like solutions, suspensions, emulsions etc. And may contain conventional adjuvants such as preservatives, stabilizers emulsifiers flavor improvers wetting agents buffers, salts etc. Infact the document mentions the use of the compound being administered in an aqueous or nonaqueous solution in a pharmaceutically acceptable oil or a mixture of liquids which may contain bacteriostatic agents, antioxidants, preservatives, buffers or other solutes to render the solution isotonic with the blood ,thickening agents suspending agents or other pharmaceutically acceptable additives which include tartarate, citrate and acetate buffers,ethanol, polyethylene glycol, polypropylene glycol, EDTA, sodium bisulphite, sodium metabisulphite ascorbic acid, high molecular weight polymers such as liquid polyethylene oxides for viscosity regulation and polyethylene derivatives of sorbitol anhydrides. Preservatives like benzoic acid methyl or propyl paraben, benzalkoniumchloride and other qurternary ammonium compounds. The example disclosed for

Parenteral solutions includes

compound of example 2	5oo mg
tartaric acid	1.5 mg
benzyl alcohol	0.1 by weight
water for injection	q.s.to 1oo ml

for nasal solutions

compound of example 2	100 mg

citric acid	1.92 g
benzalkonium chloride	0.025 percent by weight
EDTA	0.1
polyvinylalcohol	10
water	q.s.to 1oo ml

Further more documents D4 and D5 belonging to same patent family disclose about preparation of nevirapine pharmaceutical compositions inter alia suspensions.

D7 states that:

The Patent Office Chennai in examining whether a specific crystalline salt form that was being claimed was inventive over a prior generic disclosure of the free base and all "pharmaceutically acceptable salts thereof" held that because the salt form was obtained from the free base in a customary manner the subsequent claims to the specific crystalline salt formed lacked inventive step.

The applicant has specifically mentioned the use of the nevirapine hemihydrate between 1-150 microns in the composition. However, the specific advantage of this particle size is no where disclosed in the specification. The applicant mentions that this particle size is advantageous to maintain stability of the solution. The applicant claims that this particle size would result in a stable suspension for pediatric consumption. However, the complete specification no where mentions this disclosure.

It leaves me in no doubt that after going through the documents D1 to D7 a skilled person shall be able to arrive at the invention disclosed in this impugned Patent Application.

The alleged invention composition does not specifically have all the components disclosed in the cited documents and whereas all components claimed are known and whereas the established pharmaceutical excepients would produce no other effect and the effect of this disclosed pharamaceutical composition of this instant application would be of the active ingredient only and finally reducing the particle size in he range 1-150 microns by milling or other conventional known methods; therefore shall render this invention disclosed in this application obvious to the person skilled in the Art.

Furthermore, after going through the specification, I also don't see any of the process steps being novel and supported by the description for which monopoly to the applicant may be awarded.

Thus because an aqueous suspension of nevirapine hemihydrate claimed in the Application could readily be prepared in a customary manner by the person skilled in the art the claims lack inventive step.

Therefore the claims of this instant application lacks inventive step.

SECTION 3(d)

The opponents put forth their objections under section 3(d) because they alleged that claims relate to a new form of a known substance without showing the requisite of enhanced efficacy or constitute new uses of already known substances.

Section 3(d),
"the mere discovery of a new form of a known substance which does not result in the enhancement of the known efficacy of that substance or the mere discovery of any new property or new use for a known

substance ….is not considered an invention under the meaning of the Act.

Opponent continued that at a minimum the applicant must place on the record two things: 1) data relating to the therapeutic effect of the known substance and b) data relating to the therapeutic effect of the claimed substance. The applicant has failed to place on record either of these items. Firstly, the data presented in the applicant's affidavit shows stability data only for the product claimed in the application. There is no data upon which one can conclude that particle size stability is significantly enhanced over the known substance. Secondly, the data, at most, shows the stability of the nevirapine hemihydrate suspension under various storage conditions. There is no data upon which one can conclude that improved particle size stability translates into better therapeutic effect. Given this lack of data, there is no basis upon which the Patent Controller can conclude that there is the requisite enhancement in therapeutic efficacy.

The opponent also mentioned that the way in which the Madras High Court has defined 'efficacy' the Opponents submitedt that it is impossible for alleged improvements in particle size stability, no matter how comprehensively proved and placed on record, to be sufficient to meet the efficacy requirement of Section 3(d). The Court stated:

"The position therefore is, if the discovery of a new form of a known substance must be treated as an invention, then the patent applicant should show that the substance so discovered has a better therapeutic effect. Dorland's Medical Dictionary defines the expression "efficacy" in the field of pharmacology as " the ability of a drug to produce the desired therapeutic effect, and "efficacy" is independent of potency of the drug. Dictionary meaning of

"Therapeutic" is healing of disease – having a good effect on the body".

Going by the meaning for the word "efficacy" and "therapeutic" extracted above, what the patent applicant is expected to show is, how effective the new discovery made would be in healing a disease/having a good effect on the body. Novartis, Annexure 1 at para 13. Improved particle size stability, at most, means that someone who chooses to manufacture nevirapine in an aqueous solution would benefit from being able to store the medicine for longer periods of time. However, the therapeutic effect of nevirapine, whether in hemihydrate form or anhydrous form, or whether administered in aqueous, tablet, parental or any other dosage form, would remain unchanged. The applicant has failed to place on record any evidence to show that the therapeutic effect of nevirapine hemihydrate in aqueous solution is significantly enhanced over other known forms of nevirapine. As such, Claims 1, 2, and 5 are invalid and fall under Section 3(d).

I have analyzed the above arguments and have come to the conclusion that the product (composition) claims fall under section 3(d) of the Patents Act in the absence of any data for the composition to show enhanced efficacy

Therefore, I conclude that the product claims fall under section 3(d) as they are all a combination of known substances and this section clearly mentions that only if enhanced efficacy can be established such compositions would be allowed to be claimed.

section 3(e)

The opponents alleged that the composition claims are not patentable under section 3(e) of Patent Act 1970 because all the claimed substances obtained by mere admixture resulting only in the aggregation of the properties of the components thereof and are thus not inventions within the meaning of the Act under section 3(e). The opponents alleged that the applicants had neither in the description nor during the hearing gave any evidence whatsoever to show that the pharmaceutical properties exhibited any properties above and beyond the aggregation of the constituent parts.

The applicants reiterated the fact that there exits a synergy between all the ingredients since these ingredients were not mentioned in any of the cited prior documents.

I agree with the opponent that the applicant failed to show neither in specification nor through the submissions that novel pharmaceutical composition claimed exhibits any of the properties above and beyond the aggregation of the constituent parts.
So claims fall under section 3(e) of the Act and are non-patentable.

In view of the above findings and facts on records, the present application 2485/DEL/1998 is hereby refused to proceed for grant of Patent on the grounds 25(1)(e),read with 2(1)j, and25(1)f read with 3(d),and 3(e) of the Patent Act 1970, The application stands disposed off with no cost to either party.

Dated.June11,2008
The Patent office,
New Delhi

(N.R.MEENA)
ASSISTANT CONTROLLER OF PATENTS & DESIGNS

ANNEXURE 11

POSTGRANT OPPOSITION
CASE STUDY

THE PATENTS ACT, 1970
(39 of 1970)
as amended by
THE PATENTS (AMENDMENT) ACT, 2005
(15 of 2005)
(with effect from 1-1-2005)

&

THE PATENTS RULES, 2003
as amended by
THE PATENTS (AMENDMENT) RULES, 2006

(with effect from 5-5-2006)

M/s F.HOFFMANN-LA ROCHE AG

a Swiss Company of 124 Grenzacherstrasse,

CH-4002,

Basel, Switzerland.

Represented by

Mr. Pravin Anand of Anand & Anand,

Mr. D.J.Solomon of De Penning & De Penning

.... Patentee

1. M/s Ranbaxy Laboratories Ltd.,
   A-11,Sahibzada Ajit Singh
   Nagar,Ropar District, Punjab, 160 055

   Represented by Mr. R.Parthasarathy
   of Lakshmikumaran and Sridharan

2. M/s Cipla Ltd., 289, Bellalis Road,
   Mumbai Central, Mumbai – 400 008

   Represented by Mr. S.Majumdar,

   Dr. Sanchita Ganguli of S.Majumdar &
   Co.,

   Mr. A.Ramesh Kumar

3. M/s Bakul Pharma Pvt. Ltd., of Sterling Centre, 4th Floor, Dr. A.B. Road, Worli, Mumbai – 400 018

   Represented by Mr. S.Majumdar,

   Dr. Sanchita Ganguli of S.Majumdar & Co.,

4. M/s Matrix Laboratories Limited, 1-1-151/1, IV Floor, Sairam Towers, Alexander Road, Secunderabad – 500 003

   Represented by Mr. K. Feroz Ali

5. Delhi Network of Positive People, Galli No. 3, House No. 64, Village Neb Sarai, New Delhi – 110 068

   Represented by Mr. Anand Grover

6. Indian Network for People living with HIV/AIDS & The Tamil Nadu Networking People with HIV/AIDS, New No. 41 (old No 42/3), Second Main Road, Kalaimagal Nagar, Ekkaduthangal, Chennai – 600 097. (Rejoinder)

   Represented by Mr. Anand Grover

.... Opponents

Dr. Bindu Jacob   Examiner of Patents & Designs

1. History of the proceedings

1. M/s F.HOFFMANN-LA ROCHE AG a Swiss Company of 124 Grenzacherstrasse, CH-4002, Basel, Switzerland, hereinafter referred as 'patentee', have filed an application for patent for their invention titled '2-(2-AMINO-1,6-DIHYDRO-6-OXO-PURIN-9-YL)METHOXY-1,3-PROPANEDIOL DERIVATIVE' on 27th day of July 1995 through their agent M/s De Penning and De Penning and it was numbered as 959/MAS/1995 having priority of United States of America (US).

2. The agent filed a request for examination of application for patent on 27th July 2004 and the application was published under section 11(A) of the Patents (Amendment) Act, 2005, herein after referred as 'Act' in the Patent Journal No. 06/2005 dated 25th February 2005.

3. The application was taken up for the examination and the First Examination Report (FER) was issued on 17th May 2006.

4. The patent was granted with patent number 207232 and published on 29.06.2007 in the Journal of the Patent Office. M/s Ranbaxy Laboratories Ltd., M/s Cipla Ltd., M/s Bakul Pharma Pvt. Ltd., M/s Matrix Laboratories Limited, Delhi Network of Positive People and Indian Network for People living with HIV/AIDS & The Tamil Nadu Networking People with HIV/AIDS (Rejoinder) hereinafter referred as 'opponents' have filed a post-grant opposition through their attorneys under section 25 (2) of the Act within the time limit.

2. Grounds of opposition

5. The Grounds of opposition filed under section 25(2) (b), 25(2) (d), 25(2) (e), 25(2) (f), 25(2) (g), 25(2) (h) and 25(2) (i).

6. Documents submitted in the opposition
   - (i).   EP0375329
   - (ii). US 5043339
   - (iii). US6083953
   - (iv). Prosecution history of US6083953 in the USPTO
   - (v).   US 4355032
   - (vi). US 4957924
   - (vii). EP0187297
   - (viii). EP 0141927
   - (ix). US 5840891
   - (x).   US 5856481
   - (xi). Gazette Notification dt 3rd Jan 1995

(xii). EP099493

(xiii). EP167385

(xiv). GB2104070

(xv). Beauchamp et.al, Antiviral chemistry and Chemotherapy (1992), 3(3), 157-164.

(xvi). Beauchamp et.al, Drugs of the Future, 1993, 18(7): 619-628

(xvii). J.Pharm.Sci.,vol.76.No.2,Feb 1987

(xviii). Martin et al.; Journal of Pharmaceutical Sciences 1987 76:180-184

(xix). British Journal of Pharmacology(2006), 147, 1-11

(xx). J.Med.Chem., 26, 602 – 604

3. Subject matter of the Invention

7. The specification describes the invention relates to mono L-valine ester of ganciclovir and its pharmaceutically acceptable salt. The object of the invention was to provide a compound with improved bioavailability when administered orally, set out by a formula I with a number of variables. The specification further describes the advantages of L-valine ester of ganciclovir and its pharmaceutically acceptable salt and compared with many other related compounds.

4. Novelty

8. The counsel for the opponents argued that the invention is not novel in view of US '339 which discloses various esters of ganciclovir at column 1, line 39

> i. "According to one feature of the present invention there is provided a formula I:

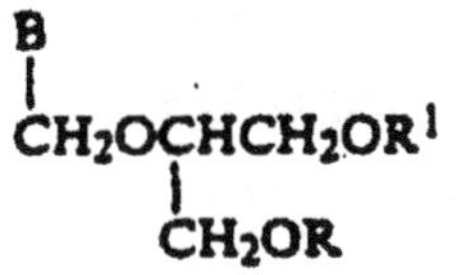

$$\overset{\displaystyle B}{|}$$
$$CH_2OCHCH_2OR^1 \qquad (I)$$
$$\underset{\displaystyle CH_2OR}{|}$$

ii. wherein R and R^1 are independently selected from a hydrogen atom and a naturally occurring neutral amino acid acyl residue providing at least one of R and R^1 represents an amino acid acyl residue and B represents a group of formula

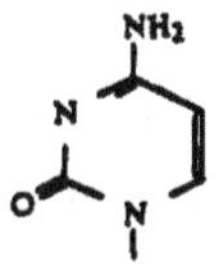

(A)

or

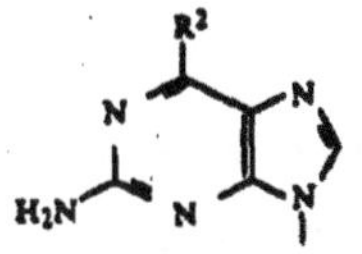

(B)

iii. in which R^2 represents a C_{1-6} straight chain, C_{3-6} branched chain or C_{3-6} cyclic alkoxy group, or a hydroxyl or amino group or a hydrogen atom and the physiologically acceptable salts thereof.

And column 2, line 17

'The amino acid acyl residue of the above compounds according to the invention may be derived for example from naturally occurring amino acids, preferably neutral amino acids i.e. amino acids with one amino group and one carboxyl group. Examples of preferred amino acids include aliphatic acids, e.g., containing up to 6 carbon atoms such as glycine, alanine, valine and isoleucine. The amino acid esters according to the invention include the mono- and di-esters of the compound of formula (I). The amino acids may be D-, L- and DL-amino acids, with the L-amino acids being most preferred.'

'The above-mentioned physiologically acceptable salts are preferably acid addition salts derived from an appropriate acid, e.g., hydrochloric, sulphuric, phosphoric, maleic, fumaric, citric, tartaric, and lactic or acetic acid.'

According to the compound of Claim 1 of '339, B is hydroxyl and the preferred amino acid valine ester is mono form, R is H and R^1 is L-valine, the compound accomplished is valganciclovir and the preferred salt is hydrochloride salt. Therefore, the 339 document clearly discloses the L-valinate ester of ganciclovir hydrochloride.

9. Further EP '329 patent discloses the amino acid esters which includes the mono- and di-esters, the (R)- and (S)- form, list of amino acids for making said mono- and di-esters and salt making acids. Example 5 of EP'329 teaches a bis-(L-valinate) ester of ganciclovir and example 6(b) teaches the process to get mono-(L-alaninate) ester of ganciclovir along with bis-(L-alaninate) ester of ganciclovir in the ratio of 1:9. It is very clear from example 6(b) that the monoester was prepared and isolated. The counsel referred the patentee's submission that in all examples of EP'329 a threefold excess of the activated amino acid was used. A skilled person reading the above processes and aiming to make mono-ester compounds would readily appreciate that by reducing the amount of the amino acid added to the reaction to less than one stoicheometric amount, relative to the diol moiety (ganciclovir, in this case) the formation of substantial amount of mono-esterified compounds will occur.

10. Further the counsel stated that a Supplementary Protection Certificate has been granted to the applicant (Glaxo) for the EP '329 patent claiming valganciclovir hydrochloride for the UK authorized medicinal use

(treatment of cytomegalovirus retinitis in AIDS patients) which includes formulation, synthetic methods are covered by at least claims 1, 2, 5, 6, 7, and 9 to 14 and possibly claim 8 of the EP '329. It is very clear that valganciclovir is disclosed and enabled by EP'329 and the Patentee (Roche) was also aware of the fact that SPC which anticipates the invention as claimed in patent 207232.

11. The corresponding US Patent 6,083,953 to Indian Patent 207232 was granted for crystalline form of valganciclovir hydrochloride and not for valganciclovir in its (R) - or (S) - form. During prosecution all the claims relating to product, process and composition were rejected referring US'339 patent by the USPTO. Several identical claims with respect to the corresponding patent applications filed in the United States, including US Patent Application No.08/812991 and 10/603503 were rejected by USPTO in light of disclosures contained in the '339 patent. Therefore, claims of the claimed invention lack novelty.

12. Claims 1-9 and 12 lacks novelty in light of disclosures contained in US '339 and equivalent EP '329. '339 Patent discloses HCl and acetate salts of mono- and di- valine esters of ganciclovir with improved oral bioavailability. Also R- & S- diastereomers of L-monovaline ester of ganciclovir inherently disclosed in '339 patent.

13. US Patent '339 and EP '329 discloses mono and divalyl esters of ganciclovir and pharmaceutically acceptable salt which exhibits enhanced oral bioavailability. Therefore, Claim 1 and the dependent claims are not novel.

14. The counsel for the patentee argued that every opponent has relied upon US '339 or EP '329 to support the ground of anticipation, it is important to note that A2 publication of EP 0375329 was published on 27 June 1990 and B1 publication of EP 0375329 was published on 31 May 1995. Accordingly, only EP 0375329A2 (herein after referred to EP'329) is a valid prior art and

not EP 0375329B1, since the disclosure of US' 339 and EP'329 are identical, they are used interchangeably in this argument. US '339 patent discloses a compound of Formula (I)

$$\underset{\text{CH}_2\text{OR}}{\underset{|}{\text{CH}_2\text{OCHCH}_2\text{OR}^1}}\overset{\overset{\text{B}}{|}}{}$$

wherein B is a cytosine or certain purine residues, and R and R1 are independently selected from a hydrogen atom and an amino acid acyl residue providing at least one of R and R1 represents an amino acid acyl residue. It also describes in broad generic terms a genus of thousands of compounds, but it contains no specific description of the mono L-valine ester of ganciclovir nor does it include any teaching that would motivate, direct or enable a person of ordinary skills in the art to make the said compound. According to US '339 col 2, lines 17 to 31. The amino acid acyl residue may be derived for example from naturally occurring amino acids, preferably neutral amino acids. Examples of preferred amino acids include aliphatic acids, e.g. ., containing up to 6 carbon atoms such as glycine, alanine, valine and isoleucine. The amino acid esters include mono and di-esters of the compound of formula 1. Accordingly, even the preferred embodiments of US '339 will encompass well over 400 compounds.

15. There are six examples in the US '339 patent demonstrating the preparation of preferred compounds of Formula (I). The examples employ an excess of esterifying agent which would not result in the production of mono-esters.

16. Example 1 is for the preparation of the bis-(L-isoleucinate) ester of the cytosine-derived nucleotide as the bis-acetate salt. Example 2 is for the preparation of the bis-(L-valinate) ester of the cytosine-derived nucleoside as the bis-acetate salt. Example 3 is for the preparation of the bis-(L-isoleucinate) ester of ganciclovir as the bis-acetate salt. Example 4 is for the preparation of the bis-(glycinate) ester of ganciclovir as the bis-acetate salt. Example 5 is for the preparation of the bis-(L-valinate) ester of

ganciclovir as the bis-acetate salt and Example 6 is for the bis-(L-alaninate) ester of ganciclovir as the bis-acetate salt. While the reference US' 339 mentions in Col. 2 Line 26 that the amino acid esters can include mono- and di-esters of the compound of formula (I), the US' 339 patent did not disclose mono-esters leave alone mono-(L)-valine ester of ganciclovir.

17. The genus of compounds disclosed in the US '339 patent is too broad and there is no landmark in the said US patent suggesting or disclosing the mono-(L)-valine ester of ganciclovir or any other monoester of ganciclovir. The said US patent does not even make any reference and teach that mono-ester of ganciclovir is a useful or desirable compound. Infact, the inventors of the US '339 patent teach that a free hydroxyl group in the prodrug is undesirable. The examples provided teach only the diesters and the monoester would not be expected to be formed using the procedures/process disclosed in the US' 339 patent which all utilize three-fold excess of ·the activated amino acid.

18. Further the counsel argued that the IPAB held in Gleevec order that working example is required in the prior art in order to establish the ground of anticipation.

> "We have carefully studied forming acids. The said compounds of formula I and salts there of are stated to be prepared in accordance with processes known per se. However, 1993 patent has not given any working example as to how a salt of imatinib could he made including imatinib mesylate", (pages 167 & 168 of IPAB order).

19. European Patent No.375329 discloses ester prodrug of ganciclovir and physiologically acceptable salts thereof having advantageous bioavailability when administered by an oral route. The patent however, does not disclose the utility as well as process for the preparation of mono esters of ganciclovir. Therefore it is an established position of law that an anticipating prior art document should name the claimed compound individually and should contain sufficient description, which should enable a person of

ordinary skilled in the art to arrive at the claimed invention without any further experimentation. Therefore, neither US'339 nor EP'329 disclose or contain "enabling disclosure" to carry out the claimed invention so as to render the US '339 as anticipating the claimed invention.

20. Also in **Synthon BV Vs. Smithkline Beecham Plc [2005] UKHL 59**, the courts held

> "30. Nevertheless, in deciding whether there has been anticipation, there is a serious risk of confusion if the two requirements are not kept distinct. For example, I have explained that for the purpose of disclosure, the prior art must disclose an invention which, if performed, would necessarily infringe the patent. It is not enough to say that, given the prior art, the person skilled in the art would without undue burden he able to come up with an invention which infringed the patent. But once the very subject-matter of the invention has been disclosed by the prior art and the question is whether it was enabled, the person skilled in the art is assumed to be willing to make trial and error experiments to get it to work. If therefore, one asks whether some degree of experimentation is to be assumed, it is very important to know whether one is talking about disclosure or about enablement"

21. Further to the Ranbaxy counsel's argument the counsel for the patentee contented that the Supplemental Protection Certificate (SPC) issued to Glaxo for EP patent '329B based on Roche clinical trails of Valganciclovir amounts to anticipation is totally false and baseless and is based on an incorrect understanding of SPC's vis-a-vis patents. Grant of patent and grant of SPC are two distinct issues. As EP 329 protects/ covers but does not specifically disclose valganciclovir, it is incorrect to state that the grant of SPC anticipates the IN '232 patent.

22. Further argued, IPAB had held that the documents related to the application to U.S. drug authority and U.S. term extension certificate and the test report of IIT and IICT were not knowledge available before the priority

date i.e.18.07.1997 of the instant application. We, therefore, cannot accept these as prior publications for consideration and cannot agree with R4 that these documents anticipate the appellant's subject compound. (page 168 of IPAB order).

23. In view of the above arguments, US '339 or EP '329 does not specifically disclose the mono-(L)-valinate ester of ganciclovir either expressly or inherently.

24. I am in an opinion that US'339 and the corresponding EP'329 do not explicitly disclose the compound of the claimed invention. The documents do not ascertain that the patents describe clear and unambiguous directions to make the compound of the claimed invention. Although the '339 and '329 patent generally discloses the existence of mono esters as part of a large class of compounds, it does not particularly disclose the compound or other property of the said compound. The information provided may be relevant but not appropriate to obtain the compound of the claimed invention. The prior art teachings would have been understood by the skilled person the date on which it was disclosed but not with the later invention. **The Technical Board of Appeal held in T/396/89 Union Carbide [1992] EPOR 312 at para 4.4:**

> "It may be easy, given a knowledge of a later invention, to select from the general teachings of a prior art document certain conditions, and apply them to an example in that document, so as to produce an end result having all the features of the later claim. However, success in so doing does not prove that the result was inevitable. All that it demonstrates is that, given knowledge of the later invention, the earlier teaching is capable of being adapted to give the same result. Such an adaptation cannot be used to attack the novelty of a later patent."

25. The examples provided in the said US'339 and EP'329 are related to diesters of ganciclovir, but not provided any hint to make the monoester.

Even though monoester is obtained as mono-(L-alaninate) ester of ganciclovir along with bis-(L-alaninate) ester of ganciclovir, it does not anticipate the mono-valinate ester of ganciclovir. The preferred compound in both the prior art documents are bis esters of amino acids such as glycine, alanine, valine and isoleucine. There was no teaching or direction in the prior art documents for making monoester of the present invention.

26. The filing date for obtaining the SPC is 27.8.2002 which is a subsequent information/knowledge that cannot be considered as a basis for determining anticipation of the present case.

5. Inventive step

27. The counsels for the opponents argued that US '924 disclose valine esters of acyclovir and pharmaceutically acceptable salts that exhibits more bioavailability than acyclovir. Acyclovir poorly absorbed when orally administered and large doses are needed to increase the oral bioavailability. Drugs having poor absorption are converted into ester to make the drug more bioavailable when administered orally. The amino acids ester of ganciclovir disclosed in EP '329 which includes mono- and di-esters, preferably D- L- and DL amino acids, more preferrably L-amino acids. It also teaches bis-(L-valinate) ester of ganciclovir and example 6(b) teaches the process to get mono-(L-alaninate) ester along with bis-(L-alaninate) ester of ganciclovir in the ratio of 1:9.

28. US '032 discloses ganciclovir and pharmaceutically acceptable salts thereof, which is highly active antiviral compound, particularly against Herpes Simplex Virus I and II and related viruses such as cytomegalovirus, Epstein-Barr virus and Varicella Zoster virus.

29. The oral form of parent drug ganciclovir has been commercially known from the US Patent '032. The L-valine ester of acyclovir has improved bioavailability than the acyclovir after oral administration. Ester forming amino acids, salt of the said esters, function of the ester salts and disease

targeted are known for the structurally similar acyclovir and ganciclovir. Therefore, person skilled in the art follows the route of L-valine ester of acyclovir i.e., Valacyclovir and apply same to ganciclovir to get valganciclovir. Valacyclovir and valganciclovir are nucleoside analogs having similar structure and used for the similar treatment.

30. Publications of Beauchamp in 1992 and 1993 disclosed the best amino-acid ester for acyclovir. There were 18 amino acid esters synthesized and tested as potential prodrugs, among those amino acid esters L-amino acid esters were better prodrugs than the corresponding D- or DL-isomers, particularly L-valyl ester was the best prodrug. Valacyclovir, the prodrug of acyclovir is more bioavailable than acyclovir that is proved to be rapid hydrolysis in vivo than the parent compound. Properties like aqua solubility, stability, antiviral activity and toxicological testing of the valine for making ester proved to be the choice of drug. Beauchamp have published many research publications in the field of antivirals, also inventor of valacyclovir and bisester form of ganciclovir. In the article Drugs Fut., 1993,18(7) page 627 said,

> 'Over many years of scientific exploration, the various attempts to develop an oral prodrug of acyclovir have revealed certain basic principles that should be applicable to other nucleoside analogs.'

31. Various forms of esters are prepared using hydroxyl group of the purine ring and side chain of acyclovir with amino acids. The modifications made to the purine ring was toxic and the modifications made to the acyclic chain resulted in improved effect.

32. Acyclovir and ganciclovir are structurally similar and functionally similar nucleoside analog. So it is obvious to a person would try for the similar ester which is already proved with improved effect. US '924 patent discloses the L-valinate ester of acyclovir and hydrochloride salt of the L-valinate ester. The diseases targeted by the two drugs L-valinate ester of acyclovir and ganciclovir are similar. L-valine is a chiral compound, its

derivative L-valinate ester of ganciclovir inherently will be a chiral molecule, therefore (R) or (S) diastereoisomers can be expected by a skilled artisan.

33. US '339 disclosed mono and di-esters of ganciclovir wherein ester forming group is selected from amino acids including glycine, alanine, valine and isoleucine, preferred amino acids are L-amino acids among D, L and DL – amino acids.

34. Using L- valine to prepare an ester with purine drugs is known in the art. Ganciclovir is structurally similar to acyclovir and both are anti-viral drugs. Valacyclovir was developed as a successful prodrug of acyclovir and its hydrochloride salt was marketed as a successful medicine. Beauchamp et. al disclosed L-valyl esters of acyclovir were the best prodrug of the esters investigated. A person skilled in the art would combine the teachings of Beauchamp's publications, US '032, US '339, EP '329 and US '924 to prepare the compound of the alleged invention viz., the L-valine ester of ganciclovir. Thus, it would have been obvious to a person skilled in the art of medicinal chemistry to prepare the hydrochloride salt of L-valine esters of ganciclovir with a more than reasonable expectation of success with the teachings of the said prior art.

35. The counsel for the patentee contented that none of the documents US'339, EP'329, Beauchamp, 1992 Article, US'032, US'924 and Martin 1987 Article cited by all the opponents for the ground of obviousness either alone or in combination render the claimed invention as obvious. Further, all the above documents have been cited in the specification as prior art documents.

36. The genus disclosed in the U Beauchamp in 1992 article discussed about toxicity associated with phosphorylation of the unconverted prodrug and a stereo-specific transporter which may contribute to the improved absorption of the amino acid in the prodrug esters, more particularly L-amino acid esters were better prodrugs that the corresponding D- or DL-isomers. In 1993 article of Beauchamp again reiterates about the toxicity

associated with the phosphorylated forms of the unconverted prodrugs. US '032 disclose ganciclovir, but there was no information on bio-availability related information, particularly oral bioavailability of monoesters of ganciclovir.

37. US'339 discloses only the di-esters wherein the preparation involves utilizing three-fold excess of the activated amino acid and the monoester would not be expected to be formed using the said six procedures in six examples. Example 6b describes a process for preparing bis-ester of an alaninate as a desired product with 10% of monoester as impurity. There is no motivation or suggestion whatsoever to make mono L valine ester of ganciclovir in US'339. US '924 relates to L valine ester of acyclovir, which does not teach about ganciclovir or esters of ganciclovir. Combining the teaching of Beauchamp's publication 1992 and 1993 with US '924, a person ordinarily skilled in the art will be motivated to block all the free OH group resulting in bisester.

38. The counsel further argued that the opponents cannot selectively choose the file wrapper of one country. The corresponding patents of '232 were filed in over 60 jurisdictions and it has been granted in over 50 jurisdictions. The nature and scope of the present claims in other countries including EP is very much similar to Indian patent '232. Therefore, it would be illogical for the opponents to rely only on the file wrapper of the US application. None of the documents either alone or in combination teach or suggest or enable a process for selective esterification of ganciclovir to obtain a prodrug having high oral bioavailability for ganciclovir that maintains the antiviral characteristics of ganciclovir. It was found by the present inventors that the monoesters of L-valine amino acid of ganciclovir are far more bioavailable than the bis-ester and despite Beauchamp's teaching away from the said monoester and despite its chirality which leads to existence of diastereomers it was a preferred compound. Thus the claimed invention possess inventive step and is non-obvious.

39. Section 2(1)ja defines "Inventive step" as follows:

> "Section 2 (ja) "Inventive step" means a feature of an invention that involves technical advance as compared to the existing knowledge or having economic significance or both and that makes the invention not obvious to a person skilled in the art;"

40. I agree with the counsels for the opponents that the nucleosides such as acyclovir, penciclovir are low aqueous solubility and low bioavailability when administered orally. To increase the oral bioavailability many modifications were done to purine ring and acyclic side chain, interestingly, ester of the said molecules shown improved bioavailability. Many esterifying agents were used and tested. Conversion of acyclovir into L-valine ester of acyclovir is suggested by '924 patent, such a modification makes the molecule more bioavailable than the base. The '329 patent discloses di- valyl amino acid ester of ganciclovir. The problem associated with the ganciclovir is poor solubility and low oral bioavailability. The prior art suggests that many similar nucleosides are converted into ester of amino acids, preferably L-valine to increase the oral bioavailability.

41. I am in an opinion that the comparative table shows the improvement in oral bioavailability of the esters of ganciclovir in example 9 of the specification is not proper. The comparison would have been made with the hydrochloride salt of other esters and monovaline ester of ganciclovir listed in the table. It is obvious that the solubility of salt, particularly hydrochloride salt is comparatively more to that of esters listed therein. Generally, esters are fairly soluble in water but salt of the ester is more soluble than the ester. Therefore, the comparison made between esters and salt in the table as an improvement with regards to bioavailability is not scientific and the results provided are not proper to meet the patentability requirement. There is no comparison between base and the salt. Since the object of the invention is to provide a prodrug of ganciclovir with improved oral bioavailability, the comparison provided in the specification to show such an improvement is not scientific. Thus the

applicant failed to provide a proper support in the complete specification for improved oral bioavailability.

42. The improved oral bioavailability of valganciclovir may be due to the addition of the L valyl ester, which allows the molecule to be actively transported but the salt form plays important role to influence the transportation. Most of the drugs listed in the pharmacopoeias are in the salt form, because the salt form of the drugs influences the solubility for better therapeutic effect.

43. The preferred ester forming compounds suggested by '329 patent and '924 patent are amino acids, particularly valine, more particularly L-valine to overcome the problem of oral drug delivery.

44. Beauchamp suggests and motivates the involvement of stereospecific (L- vs D-) transport process using common branched chain amino acids, L-valine and L-isoleucine, particularly L-valine ester which makes the drug more oral bioavailble.

In **Pfizer v. Apotex (U.S.Court of Appeal, 20061261)**, observed that for the test of obviousness only a reasonable expectation of success and not a guarantee is needed.

In **Aventis v. Lupin (U.S.Court of Appeal, 20061530)** the court held that "where the prior art gives the reason or motivation to make the claimed compositions, creates a prima facie case of obviousness."

45. The skilled person would have been motivated to prepare mono L-valine ester of ganciclovir from the teachings of the '329, '924 and the Beauchamp articles. Therefore, Claim 1 and dependent claims are not inventive.

46. Neither '339 patent nor '329 patent specifically mentioned the process for the preparation of the compound of the claimed invention. Identification of the compound of the invention from '329 is obvious, but the method for the preparation of such a compound requires extensive research work. Even though the method for hydrolyzing one of the ester group of '329 patent or any other steps involved in the preparation is by conventional method it could not have been ascertained before it was produced. Therefore I allow the process claim(s) but restricted to single process.

6. Not an Invention

47. The counsels for the opponents argued that the compound claimed in claims 1-9 and 12 relates to a new form of a known substance which is already disclosed in US '339 patent. Data provided in the complete specification is an alleged increase in bioavailability of acetate and hydrochloride salts of the L-monovaline ester in rats and monkeys wherein the increase in bioavailability in not sufficient to meet the requirement of significant enhancement in therapeutic efficacy. The table provided in example 9 of the specification with bioavailability data did not provide any comparison between salt and base of valganciclovir. Therefore the comparative table is not proper.

48. Valganciclovir is a prodrug of ganciclovir, however, the pro drug is also used for the purpose for which original drug is used. Acyclovir and L-valine-ester of acyclovir, i.e., valaciclovir are antiviral drug of similar class is also known in the art. Prodrug will be developed in order to enhance the bioavailability when given orally. The prodrug achieves the same as that of the drug.

49. Ester of the known substance prima facie will get a patent only if it shows significant enhancement of efficacy. The Hon'ble High Court of Madras in Novartis Judgment held the constitutional validity of section 3(d) as categorically that efficacy means therapeutic efficacy followed by IPAB

judgment. In the present case, mono ester demonstrated to have more bioavailability compared to that of bis ester of ganciclovir that is not considered as efficacy. The Hon'ble IPAB had also stated that 'Efficacy' and 'bio-availability' are two different concepts and are not the same. The Hon'ble IPAB has also stated that this difference is also proved from the definition of efficacy, which states that therapeutic effect is independent of property (i.e. bio-availability). Claim 4 is not clearly and particularly described and in the absence of any improved effect the crystalline form considered as another form of a known substance u/s 3(d) of the Act.

50. Since claim 1 is not novel and inventive, making a composition of known drug with known excipients cannot be considered as an invention. Therefore, claim 9 is a mere admixture resulting only in the aggregation of the properties of the components thereof.

> Section 3 (d): the mere discovery of a new form of a known substance which does not result in the enhancement of the known efficacy of that substance or the mere discovery of any new property or new use for a known substance or of the mere use of a known process, machine or apparatus unless such known process results in a new product or employs at least one new reactant.

> Explanation to Section 3 (d): "Salts, esters, ethers, polymorphs, metabolites, pure form, particle size, isomers, mixtures of isomers, complexes, combinations, and other derivatives of known substance shall be considered to be the same substance, unless they differ significantly in properties with regard to efficacy.

51. The counsels for the opponents further argued that the complete specification does not disclose any synergistic effect for the substance with a pharmaceutically acceptable excipient or carrier material. Therefore, claim 9 falls under section 3(e) of the Act.

52. The counsel for the patentee submitted that valganciclovir is not only more "efficacious" having regard to compounds known for treatment of CMV but even "therapeutic" and "curative". The enhancement in oral bioavailability has resulted in direct control over dosage administered to the patient, thereby minimizing the risks associated with prior art intravenous treatments, particularly for immune compromised patients as well as reduction in any side effects that the drug molecule itself may cause in a patient due to over dosage.

53. Further the counsel referred Per Ljungman's affidavit which explains in detail about the effects of low resistance, no mutations, and systemic exposure, which are achieved by valganciclovir and in paragraph 40,

> "Valganciclovir has a bioavailability of approximately 10 times that of oral ganciclovir, with one daily dose of 450 mg of valganciclovir giving a similar area under the concentrative curve (AUC) as Ig three times daily of oral ganciclovir. In contrast to oral ganciclovir, the <u>systemic exposure</u> increases with the dose of valganciclovir. The maximum concentration when given in one daily dose of 900 mg is typically 5-6 mg/ml and the AUC up to twice what can be achieved by oral ganciclovir given 3 times/day. "

In paragraph 23 at page 9 of the said affidavit equates the increased bioavailability of valganciclovir with the positive existence of clinical efficacy in the following words:-

> "<u>Clinical efficacy</u> results from many important aspects of both the chosen drug and the status of the treated patient. Important aspects of the drug influencing clinical efficacy include the side effect profile, bioavailability, and drug interactions. Clinical efficacy is also influenced by the concentration of the antiviral drug that can be delivered to the relevant site of infection or disease, such as through the blood for preemptive therapy or into the eye for treatment of CMV retinitis. Examples of patient factors influencing clinical efficacy are gut graft-vs-host diseases that can influence absorption of an oral drug

and the degree of immune-suppression of the patient. The more severely a patient is immune-suppressed, the more difficult it is to effectively decrease CMV replication.

54. The counsel further submitted that the bioavailability and therapeutic efficacy are not one and the same but closely related in such a way that one affects the other. The increased bioavailability is a property and the effect of the same is low resistance, no mutations, system exposure and avoidance of the drawbacks of the intravenous treatment which are nothing but therapeutic efficacy as explained in Per Ljungman affidavit, particularly in paragraphs 30 to 48 .

55. The counsel submitted that opponent's argument on the comparative data provided in Example 9 of the specification for the oral bio availability cannot be accepted since valganciclovir is in hydrochloride or acetate salt form where as ganciclovir and bis esters are not in salt form do not contain any merit. All bioavailability experiments for mono esters of '232 patent were conducted with either the hydrochloride or the acetate (salt of acetic acid) salts, which was done for chemical stability reasons. In fact, the improved oral bioavailability of valganciclovir is not because of the particular salt form, but due to the addition of the L valyl ester, which allows the molecule to be actively transported and is not dependent on the particular salt form or the solid state characteristics of the molecule.

56. Claim 9 is directed to a composition comprising a novel and inventive compound, which is being a dependent claim, derives novelty and inventive step from the compound claimed in claims 1 to 8. Hence, claim 9 does not fall within the scope of Section 3(e) of the Patent Act.

57. I agree with the arguments of the counsels for the opponents that the oral bioavailability is not therapeutic efficacy under the provisions of the Act. Data provided in example 9 of the specification is pertaining to the bioavailability, but not for the therapeutic efficacy. The improved bioavailability may increase the clinical efficacy in turn it may influence the therapeutic efficacy for which there is no support is provided in the specification. Clinical efficacy and therapeutic efficacy is not considered as

one and the same, but it is different. In general, it is obvious that the prodrug of compound exhibit improved solubility, low resistance, no mutations, system exposure and avoidance of the drawbacks of the intravenous treatment which are inherent and expected properties of the prodrug. The composition claimed in specification is a mere statement without any scientific work or without any support showing synergistic property. Therefore the compound and its pharmaceutically acceptable salts, isomers, crystalline form and composition do not fulfill the requirement under the provision of the Act.

7. Statement and undertaking regarding foreign applications

58. The counsels for the opponents argued that the applicant failed to furnish the information required under section 8 of the Act. The patentee filed Form 4 on 27-7-1995 declaring only US Patent Application No.08/281893 as a corresponding foreign application pending and Annex to Form 4 was filed on 8-6-1996, but still further information about foreign filing on 23-05-2006 which was beyond the time limit. It is evident from the application data and transaction history of US Patent Application No.08/281893 available in the website of USPTO that a non-final rejection had been mailed on 16-6-1995, over a month before the filing of the present application. Annex to Form 4 submitted subsequently on 8-6-1996 lists US Patent Application No.08/281893 as 'pending', whereas the application was abandoned on 16-6-1995. Therefore the patentee has furnished false information.

59. The counsel for the patentee submitted that the all the relevant information required under the said section 8 have been submitted to the Patent Office. Accordingly, no false information has been submitted pertaining to the status of the application filed in other jurisdictions.

60. Section 8. (1) Where an applicant for a patent under this Act is prosecuting either alone or jointly with any other person an application for a patent in any country outside India in respect of the same or

substantially the same invention, or where to his knowledge such an application is being prosecuted by some person through whom he claims or by some person deriving title from him, he shall file along with his application-

(i). a statement setting out detailed particulars of such application is being prosecuted, the serial number and date of filing of the application and such other particulars may be prescribed; and

(ii).an undertaking that, up to the date of the acceptance of his complete specification filed in India, he would keep the Controller informed in writing, from time to time, of details of the nature referred into clause (a) in respect of every other application relating to the same or substantially the same invention, if any, filed in any country outside India substantially the same invention, if any, filed in any country outside India subsequently to the filing of the statement referred to in the aforesaid clause, within the prescribed time.

Rule 13 (1) Statement and undertaking regarding foreign applications.-

(1). The statement and undertaking required to be filed by an applicant for a patent under sub-section (1) of section 8 shall be made in Form 4.

(2) The time within which the applicant for a patent shall keep the Controller informed of the details in respect of other applications filed in any country outside India in the undertaking to be given by him under clause (b) of sub-section (1) of section 8 shall be three months from the date of such filing.

61. The ground for opposition under section 25(2) (h) of the Act as follows:

    (i). the patentee has failed to disclose to the Controller the information required by Section 8, or

    (ii). has furnished the information which in any material particular was false to his knowledge.

62. Photocopy of the prosecution history of US application which is taken from the website of the USPTO submitted during the proceedings as evidence not an authenticated document, therefore it is not considered. Different countries have different provisions in different jurisdictions. The patentee has met all the requirements under the provisions of the Act during prosecution of the application.

8. Locus standi

63. The counsel for the opponents (5) and (6) submitted that the provision includes an organization representing persons living with HIV and come within the meaning of section 2(1) (t) of the Patents Act and has locus to file this post-grant opposition, especially in valganciclovir.

64. The counsel for the patentee argued that DNP+ has no manufacturing, trading or research interest and is, therefore, not a person interested within the meaning of Section 25(2) of the Patents Act, 1970. It is stated that under Section 25(2), the language used "person interested" as opposed to Section 25(1) which uses the language "any person". The person interested must be a person with a direct tangible commercial or research interest. The person must have, therefore, either a manufacturing, trading or research interest or must own patents in the field or must suffer some threat, injury or otherwise had affected by the presence of the patent.

65. The provision of the Act as follows:

    2(t) "person interested" includes a person engaged in, or in promoting, research in the same field as that to which the invention relates;

In **Ajay Industrial Corpn. Vs Shiro Kanso, AIR 1983 Delhi, 496,**

"In our opinion, a 'person interested' within the meaning of section 64 must be a person who has a direct, present and tangible commercial interest or public interest which is injured or affected by the continuance of the patent on the register."

66. DNP+, in my opinion, is a person affected or injured and well within the provision of section 2(1) (t). The transitional word 'including' is open term, which 'including the persons provided therein but not excluding others'. Therefore, I allow DNP+ as an opponent in the present case.

9. Conventional application

67. The counsels for the opponents contented that the application has to be made within twelve months from the date of filing of the application in a convention country. This application claims priority date from patent application No.08/281893 filed at the USA on 28-07-1994. U.S.A. was not declared as a convention country by India at the time of filing of the basic application. Section 135 of the Patents Act strictly requires this. On 28-07-1994 when the basic application was filed in U.S.A. it was not a convention country.   Only by a notification issued on January 3rd, 1995 U.S.A. was declared as a convention country. Indian Patents Act does not protect product patent of drugs before 1st January, 1995 and so this alleged invention is not valid. The counsels referred the Daniel AC v/s. Controller of Patents.

68. The counsel for the patentee submitted that the ground of opposition by way of application for amending the notice of opposition and statement of opposition filed on 3rd April 2009, which was filed much after the prescribed time period of one year from the date of publication of grant of patent that expired on 29th June 2008. Thus, the amendment should not be allowed.

69. The counsel for the patentee refers to the Controller's decision in **Eli Lilly & Co. vs. Ranbaxy Laboratories Limited in respect of Indian Patent Application No. 85/DEL/1995 where the Controller held the following:**

> "I find that as such the issue of validity of priority does not fall within the ambit of any grounds of opposition as stipulated in Section 25(1) of the Patents (Amended) Act, 2005. Needless to mention that the applicant & opponent are required to limit their submissions only on the grounds specified u/s 25(1) (a) to 25 (1) (k) but on no other ground"

> The grounds of pre-grant opposition provided under Section 25(1) are identical to the grounds of post-grant opposition provided under Section 25(2). Hence, the intervener's arguments or submissions do not fall within the ambit of the ground specified under Section 25(2) (i).

70. USA had been notified as convention country well before the date of filing of this application in India. In Novartis decision, the respondents objected to the grant of priority date to Novartis as Switzerland being the basic country was not a convention country on the date of filing of the application. The IPAB held as follows:-

> "In the decision dated 07.09.2005 in the case of **Agouron Pharmaceuticals Inc. V Controller of Patents in the High Court at Calcutta (special jurisdiction. Original side) (AID NO. 2 of 2001) Hon'ble S.K. Mukherjee, J** has observed "It is well settled that the appellate court is entitled to take into consideration any change in law and give proper relief on that basis". Accordingly, we do not agree with the arguments of the respondents and find that the appellant is fully justified and entitled to get the convention priority date 18.07.1997 under the amended section 133 of the Act. Provision of section 6 of General Clauses Act, 1897 does not apply here as the original Act has not been repeated. "

71. Further the counsel contented that the Calcutta High Court order of Justice **Ruma Pal in Daniel vs Controller of Patents** will not be applicable to the present case because the order was under Section 15 of the Patents Act and not under the ground of opposition of Section 25 and section 133 of the Patents Act has been amended since then the order is passed. Therefore, this ground of opposition is not maintainable as on the date of filing of the application in India, US was a convention country under Section 133 of the Indian Patents Act.

72. I am in an opinion that US was a conventional country when the application was filed in India. Even though Government of India notified US as a conventional country after the filing date of the US application, the door was opened for the applicant when the application was filed in India. Nowhere in the Patent Act mentioned that the invention relating to product carried out or application filed before 1995 are not patentable. Therefore I allow the conventional status of the present application.

73. I agree with the counsel for the patentee that new ground of opposition by way of amending much after prescribed time limit not allowed.

> **Kawal Singh Akbar v. Baldeo Singh Akbar, AIR 1957 Nagpur 57,** the Nagpur High Court held: "It was held that the application to take the additional ground should be treated as a new application to set aside the award and must be dismissed as it was barred by limitation. No quarter can, therefore, be given to the latches and delay, which the appellant has been guilty of".

74. The additional ground added to the opposition is not allowed.

75. I have not considered any other ground filed by way of opposition in this case, which is irrelevant.

76. In view of the discussion in the preceding paragraphs, considering the relevant arguments put forward by the Counsels for the opponents and counsel for the patentee at the hearing, the documents on record and the relevant written submissions made by all the parties and all the circumstances of the case, the post-grant opposition filed by the opponents under section 25(2) of the Act is accordingly order to amend the patent to process claims restricted to single process, if the patentee wish to proceed, can make a request within 15 days from the date of receipt of this decision.

Dated this 30th day of April, 2010.

(Dr. S.P.SUBRAMANIYAN)
Assistant Controller of Patents & Designs

ANNEXURE 12

NOTICE OF WORKING OF PATENT

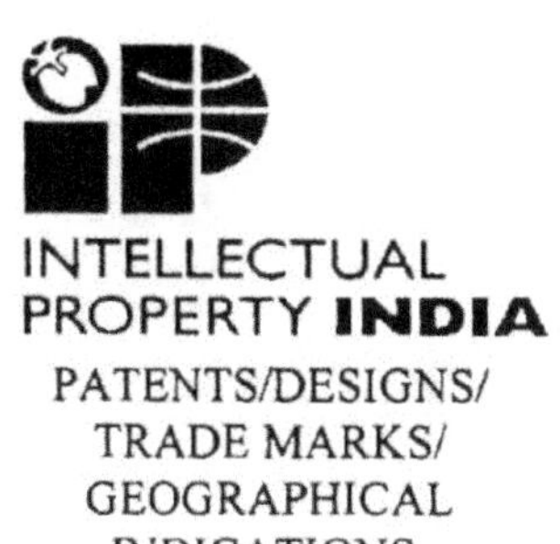

INTELLECTUAL PROPERTY INDIA
PATENTS/DESIGNS/
TRADE MARKS/
GEOGRAPHICAL
INDICATIONS.

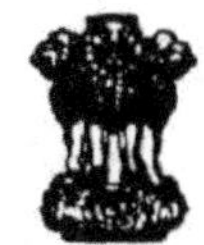

सत्यमेव जयते
Government of India
Office of The Controller General,
Patents, Designs & Trade Marks,
Boudhik Sampada Bhavan,
S.M. Road, Antop Hill,
Mumbai-400 037 (India)

(Tel):   ☎   022-24132735
                022-24123388
(Fax):   ☒   022-24123322
(Email): **cgoffice-mh@nic.in**
(Website): **www.ipindia.nic.in**

CG/Public Notice/2014/ 292   **Dated: 28.02.2014**

PUBLIC NOTICE

In accordance with the provisions contained in sub-section (2) of section 146 of the Patents Act, 1970 read with rule 131 of the Patents Rules, 2003, all Patentees and Licensees (whether exclusive or otherwise) are required to furnish information in Form-27 in respect of each calendar year, within three months of the end of each year.

All the Patentees and Licensees are hereby called upon to comply with the above provisions with regard to information for the year 2013. Attention is also invited to the provisions contained in section 122 of the Patents Act, 1970.

The Patent Office appeals to all that e-filing service available on the official website www.ipindia.nic.in may be used for this purpose, as far as possible.

(Chaitanya Prasad)
Controller General of Patents, Designs & Trade Marks

ANNEXURE 13

REVOKING OF PATENT BY GAZETTE NOTIFICATION

रजिस्ट्री सं० डी० एल०-33004/99

REGD. NO. D. L.-33004/99

भारत का राजपत्र
The Gazette of India

असाधारण

EXTRAORDINARY

भाग II—खण्ड 3—उप-खण्ड (ii)

PART II—Section 3—Sub-section (ii)

प्राधिकार से प्रकाशित

PUBLISHED BY AUTHORITY

सं. 2085]	नई दिल्ली, बृहस्पतिवार, अक्तूबर 18, 2012/आश्विन 26, 1934
No. 2085]	NEW DELHI, THURSDAY, OCTOBER 18, 2012/ASVINA 26, 1934

वाणिज्य और उद्योग मंत्रालय

(औद्योगिक नीति और संवर्धन विभाग)

अधिसूचना

नई दिल्ली, 18 अक्तूबर, 2012

का.आ. 2517(अ).—केन्द्रीय सरकार, पेटेंट अधिनियम, 1970 (1970 का 39) की धारा 66 द्वारा प्रदत्त शक्तियों का प्रयोग करते हुए, यह घोषित करती है कि मै. अवेस्थाजन लि., डिस्कवरर 9वाँ तल, इंटरनेशनल टैक पार्क, व्हाइटफील्ड रोड, बंगलौर-560066 को प्रदत्त पेटेंट सं. 252093, जिसका शीर्षक "एक सहक्रियशील, अयुर्वेदिक/कार्यशील खाद्य जैव सक्रिय संयोजन (सिनाटा) है और उसकी निर्मिति की प्रक्रिया" साधारणतः जनता पर प्रतिकूल प्रभाव डालने वाला है ।

2. उपर उल्लिखित धारा 66 के अधीन, उक्त पेटेंट को प्रतिसंहृत किया गया समझा जाएगा ।

[फा. सं. 12/35/2012-आईपीआर-III]

डी. वी. प्रसाद, संयुक्त सचिव

MINISTRY OF COMMERCE AND INDUSTRY

(Department of Industrial Policy and Promotion)

NOTIFICATION

New Delhi, the 18th October, 2012

S.O. 2517(E).—In exercise of the powers conferred by Section 66 of the Patents Act, 1970 (39 of 1970), the Central Government hereby declares that Patent No. 252093, entitled "a Synergistic, Ayurvedic/functional food bioactive composition (Cinata) and a process of preparation thereof" granted to M/s. Avesthagen Ltd., Discoverer, 9th Floor, International Tech Park, Whitefield Road, Bangalore-560066 is generally prejudicial to the public.

2. Under Section 66 mentioned above, the said patent shall be deemed to be revoked.

[F. No. 12/35/2012-IPR-III]

D. V. PRASAD, Jt. Secy.

3977 GI/2012

Printed by the Manager, Government of India Press, Ring Road, Mayapuri, New Delhi-110064 and Published by the Controller of Publications, Delhi-110054.

ANNEXURE 14

FEE FOR PATENT APPLICATION, OFFICE PROCEDURE AND MAINTENANCE

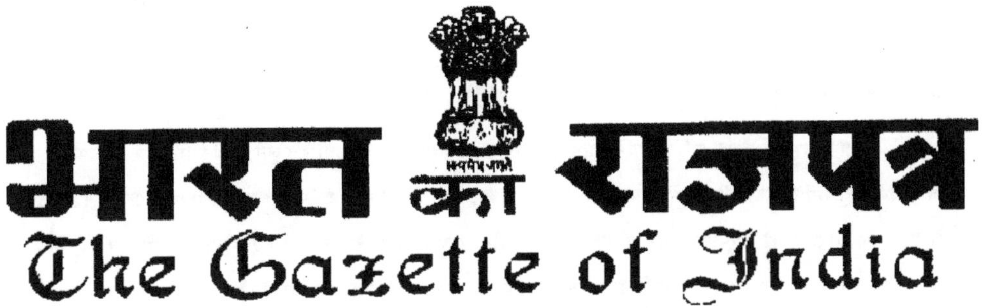

असाधारण

EXTRAORDINARY

भाग II—खण्ड 3—उप-खण्ड (i)

PART II—Section 3—Sub-section (i)

प्राधिकार से प्रकाशित

PUBLISHED BY AUTHORITY

सं. 91]	नई दिल्ली, शुक्रवार, फरवरी 28, 2014/फाल्गुन 9, 1935
No. 91]	NEW DELHI, FRIDAY, FEBRUARY 28, 2014/PHALGUNA 9, 1935

वाणिज्य और उद्योग मंत्रालय

(औद्योगिक नीति और संवर्द्धन विभाग)

अधिसूचना

नई दिल्ली, 28 फरवरी, 2014

सा.का.नि. 125(अ).—पेटेंट अधिनियम, 1970 (1970 का 39) की धारा 159 की उप-धारा (3) के अधीन यथा अपेक्षित कतिपय प्रारूप नियम, अर्थात् पेटेंट (संशोधन) नियम, 2013 को ऐसे सभी व्यक्तियों से, जिनके उससे प्रभावित होने की संभावना है, उस तारीख से, जिसको अधिसूचना वाले राजपत्र की प्रतियाँ जनसाधारण को उपलब्ध कराई गई थी, पैंतालीस दिनों की अवधि की समाप्ति से पूर्व आक्षेप और सुझाव आमंत्रित करने के लिए भारत के राजपत्र, असाधारण, भाग-II, खण्ड 3, उपखण्ड (i) में भारत सरकार, वाणिज्य और उद्योग मंत्रालय, (औद्योगिक नीति और संवर्द्धन विभाग) की अधिसूचना संख्यांक सा.का.नि. 286 (अ), तारीख 6 मई, 2013 द्वारा प्रकाशित किए गए थे;

और उक्त अधिसूचना वाले राजपत्र की प्रतियाँ तारीख 12 जून, 2013 को जनसाधारण को उपलब्ध करा दी गई थी;

और उक्त प्रारूप नियमों के संबंध में जनसाधारण से प्राप्त आक्षेप और सुझावों पर केन्द्रीय सरकार द्वारा विचार किया गया है;

अत: अब, केन्द्रीय सरकार, पेटेंट अधिनियम, 1970 (1970 का 39) की धारा 159 द्वारा प्रदत्त शक्तियों का प्रयोग करते हुए, पेटेंट नियम, 2003 का और संशोधन करने के लिए निम्नलिखित नियम बनाती है, अर्थात्-

1. (1) इन नियमों का संक्षिप्त नाम पेटेंट (संशोधन) नियम, 2014 है ।

    (2) ये राजपत्र में उनके प्रकाशन की तारीख को प्रवृत्त होंगे ।

2. पेटेंट नियम, 2003 (जिसे इसमें इसके पश्चात् मूल नियम कहा गया है) के नियम 2 में ---

(i) खंड (घ) के पश्चात् निम्नलिखित खंड अंतःस्थापित किया जाएगा, अर्थात:

'(घक) "प्रकृत व्यक्ति से भिन्न" में "लघु अस्तित्व" शामिल होगी।'

(ii) खंड (च) के पश्चात् निम्नलिखित खंड अंतःस्थापित किया जाएगा, अर्थात्:

'(चक) "लघु अस्तित्व" से निम्न अभिप्रेत है- (i) वस्तुओं का विनिर्माण या उत्पादन लगे हुए किसी उद्यम के मामले में, एक उद्यम जहाँ संयंत्र और मशीनरी में किया गया निवेश "सूक्ष्म, लघु और मध्यम उद्यम विकास अधिनियम, 2006 (2006 का 27)" की धारा 7 की उप–धारा (1) के खंड (क) के अधीन मध्यम उद्यम के लिए निर्दिष्ट सीमा से अधिक न हो; और (ii) सेवा प्रदान या उपलब्ध कराने वाले किसी उद्यम के मामले में, एक उद्यम जहाँ उपस्कर में किया गया निवेश "सूक्ष्म, लघु और मध्यम उद्यम विकास अधिनियम, 2006" की धारा 7 की उप–धारा (1) के खंड (ख) के अधीन मध्यम उद्यम के लिए निर्दिष्ट सीमा से अधिक न हो ।

स्पष्टीकरण : 1.- इस खंड के प्रयोजन के लिए, "उद्यम" से ऐसा कोई औद्योगिक उपक्रम या कोई व्याबसायिक समुत्थान या कोई अन्य स्थापन अभिप्रेत है, चाहे वह किसी भी नाम से ज्ञात हो, जो उद्योग (विकास और विनियमन) अधिनियम, 1951 (1951 का 65) की पहली अनुसूची में विनिर्दिष्ट किसी उद्योग से संबंधित वस्तुओं के विनिर्माण या उत्पादन में, किसी रीति से लगा हुआ है या किसी ऐसे उद्योग में कोई सेवा या सेवाओं को उपलब्ध कराने या उन्हें प्रदान कराने में लगा हुआ है ।

स्पष्टीकरण: 2.- संयंत्र और मशीनरी में किए गए निवेश की संगणना में प्रदूषण नियंत्रण, शोध और विकास, औद्योगिक सुरक्षा उपकरण तथा सूक्ष्म, लघु और मध्यम उद्यम विकास अधिनियम, 2006 (2006 का 27) के तहत अधिसूचना द्वारा यथा विनिर्दिष्ट ऐसी अन्य वस्तुओं को सम्मिलित नहीं किया जाएगा।

स्पष्टीकरण: 3.- भारतीय रिजर्व बैंक की विदेशी मुद्रा की निर्देश दर अभिभावी होगी।'

3.   मूल नियम के नियम 7 में - उप-नियम (3) के पश्चात् निम्नलिखित उप-नियम अंतःस्थापित किया जाएगा, अर्थात्:

(i) उप-नियम (1) के पश्चात् निम्नलिखित उपबंधों को अंतःस्थापित किया जाएगा, अर्थात्:

"परन्तु यह कि जब कोई पेटेंट के लिए आवेदन या अन्य कोई दस्तावेज़ भौतिक रूप में अर्थात् मुद्रित प्रति के रूप विधान में फाइल किया जाता है, तो दस प्रतिशत अतिरिक्त फीस संदेय होगा ।

परन्तु यह और कि किसी लघु अस्तित्व के संदर्भ में प्रत्येक दस्तावेज़, जिसके लिए कोई फीस विहित है, प्ररूप-28 के साथ संलग्न होगा।"

(ii) "(3क) किसी लघु अस्तित्व द्वारा प्रक्रियागत आवेदन को पूर्णतः या अंशतः किसी प्रकृत व्यक्ति के अतिरिक्त किसी अन्य व्यक्ति (लघु अस्तित्व के सिवाय) को हस्तांतरित करने की स्थिति में उसी मामले में किसी लघु अस्तित्व से प्रभारित फीस (फीसों) और किसी प्रकृत व्यक्ति के अतिरिक्त किसी अन्य व्यक्ति (लघु अस्तित्व के सिवाय) से प्रभार्य फीस (फीसों) के परिमाण में अंतर, यदि कोई हो, का भुगतान नए आवेदक द्वारा हस्तांतरण के अनुरोध के साथ किया जाएगा ।"

4.   मूल नियम के नियम 55 के उप-नियम (1) में "फाइल किए जाएंगे" शब्द के पश्चात् "प्ररूप 7 (क) में" शब्द, कोष्ठक और अक्षर अंतःस्थापित किये जाएंगे ।

5.   मूल नियम की पहली अनुसूची के स्थान पर निम्नलिखित अनुसूची रखी जाएगी, अर्थात्:-

"पहली अनुसूची
(नियम 7 देखें)
फीस

प्रविष्टि संख्यांक	जिस पर संदेय है	सुसंगत प्ररूप संख्यांक	ई-फाइलिंग के लिए			भौतिक रूप में फाइल करने के लिए		
			प्रकृत व्यक्ति (व्यक्तियों) के लिए	या तो अकेले या प्रकृत व्यक्ति (व्यक्तियों) के साथ संयुक्त रूप में प्रकृत व्यक्ति (व्यक्तियों) से भिन्न व्यक्ति के लिए		प्रकृत व्यक्ति (व्यक्तियों) के लिए दस प्रतिशत अतिरिक्त फीस	या तो अकेले या प्रकृत व्यक्ति (व्यक्तियों) के साथ संयुक्त रूप में प्रकृत व्यक्ति(व्यक्तियों) से भिन्न व्यक्ति के लिए दस प्रतिशत अतिरिक्त फीस	
				लघु अस्तित्व के लिए	लघु अस्तित्व के अतिरिक्त अन्य के लिए		लघु अस्तित्व के लिए	लघु अस्तित्व के अतिरिक्त अन्य के लिए
1	2	3	4	5	6	7	8	9
			रुपए	रुपए	रुपए	रुपए	रुपए	रुपए
1.	अनंतिम/सम्पूर्ण विनिर्देश के साथ धारा 7, धारा 54 और धारा 135 और नियम 20(1) के अधीन किसी पेटेंट के लिए आवेदन पर - (i) 30 के अतिरिक्त प्रत्येक विनिर्देश पत्रे के लिए; (ii) 10 के अतिरिक्त प्रत्येक दावे के लिए।	1	1600 प्रत्येक गुणज पूर्विकता की दशा में 1600 के गुणजों में (i) 160 (ii) 320	4000 प्रत्येक गुणज पूर्विकता की दशा में 4000 के गुणजों में (i) 400 (ii) 800	8000 प्रत्येक गुणज पूर्विकता की दशा में 8000 के गुणजों में (i) 800 (ii) 1,600	1760 प्रत्येक गुणज पूर्विकता की दशा में 1760 के गुणजों में (i) 176 (ii) 352	4400 प्रत्येक गुणज पूर्विकता की दशा में 4400 के गुणजों में (i) 440 (ii) 880	8,800 प्रत्येक गुणज पूर्विकता की दशा में 8,800 के गुणजों में (i) 880 (ii) 1760
2.	अनंतिम विनिर्देश के पश्चात् सम्पूर्ण विनिर्देश फाइल करने पर 30 पृष्ठ तक जिसमें 10 दावे तक हों - (i) 30 के अतिरिक्त प्रत्येक विनिर्देश पत्रे के लिए; (ii) 10 के अतिरिक्त प्रत्येक दावे के लिए के।	2	कोई फीस नहीं (i) 160 (ii) 320	कोई फीस नहीं (i) 400 (ii) 800	कोई फीस नहीं (i) 800 (ii) 1600	कोई फीस नहीं (i) 176 (ii) 352	कोई फीस नहीं (i) 440 (ii) 880	कोई फीस नहीं (i) 880 (ii) 1760
3.	धारा 8 के अधीन विवरण और वचनबंध फाइल करने पर।	3	कोई फीस नहीं	कोई फीस नहीं	कोई फीस नहीं	कोई फीस नहीं	कोई फीस नहीं	कोई फीस नहीं
4.	धारा 53(2) और धारा 142(4), नियम 13(6), नियम 80(1क) और नियम 130 के अधीन समय विस्तार के अनुरोध पर।	4	480 प्रति मास	1200 प्रति मास	2400 प्रति मास	528 प्रति मास	1320 प्रति मास	2640 प्रति मास

Table Contd...

5.	नियम 13(6) के अधीन आविष्कारवृत्ति के हैसियत में घोषणा फाइल करने पर।	5	कोई फीस नहीं	कोई फीस नहीं	कोई फीस नहीं	कोई फीस नहीं	कोई फीस नहीं	कोई फीस नहीं
6.	अगली तारीख के लिए आवेदन पर।	-	800	2000	4000	880	2200	4400
7.	धारा 19(2) के अधीन निर्देश को हटाने के लिए आवेदन पर।	-	800	2000	4000	880	2200	4400
8.	(i) धारा 20(1) के अधीन दावे पर;	6	800	2000	4000	880	2200	4400
	(ii) धारा 20(4) या धारा 20(5) के अधीन निदेश के लिए अनुरोध पर।	6	800	2000	4000	880	2200	4400
9.	(i) धारा 25(1) के अधीन पेटेंट अनुदान का विरोध करने के लिए आवेदन फाइल करने पर;	7क	कोई फीस नहीं	कोई फीस नहीं	कोई फीस नहीं	कोई फीस नहीं	कोई फीस नहीं	कोई फीस नहीं
	(ii) धारा 25(2) के अधीन पेटेंट को मंजूर करने का विरोध की सूचना पर।	7	2400	6000	12000	2640	6600	13200
10.	नियम 62(2) के अधीन यह सूचना देने पर कि नियंत्रक के समक्ष सुनवाई में उपस्थित रहा जाएगा।	--	1500	3750	7500	1650	4125	8250
11.	धारा 28(2), धारा 28(3) या धारा 28(7) के अधीन आवेदन पर।	8	800	2000	4000	880	2200	4400
12.	धारा 11क(2) और नियम, 24क के अधीन प्रकाशन हेतु अनुरोध।	9	2500	6250	12500	2750	6875	13750
13.	आवेदन के प्रकाशन के पूर्व धारा 11ख(4) और नियम 26(1) के अधीन आवेदन के प्रत्याहरण के लिए आवेदन।	--	1600	4000	8000	1760	4400	8800
14.	पेटेंट आवेदन के परीक्षण हेतु अनुरोध पर - (क) धारा 11ख और नियम 24(1) के अधीन;	18	4000	10000	20000	4400	11000	22000
	(ख) नियम 20(4)(ii) के अधीन।		5600	14000	28000	6160	15400	30800
15.	धारा 44 के अधीन पेटेंट के संशोधन के लिए आवेदन पर।	10	2400	6000	12000	2640	6600	13200
16.	धारा 51(1) या धारा 51(2) के अधीन निदेश के लिए आवेदन पर।	11	2400	6000	12000	2640	6600	13200
17.	धारा 26(1) या धारा 52(2) के अधीन पेटेंट मंजूर करने के लिए अनुरोध पर।	12	2400	6000	12000	2640	6600	13200

Table Contd...

18.	धारा 55(1) के अधीन पेटेंट के परिवर्धन को एक स्वतंत्र पेटेंट में संपरिवर्तित करने के अनुरोध पर।	--	2400	6000	12000	2640	6600	13200
19.	धारा 53 के अधीन पेटेंट के नवीनीकरण हेतु-							
(i)	पेटेंट की तारीख से दूसरे वर्ष की समाप्ति से पूर्व तीसरे वर्ष की बाबत;	--	800	2000	4000	880	2200	4400
(ii)	तीसरे वर्ष की समाप्ति से पूर्व चौथे वर्ष की बाबत;	--	800	2000	4000	880	2200	4400
(iii)	चौथे वर्ष की समाप्ति से पूर्व पांचवे वर्ष की बाबत;	--	800	2000	4000	880	2200	4400
(iv)	पांचवे वर्ष की समाप्ति से पूर्व छठे वर्ष की बाबत;	--	800	2000	4000	880	2200	4400
(v)	छठे वर्ष की समाप्ति से पूर्व सातवें वर्ष की बाबत;	--	2400	6000	12000	2640	6600	13200
(vi)	सातवें वर्ष की समाप्ति से पूर्व आठवें वर्ष की बाबत;	--	2400	6000	12000	2640	6600	13200
(vii)	आठवें वर्ष की समाप्ति से पूर्व नवें वर्ष की बाबत;	--	2400	6000	12000	2640	6600	13200
(viii)	नवें वर्ष की समाप्ति से पूर्व दसवें वर्ष की बाबत;	--	2400	6000	12000	2640	6600	13200
(ix)	दसवें वर्ष की समाप्ति से पूर्व ग्यारहवें वर्ष की बाबत;	--	4800	12000	24000	5280	13200	26400
(x)	ग्यारहवें वर्ष की समाप्ति से पूर्व बारहवें वर्ष की बाबत;	--	4800	12000	24000	5280	13200	26400
(xi)	बारहवें वर्ष की समाप्ति से पूर्व तेरहवें वर्ष की बाबत;	--	4800	12000	24000	5280	13200	26400
(xii)	तेरहवें वर्ष की समाप्ति से पूर्व चौदहवें वर्ष की बाबत;	--	4800	12000	24000	5280	13200	26400
(xiii)	चौदहवें वर्ष की समाप्ति से पूर्व पन्द्रहवें वर्ष की बाबत;	--	4800	12000	24000	5280	13200	26400
(xiv)	पन्द्रहवें वर्ष की समाप्ति से पूर्व सोलहवें वर्ष की बाबत;	--	8000	20000	40000	8800	22000	44000
(xv)	सोलहवें वर्ष की समाप्ति से पूर्व सतरहवें वर्ष की बाबत;	--	8000	20000	40000	8800	22000	44000
(xvi)	सतरहवें वर्ष की समाप्ति से पूर्व अठारहवें वर्ष की बाबत;	--	8000	20000	40000	8800	22000	44000
(xvii)	अठारहवें वर्ष की समाप्ति से पूर्व उन्नीसवें वर्ष की बाबत;	--	8000	20000	40000	8800	22000	44000
(xviii)	उन्नीसवें वर्ष की समाप्ति से पूर्व बीसवें वर्ष की बाबत।	--	8000	20000	40000	8800	22000	44000

Table Contd...

20.	धारा 57 के अधीन पेटेंट के लिए आवेदन/सम्पूर्ण विनिर्देश/अन्य संबद्ध दस्तावेजों के संशोधन के लिए आवेदन पर -	13						
(i)	पेटेंट मंजूर करने से पूर्व;		800	2000	4000	880	2200	4400
(ii)	पेटेंट मंजूर करने के पश्चात् ;		1600	4000	8000	1760	4400	8800
(iii)	जहाँ संशोधन नाम/पता/राष्ट्रीयता/सेवार्थ पता में संशोधन होना है।		320	800	1600	352	880	1760
21.	धारा 57(4), धारा (61)1 और धारा 87(2) के अधीन किसी आवेदन के विरोध या धारा 63(3) के अधीन पेटेंट के अभ्यर्पण या धारा 78(5) के अधीन अनुरोध की सूचना पर।	14	2400	6000	12000	2640	6600	13200
22.	धारा 60 के अधीन पेटेंट के प्रत्यावर्तन के लिए आवेदन पर।	15	2400	6000	12000	2640	6600	13200
23.	प्रत्यावर्तन के लिए अतिरिक्त फीस।	--	4800	12000	24000	5280	13200	26400
24.	धारा 63 के अधीन पेटेंट के अभ्यर्पण की प्रस्थापना की सूचना पर।	--	1000	2500	5000	1100	2750	5500
25.	धारा 69(1) या धारा 69(2) और नियम 90(1) या नियम 90(2) के अधीन किसी व्यक्ति के किसी पेटेंट या उसके अंश के हकदार या बन्धकदार के रूप में या किसी व्यक्ति के अनुज्ञप्तिधारी के रूप में या अन्यथा के रूप में पेटेंट रजिस्टर में नाम की प्रविष्टि के लिए या किसी दस्तावेज़ की अधिसूचना की पेटेंट रजिस्टर में प्रविष्टि के लिए आवेदन पर।	16	1600 (प्रत्येक पेटेंट की बाबत)	4000 (प्रत्येक पेटेंट की बाबत)	8000 (प्रत्येक पेटेंट की बाबत)	1760 (प्रत्येक पेटेंट की बाबत)	4400 (प्रत्येक पेटेंट की बाबत)	8800 (प्रत्येक पेटेंट की बाबत)
26.	नियम 94(1) या नियम 118(1) के अधीन पेटेंट रजिस्टर या पेटेंट अभिकर्त्ता रजिस्टर में किसी प्रविष्टि के परिवर्तन के लिए आवेदन पर।	--	320	800	1600	352	880	1760
27.	नियम 94(3) के अधीन पेटेंट रजिस्टर में किसी अतिरिक्त सेवार्थ पते की प्रविष्टि करने के लिए अनुरोध पर।	--	800	2000	4000	880	2200	4400

Table *Contd…*

28.	धारा 84(1), धारा 91 (1), धारा 92(1) और धारा 92क के अधीन अनिवार्य अनुज्ञप्ति के लिए आवेदन पर।	17	2400	6000	12000	2640	6600	13200
29.	धारा 85(1) के अधीन पेटेंट के प्रतिसंहरण के लिए आवेदन पर।	19	2400	6000	12000	2640	6600	13200
30.	धारा 88(4) के अधीन अनुज्ञप्ति के निबंधनों और शर्तों के पुनरीक्षण के लिए आवेदन पर।	20	2400	6000	12000	2640	6600	13200
31.	धारा 94 के अधीन अनिवार्य अनुज्ञप्ति की समाप्ति के लिए अनुरोध पर।	21	2400	6000	12000	2640	6600	13200
32.	नियम 109 (1) या नियम 112 के अधीन पेटेंट अभिकर्ता के रूप में रजिस्ट्रीकरण के लिए आवेदन पर।	22	3200	--	--	3520	--	--
33.	नियम 109(3) के अधीन अर्हक परीक्षा में बैठने के लिए अनुरोध पर।	--	1600	--	--	1760	--	--
34.	पेटेंट अभिकर्ता रजिस्टर में किसी व्यक्ति के नाम के बने रहने के लिए:- (i) पहले वर्ष के लिए रजिस्ट्रीकरण के साथ संदत्त की जानी वाली; (ii) प्रत्येक वर्ष के लिए पहले वर्ष को छोड़कर प्रत्येक वर्ष की पहली अप्रैल को संदत्त की जाने वाली।	-	800 800	-- --	-- --	880 880	-- --	-- --
35.	नियम 111क के अधीन पेटेंट अभिकर्ता के द्वितीय प्रमाण-पत्र के लिए आवेदन पर।	--	1600	--	--	1760	--	--
36.	नियम 117(1) के अधीन पेटेंट अभिकर्ता रजिस्टर में किसी व्यक्ति के नाम के प्रत्यावर्तन के लिए आवेदन पर।	23	1600 (योग प्रविष्टि संख्यांक 34 के अधीन निरंतरता फीस)	--	--	1760 (योग प्रविष्टि संख्यांक 34 के अधीन निरंतरता फीस)	--	--
37.	धारा 78(2) के अधीन लिपिकीय त्रुटियों की शुद्धि के लिए अनुरोध पर।	--	800	2000	4000	880	2200	4400

Table Contd...

38.	धारा 77(1)(च) या धारा 77(1) (छ) के अधीन नियंत्रक के विनिश्चय या आदेश के पुनर्विलोकन या उसे अपास्त करने के लिए आवेदन पर।	24	1600	4000	8000	1760	4400	8800
39.	धारा 39 और नियम 71(1) के अधीन भारत से बाहर पेटेंट के आवदेन के लिए अनुज्ञा हेतु आवेदन पर।	25	1600	4000	8000	1760	4400	8800
40.	धारा 154 और नियम 132 के अधीन पेटेंट की द्वितीय प्रति के लिए आवेदन पर।	--	1600	4000	8000	1760	4400	8800
41.	धारा 72 के अधीन प्रमाणित प्रतियों के लिए या धारा 147 और नियम 133 के अधीन प्रमाण-पत्र के लिए अनुरोध पर।	--	1000 (30 पृष्ठ तक और उसके पश्चात् प्रत्येक अतिरिक्त पृष्ठ के लिए 30)	2500 (30 पृष्ठ तक और उसके पश्चात् प्रत्येक अतिरिक्त पृष्ठ के लिए 75)	5000 (30 पृष्ठ तक और उसके पश्चात् प्रत्येक अतिरिक्त पृष्ठ के लिए 150)	1100 (30 पृष्ठ तक और उसके पश्चात् प्रत्येक अतिरिक्त पृष्ठ के लिए 30)	2750 (30 पृष्ठ तक और उसके पश्चात् प्रत्येक अतिरिक्त पृष्ठ के लिए 75)	5500 (30 पृष्ठ तक और उसके पश्चात् प्रत्येक अतिरिक्त पृष्ठ के लिए 150)
42.	प्रत्येक मुद्रित, कार्यालय प्रतियों के प्रमाणन के लिए।	--	800	2000	4000	880	2200	4400
43.	धारा 72 के अधीन रजिस्टर के निरीक्षण, नियम 27 या नियम 74 (क) के अधीन निरीक्षण के लिए अनुरोध पर।	--	320	800	1600	352	880	1760
44.	धारा 127, धारा 132 और धारा 153 और नियम 134 के अधीन सूचना हेतु अनुरोध पर।	--	480	1200	2400	528	1320	2640
45.	पेटेंट अभिकर्ता के प्राधिकार के प्ररूप पर।	26	कोई फीस नहीं	कोई फीस नहीं	कोई फीस नहीं	कोई फीस नहीं	कोई फीस नहीं	कोई फीस नहीं
46.	ऐसी याचिका पर जो अन्यथा उपलब्ध नहीं है।	--	1600	4000	8000	1760	4400	8800
47.	दस्तावेजों की फोटो प्रतियों के प्रदाय के लिए प्रति पृष्ठ।	--	8	8	8	8	8	8
48.	अंतर्राष्ट्रीय आवेदन के लिए पारेषण फीस।	--	3200	8000	16000	3250	8800	17600

Table *Contd…*

| 49. | पूर्विकिता दस्तावेज़ की प्रामाणिक प्रति तैयार करने और उसे विश्व बौद्धिक सम्पदा संगठन के अंतर्राष्ट्रीय ब्यूरो को पारेषित करने के लिए। | -- | 1000 (30 पृष्ठ तक और उसके पश्चात् प्रत्येक अतिरिक्त पृष्ठ के लिए 30) | 2500 (30 पृष्ठ तक और उसके पश्चात् प्रत्येक अतिरिक्त पृष्ठ के लिए 75) | 5000 (30 पृष्ठ तक और उसके पश्चात् प्रत्येक अतिरिक्त पृष्ठ के लिए 150) | 1100 (30 पृष्ठ तक और उसके पश्चात् प्रत्येक अतिरिक्त पृष्ठ के लिए 30) | 2750 (30 पृष्ठ तक और उसके पश्चात् प्रत्येक अतिरिक्त पृष्ठ के लिए 75) | 5500 (30 पृष्ठ तक और उसके पश्चात् प्रत्येक अतिरिक्त पृष्ठ के लिए 150) |
| 50. | धारा 146(2) और नियम 131(1) के अधीन भारत में पेटेंट प्राप्त आविष्कार के वाणिज्यिक स्तर पर कार्यकरण के संबंध में विवरण पर। | 27 | कोई फीस नहीं | कोई फीस नहीं | कोई फीस नहीं | कोई फीस नहीं | कोई फीस नहीं | कोई फीस नहीं |

टिप्पण : सभी प्ररूप, आवेदन, अनुरोध, सूचना, अभ्यावेदन को अनुलिपि रूप में दाखिल किया जाना चाहिए, परंतु यह कि नियमों में अन्यथा विनिर्दिष्ट न हो।"

6. मूल नियम की दूसरी अनुसूची में, "प्ररूपों की सूची" में –

(i) "प्ररूप संख्या 27", संख्या 7 के पश्चात्, निम्नलिखित अंतःस्थापित किया जाएगा, अर्थात्:-

| "7क | धारा 25(1) और नियम 55(1) | धारा 25 की उप-धारा (1) के अधीन किसी पेटेंट अनुदत्त किए जाने का विरोध करने के लिए आवेदन फाइल करने के लिए।" |

(ii) "प्ररूप संख्या 27" के पश्चात्, निम्नलिखित अंतःस्थापित किया जाएगा, अर्थात्:-

| "28 | नियम 2(च क) और 7 | किसी लघु अस्तित्व द्वारा उस प्रत्येक दस्तावेज़ के साथ फाइल जिसके लिए फीस निर्दिष्ट है।" |

7. मूल नियम की दूसरी अनुसूची में, -

(i) प्ररूप 7 के पश्चात्, निम्नलिखित प्ररूप अंतःस्थापित किया जाएगा, अर्थात्:-

"प्ररूप-7क

पेटेंट अधिनियम, 1970 (1970 का 39)

एवं

पेटेंट नियम, 2003

पेटेंट के मंजूर करने पर विरोध के लिए अभ्यावेदन

[नियम 55 देखें]

1. नाम, पता और राष्ट्रीयता

मैं/हम————————————————— को प्रकाशित

————— द्वारा किए गए दिनांक —————की आवेदन संख्या————

————— के संबंध में पेटेंट मंजूर करने के विरोध के —————

माध्यम से अभ्यावेदन करता हूँ/करते हैं।

2. एक के पश्चात् दूसरे
आधार का उल्लेख।

लिए गए आधार ————————————————

3. पूरा पता डाक सूचक संख्या/कोड
सहित और राज्य के दूरभाष और
फैक्स नंबर के साथ।

भारत में तामील के लिए मेरा/हमारा पता है ———

—————————————————————

4. विरोध करने वाले या उनकी या
उसके प्राधिकृत पंजीकृत पेटेंट
अभिकर्ता द्वारा हस्ताक्षरित किया जाय।

हस्ताक्षर ————————————————

5. प्रकृत व्यक्ति का नाम जिन्होंने (———————————————)
हस्ताक्षर किया है ।

सेवा में,

नियंत्रक, पेटेंट

पेटेंट कार्यालय,

पता ——————————

(ii) प्ररूप 27 के पश्चात्, निम्नलिखित प्ररूप अंतःस्थापित किया जाएगा, अर्थात्:-

"प्ररूप-28

पेटेंट अधिनियम, 1970 (1970 का 39)

एवं

पेटेंट नियम, 2003

किसी लघु अस्तित्व द्वारा दाखिल की जाने वाली

[नियम 2(चक) और 7 देखें]

1.नाम, पता और राष्ट्रीयता

मैं/हम—————————————————अंतःस्थापित करें ———

————————————————— पेटेंट आवेदन संख्या /

पेटेंट संख्या ——————————————————————

——————————के संबंध में

आवेदक/ पेटेंटधारी

यह घोषणा करता हूँ/करते हैं कि मैं/हम नियम 2(च क) के अनुसार एक
लघु अस्तित्व हूँ/ हैं और सबूत के रूप में निम्नलिखित दस्तावेज़ प्रस्तुत करता
हूँ/करते हैं।

2. दस्तावेज़ का विवरण दें।

(i) छोटे, लघु और मध्यम उद्यम अधिनियम, 2006 के अधीन रजिस्ट्रीकृत
होने का साक्ष्य
(भारतीय अस्तित्व के संदर्भ में)

(ii.) कोई अन्य दस्तावेज़ (विदेशी अस्तित्व के संदर्भ में)

3.   आवेदक/पेटेंटी (पेटेंटधारी) प्राधिकृत रजिस्ट्रीकृत

यहाँ प्रदत्त सूचना मेरे ज्ञान और विश्वास के अनुसार सत्य है।

पेटेंट अभिकर्ता द्वारा हस्ताक्षरित किया जाय।

4.   उस प्रकृत व्यक्ति का नाम

जिन्होंने हस्ताक्षर किया है   तारीख--------------------

5.   जिस व्यक्ति ने हस्ताक्षर किया है उनका पदनाम और शासकीय मुहर, यदि कोई हो।

हस्ताक्षर

नाम

पदनाम

सेवा में,

नियंत्रक, पेटेंट

पेटेंट कार्यालय,

पता ------------------------,

टिप्पण : लघु अस्तित्व होने का दावा करने के योग्य होने के लिए भारतीय अस्तित्व ऊपर वर्णित साक्ष्य प्रस्तुत करें।"

8.   मूल नियम की चौथी अनुसूची के स्थान पर निम्नलिखित अनुसूची स्थापित की जाएगी, अर्थात्:-

"चौथी अनुसूची
[नियम 136(1) का उपबंध देखें]

प्रविष्टि संख्यांक	मामला जिसके संबंध में लागत दी जानी है	प्रकृत व्यक्ति (व्यक्तियों) के लिए	या तो अकेले या प्रकृत व्यक्ति (व्यक्तियों) के साथ संयुक्त रूप में प्रकृत व्यक्ति (व्यक्तियों) से भिन्न व्यक्ति के लिए	
			लघु अस्तित्व के लिए	लघु अस्तित्व के सिवाय अन्य के लिए
1	2	3	4	5
1.	धारा 25, धारा 57, धारा 60, धारा 63, धारा 78, धारा 87(2) या धारा 88(4) के अधीन विरोध की सूचना के लिए।	2400	6000	12000
2.	धारा 84(1), धारा 91(1) या धारा 92(1) के अधीन अनिवार्य अनुज्ञप्ति के लिए आवेदन के लिए।	1500	3000	6000
3.	धारा 88(4) के अधीन अनुज्ञप्ति के निबंधनों और शर्तों के पुनरीक्षण के लिए आवेदन के लिए।	2400	6000	12000
4.	नियम 62(2) के अधीन सुनवाई के दौरान उपस्थित रहने के आशय की सूचना के लिए।	1500	3000	6000
5.	जहाँ किसी पेटेंट अभिकर्ता या अन्य व्यक्ति को नियुक्त किया गया है वहाँ मुखतारनामें के लिए स्टांप फीस या सुसंगत शपथ पत्रों के संबंध में स्टांप फीस।	वास्तविक रूप से संदत्त रकम	वास्तविक रूप से संदत्त रकम	वास्तविक रूप से संदत्त रकम

Table Contd...

6.	नियम 57 के अधीन लिखित कथन या नियम 58 के अधीन लिखित कथन या प्रत्येक शपथ पत्र, यदि सुसंगत हो, के लिए।	4000	4000	5000
7.	कार्यवाही में प्रस्तुत प्रकाशन के प्रत्येक दस्तावेज़, यदि सुसंगत हो, के लिए।	1600	1600	2000
8.	प्रत्येक अनावश्यक या असंगत शपथ पत्र या प्रोद्धरण के लिए।	1600	1600	2000
9.	नियंत्रक के समक्ष प्रत्येक दिन या आंशिक दिन की सुनवाई के लिए।	4000	4000	5000"।

[फा. सं. 14/6/2012-आई. पी. आर.-III]

डी. बी. प्रसाद, संयुक्त सचिव

पादटिप्पण:—मूल नियम भारत के राजपत्र में अधिसूचना संख्या का. आ. 493 (अ) तारीख 2 मई, 2003 द्वारा प्रकाशित किए गए और निम्नलिखित अधिसूचना संख्यांक द्वारा पश्चातवर्ती संशोधन किया गया -

    (i)   का. आ. 1418(अ) तारीख 28 दिसम्बर, 2004

    (ii)   का. आ. 657(अ) तारीख 5 मई, 2006;

    (iii)   का. आ. 2296(अ) तारीख 25 सितम्बर, 2012

    (iv) का. आ. 1029(अ) तारीख 23 अप्रैल, 2013

MINISTRY OF COMMERCE AND INDUSTRY

(Department of Industrial Policy and Promotion)

NOTIFICATION

New Delhi, the 28th February , 2014

    G.S.R. 125(E).— Whereas certain draft rules, namely the Patents (Amendment) Rules, 2013 were published as required under sub-section (3) of Section 159 of the Patents Act, 1970 (39 of 1970), *vide* notification of the Government of India in the Ministry of Commerce and Industry (Department of Industrial Policy and Promotion), number G.S.R. 286(E), dated the 6th May, 2013, in the Gazette of India, Extraordinary, Part II, Section 3, sub-section (i), dated the 6th May, 2013, for inviting objections and suggestions from all persons likely to be affected thereby before the expiry of a period of forty-five days from the date on which copies of the Gazette containing the notification were made available to the public;

    And whereas, the copies of the Gazette containing the said notification were made available to the public on the 12th June, 2013;

    And whereas, the objections and the suggestions received from the public on the said draft rules have been considered by the Central Government;

    Now, therefore, in exercise of the powers conferred by Section 159 of the Patents Act, 1970 (39 of 1970), the Central Government hereby makes the following rules further to amend the Patents Rules, 2003, namely:—

1.   (1) These rules may be called the Patents (Amendment) Rules, 2014.

         (2) They shall come into force on the date of their publication in the Official Gazette.

2.   In rule 2 of the Patents Rules, 2003 (hereinafter referred to as the principal rules),—

    (i) after clause (d), the following clause shall be inserted, namely:—

        '(da) " person other than a natural person" shall include a "small entity" ' ;

    (ii) after clause (f), the following clause shall be inserted, namely:—

    (i) in case of an enterprise engaged in the manufacture or production of goods, an enterprise where the investment in plant and machinery does not exceed the limit specified for a medium enterprise under clause (a) of sub-section (1) of section 7 of the Micro, Small and Medium Enterprises Development Act, 2006 (27 of 2006); and

(ii) in case of an enterprise engaged in providing or rendering of services, an enterprise where the investment in equipment is not more than the limit specified for medium enterprises under clause (b) of sub-section (1) of Section 7 of the Micro, Small and Medium Enterprises Development Act, 2006.

Explanation 1. -- For the purpose of this clause, "enterprise" means an industrial undertaking or a business concern or any other establishment, by whatever name called, engaged in the manufacture or production of goods, in any manner, pertaining to any industry specified in the First Schedule to the Industries (Development and Regulation) Act, 1951 (65 of 1951) or engaged in providing or rendering of any service or services in such an industry.

Explanation 2. - In calculating the investment in plant and machinery, the cost of pollution control, research and development, industrial safety devices and such other things as may be specified by notification under the Micro, Small and Medium Enterprises Development Act, 2006 (27 of 2006), shall be excluded.

Explanation 3. - The reference rates of foreign currency of the Reserve Bank of India shall prevail.'.

3. In rule 7 of the principal rules, -
   (i) after sub rule (1), the following provisos shall be inserted, namely:-
   " Provided that ten per cent additional fee shall be payable when the applications for patent and other documents are filed through physical mode, namely, in hard copy format:
   Provided further that in the case of a small entity, every document, for which a fee has been specified, shall be accompanied by Form-28.".
   (ii) after sub-rule (3), the following sub-rule shall be inserted, namely:---
   "(3A) In case an application processed by a small entity is fully or partly transferred to a person other than a natural person (except a small entity), the difference, if any, in the scale of fee(s) between the fee(s) charged from a small entity and the fee(s) chargeable from the person other than a natural person (except a small entity) in the same matter shall be paid by the new applicant with the request for transfer." ;
4. In sub- rule (1) of rule 55 of the principal rules, after the words "shall be filed", the words, figure, brackets and letter " in Form 7 (A)" shall be inserted.
5. For the First Schedule to the principle rules, the following Schedule shall be substituted, namely :---

"THE FIRST SCHEDULE

(See rule 7)

FEES

Number of entry	On what payable	Number of the relevant Form	For e-filing			For physical filing		
			For natural person (s)	For person other than natural person(s) either alone or jointly with natural person(s)		For natural person (s) with ten per cent additional fee	For person other than natural person(s) either alone or jointly with natural person (s) with ten per cent additional fee.	
				For small entity	For others except small entity		For small entity	For Others except small entity
1	2	3	4	5	6	7	8	9
			Rupees	Rupees	Rupees	Rupees	Rupees	Rupees

Table *Contd...*

No.								
1.	On application for a patent under sections 7, 54 or 135 and rule 20(1) accompanied by provisional or complete specification—	1	1600 Multiple of 1600 in case of every multiple priority.	4000 Multiple of 4000 in case of every multiple priority.	8,000 Multiple of 8,000 in case of every multiple priority	1760 Multiple of 1760 in case of every multiple priority.	4400 Multiple of 4400 in case of every multiple priority.	8,800 Multiple of 8,800 in case of every multiple priority.
	(i) for each sheet of specification in addition to 30; (ii) for each claim in addition to 10.		(i) 160 (ii) 320	(i) 400 (ii) 800	(i)800 (ii) 1,600	(i) 176 (ii) 352	(i) 440 (ii) 880	(i) 880 (ii) 1760
2.	On filing complete specification after provisional upto 30 pages having up to 10 claims- (i) for each sheet of specification in addition to 30; (ii) for each claim in addition to 10.	2	No fee ((i) 160 (ii) 320	No fee (i) 400 (ii) 800	No fee (i) 800 (ii) 1,600	No fee (i) 176 (ii) 352	No fee (i) 440 (ii) 880	No fee (i) 880 (ii) 1760
3.	On filing a statement and undertaking under section 8.	3	No fee	No fee	No fee	No fee	No fee	No fee
4.	On request for extension of time under sections 53(2) and 142(4), rules 13(6), 80(1 A) and 130.	4	480 per month	1200 per month	2400 per month	528 per month	1320 per month	2640 per month
5.	On filing a declaration as to inventorship under rule 13(6).	5	No fee	No fee	No fee	No fee	No fee	No fee
6.	On application for postdating.	-	800	2000	4000	880	2200	4400
7.	On application for deletion of reference under section 19 (2).	-	800	2000	4000	880	2200	4400
8.	(i) On claim under section 20(1);	6	800	2000	4000	880	2200	4400
	(ii) On request for direction under section 20 (4) or 20 (5).	6	800	2000	4000	880	2200	4400

Table *Contd...*

9.	(i) On filing representation opposing grant of patent under section 25(1);	7A	No fee	No fee	No fee	No fee	No fee	No fee
	(ii) On notice of opposition to grant of patent under section 25(2).	7	2400	6000	12000	2640	6600	13200
10.	On giving notice that hearing before Controller shall be attended under rule 62(2).	–	1500	3750	7500	1650	4125	8250
11.	On application under sections 28(2), 28(3) or 28(7).	8	800	2000	4000	880	2200	4400
12.	Request for publication under section 11A(2) and rule24A.	9	2500	6250	12500	2750	6875	13750
13.	Application for withdrawing the application under section 11B(4) and rule 26(1) before publication of the application	--	1600	4000	8000	1760	4400	8800
14.	On request for examination of application for patent— (a) under section 11B and rule24(1); (b) under rule 20(4)(ii).	18	4000 5600	10000 14000	20000 28000	4400 6160	11000 15400	22000 30800
15.	On application under section 44 for amendment of patent.	10	2400	6000	12000	2640	6600	13200
16.	On application for directions under section 51(1) or 51(2).	11	2400	6000	12000	2640	6600	13200

Table *Contd...*

17.	On request for grant of a patent under sections 26(1) and 52(2).	12	2400	6000	12000	2640	6600	13200
18.	On request for converting a patent of addition to an independent patent under section 55 (1).	--	2400	6000	12000	2640	6600	13200
19.	For renewal of a patent under section 53-							
(i)	before the expiration of the 2nd year from the date of patent in respect of 3rd year;	-	800	2000	4000	880	2200	4400
(ii)	before the expiration of the 3rd year in respect of the 4th year;	-	800	2000	4000	880	2200	4400
(iii)	before the expiration of the 4th year in respect of the 5th year;	-	800	2000	4000	880	2200	4400
(iv)	before the expiration of the 5th year in respect of the 6th year;	-	800	2000	4000	880	2200	4400
(v)	before the expiration of the 6th year in respect of the 7th year;	-	2400	6000	12000	2640	6600	13200
(vi)	before the expiration of the 7th year in respect of the 8th year;	-	2400	6000	12000	2640	6600	13200
(vii)	before the expiration of the 8th year in respect of the 9th year;	-	2400	6000	12000	2640	6600	13200
(viii)	before the expiration of the 9th year in respect of the 10th year;	-	2400	6000	12000	2640	6600	13200
(ix)	before the expiration of the 10th year in respect of the 11th year;	-	4800	12000	24000	5280	13200	26400

Table *Contd...*

(x)	before the expiration of the 11th year in respect of the 12th year;	–	4800	12000	24000	5280	13200	26400
(xi)	before the expiration of the 12th year in respect of the 13th year;	–	4800	12000	24000	5280	13200	26400
(xii)	before the expiration of the 13th year in respect of the 14th year;	–	4800	12000	24000	5280	13200	26400
(xiii)	before the expiration of the 14th year in respect of the 15th year;	–	4800	12000	24000	5280	13200	26400
(xiv)	before the expiration of the 15th year in respect of the 16th year;	–	8000	20000	40000	8800	22000	44000
(xv)	before the expiration of the 16th year in respect of the 17th year;	–.	8000	20000	40000	8800	22000	44000
(xvi)	before the expiration of the 17th year in respect of the 18th year;	–	8000	20000	40000	8800	22000	44000
(xvii)	before the expiration of the 18th year in respect of the 19th year;	–	8000	20000	40000	8800	22000	44000
(xviii)	before the expiration of the 19th year in respect of the 20th year.		8000	20000	40000	8800	22000	44000
20.	On application for amendment of application for patent or complete specification or other related documents under section 57---	13						
(i)	before grant of patent;		800	2000	4000	880	2200	4400
(ii)	after grant of patent;		1600	4000	8000	1760	4400	8800
(iii)	where amendment is for changing name or address or nationality or address for service.		320	800	1600	352	880	1760

Table *Contd...*

21.	On notice of opposition to an application under sections 57(4), 61(1) and 87(2) or to surrender a patent under section 63(3) or to a request under section 78(5).	14	2400	6000	12000	2640	6600	13,200
22.	On application for restoration of a patent under section 60.	15	2400	6000	12000	2640	6600	13,200
23.	Additional fee for restoration.	--	4800	12000	24000	5280	13200	26400
24.	On notice of offer to surrender a patent under section 63.	--	1000	2500	5000	1100	2750	5500
25	On application for the entry in the register of patents of the name of a person entitled to a patent or as a share or as a mortgage or as licensee or as otherwise or for the entry in the register of patents of notification of a document under sections 69(1) or 69(2) and rules 90(1) or 90(2).	16	1600 (In respect of each patent)	4000 (In respect of each patent)	8,000 (In respect of each patent)	1760 (In respect of each patent)	4400 (In respect of each patent)	8,800 (In respect of each patent)
26.	On application for alteration of an entry in the register of patents or register of patent agent under rules 94(1) or rule 118(1).	--	320	800	1600	352	880	1,760
27.	On request for entry of an additional address for service in the Register of Patents under rule 94(3).	--	800	2000	4000	880	2200	4,400
28.	On application for compulsory license under sections 84(1), 91 (1), 92(1) and 92A.	17	2400	6000	12000	2640	6600	13200
29.	On application for revocation of a patent under section 85(1).	19	2400	6000	12000	2640	6600	13200

Table *Contd...*

30.	On application for revision of terms and conditions of licence under section 88(4).	20	2400	6000	12000	2640	6600	13200
31.	On request for termination of compulsory licence under section 94.	21	2400	6000	12000	2640	6600	13200
32.	On application for registration as a patent agent under rule 109 (1) or 112.	22	3200	-	-	3520	-	-
33.	On request for appearing in the qualifying examination under rule 109(3).	--	1600	-	-	1760		-
34.	For continuance of the name of a person in the register of patent agent— (i) for the 1ˢᵗ year to be paid along with registration; (ii) for every year excluding the 1st year to be paid on the 1st April in each year.	- -	800 800	- -	- -	880 880	- -	- -
35.	On application for duplicate certificate of patent agent under rule 111A.	-	1600	-	-	1760		-
36.	On application for restoration of the name of a person in the register of patent agents under rule 117(1).	23	1600 (Plus continuation fee under entry number 34)	-	-	1760 (Plus continuation fee under entry number 34)	-	-
37.	On a request for correction of clerical error under section 78(2).	--	800	2000	4000	880	2200	4400

Table Contd…

No.	Description							
38.	On application for review or setting aside the decisions or order of the controller under section 77(l) (f) or 77(l) (g).	24	1600	4000	8000	1760	4400	8800
39	On application for permission for applying patent outside India under section 39 and rule 71(1).	25	1600	4000	8000	1760	4400	8800
40	On application for duplicate patent under section 154 and rule 132.	--	1600	4000	8000	1760	4400	8800
41	On request for certified copies under section 72 or for certificate under section 147 and rule 133.	--	1000 (up to 30 pages and, thereafter, 30 for each extra page)	2500 (up to 30 pages and, thereafter, 75 for each extra page)	5000 (up to 30 pages and, thereafter, 150 for each extra page) thereafter)	1100 (up to 30 pages and, thereafter, 30 for each extra page)	2750 (up to 30 pages and, thereafter, 75 for each extra page)	5500 (up to 30 pages and, thereafter, 150 for each extra page) thereafter)
42	For certifying office copies, printed each.	--	800	2000	4000	880	2200	4400
43	On request for inspection of register under section 72, inspection under rule 27 or rule 74A.	--	320	800	1600	352	880	1760
44	On request for information under sections 127, 132 and 153 and rule135.	--	480	1200	2400	528	1320	2640
45	On form of authorisation of patent agent.	26	No fee	No fee	No fee	No fee	No fee	No fee
46	On petition not otherwise provided for.	--	1600	4000	8000	1760	4400	8800

Table _Contd..._

47	For supplying of photocopies of the documents per page.	--	8	8	8	8	8	8
48	Transmittal fee for International application.	--	3200	8000	16000	3250	8800	17600
49	For preparation of certified copy of priority document and for transmission of the same to the International Bureau of World Intellectual Property Organisation.	--	1000 (up to 30 pages and, thereafter, 30 for each extra page)	2500 (up to 30 pages and, thereafter, 75 for each extra page)	5000 (up to 30 pages and, thereafter, 150 for each extra page)	1100 (up to 30 pages and, thereafter, 30 for each extra page)	2750 (up to 30 pages and, thereafter, 75 for each extra page)	5500 (up to 30 pages and, thereafter, 150 for each extra page)
50	On statement regarding working of a patented invention on a commercial scale in India under section 146(2) and rule 131(1).	27	No fee	No fee	No fee	No fee	No fee	No fee

Note: All the Forms, Applications, Requests, Notices and Petitions shall be filed in duplicate unless otherwise specified in the rules.

6. In the Second Schedule to the principle rules, in the "LIST OF FORMS"—

(i) after "Form No. 7", the following shall be inserted, namely :—

"7A.	Section 25(1) and rule 55 (1)	For filing a representation opposing grant of a patent under sub-section (1) of section 25.";

(ii) after "Form No. 27", the following shall be inserted, namely :—

"28.	Rules 2(fa) and 7	To be submitted by a small entity with every document for which a fee has been specified".

7. In the Second Schedule to the principle rules,-

(i) after Form 7, the following Form shall be inserted, namely :—

"FORM 7A

THE PATENTS ACT, 1970 (39 OF 1970)

AND

THE PATENTS RULES, 2003

REPRESENTATION FOR OPPOSITION TO GRANT OF PATENT

[see rule 55]

1. State names, address and nationality.

I/We,.....................................
....
hereby give representation by way of opposition to the grant of patent in respect of application no.................dated...............   made by........... and published on ....

2. State the grounds taken one after another.

on the grounds ....
....
....

3. Complete address including postal
....
index number/code and state along

with telephone and fax number.

My/our address for service in India is

....

....

4. To be signed by the opponent or by his/her authorized registered patent agent.

Signature

5. Name and designation of the natural person who has signed.

(............................)

To
The Controller of Patents,
The Patent Office,
At ...." ;
    (i)   after Form 27, the following Form shall be inserted, namely :

"FORM 28
THE PATENTS ACT, 1970
(39 of 1970)
AND
THE PATENTS RULES, 2003
TO BE SUBMITTED BY A SMALL ENTITY

[See rules 2(fa) and 7]

Insert name, address and nationality.

I/We ....
....
....
applicant/patentee in respect of the patent application no. ....or patent no............
hereby declare that I/we am/are a small entity in accordance with rule 2(fa) and submit the following document(s) as proof:

State the particulars of the documents.

To be signed by the applicant(s) / patentee (s) / authorised registered patent agent.

Name of the natural person who has signed.

Designation and official seal, if any, of the person who has signed.

(i.) Evidence of registration under the Micro, Small and Medium Enterprises Act, 2006 (27 of 2006 (in case of Indian entities).

(ii.) Any other document (in case of foreign entities). The information provided herein is correct to the best of my/our knowledge and belief.

Dated this ....day of .... 20...

Signature ....
(Name) ....
(Designation) ....

To
The Controller of Patents,
The Patent Office,
At.................................

Note: Indian entities shall submit the evidence mentioned above to be eligible for claiming the status of a small entity.".

8. For the Fourth Schedule to the principle rules, the following Schedule shall be substituted, namely :-

"THE FOURTH SCHEDULE

[See proviso to rule 136(1)]

Number of entry	Matter in respect of which cost to be awarded	Amount in fees (in rupees)		
		For natural person(s)	For person other than natural person(s) either alone or jointly with natural person (s)	
			For small entity	For others except small entity
1	2	3	4	5
1	For notice of opposition under sections 25, 57, 60, 63, 78, 87(2) or 88(4).	2400	6000	12000
2	For application for compulsory licence under sections 84(1), 91(1) or 92(1).	1500	3000	6000
3	For application for revision of terms and conditions of licence under section 88(4) .	2400	6000	12000
4	For notice of intention to attend the hearing under rule 62(2).	1500	3000	6000

Table *Contd...*

		The amount actually paid.	The amount actually paid.	The amount actually paid.
5	Stamp fee for power of attorney where a patent agent or other person has been appointed or stamp fee in respect of relevant affidavits.			
6	For written statement under rule 57 or reply statement under rule 58 or for each affidavit, if relevant.	4000	4000	5000
7	For each document of publication produced in the proceedings, if relevant	1600	1600	2000
8	For each unnecessary or irrelevant affidavit or citation.	1600	1600	2000
9	For every day or part day of hearing before the Controller.	4000	4000	5000".

[F.No. 14/6/2012-IPR-III]
D.V. PRASAD, Jt. Secy.

Footnote:- The principal rules were published in the Gazette of India *vide* notification number S.O.493 (E), dated the 2nd May, 2003, and subsequently amended *vide* notification number –
(i) S.O.1418 (E), dated the 28th December, 2004;
(ii) S.O. 657 (E), dated the 5th May, 2006; and
(iii) S.O. 2296 (E), dated the 25th September, 2012.
(iv) S.O. 1029 (E), dated 23rd April, 2013.

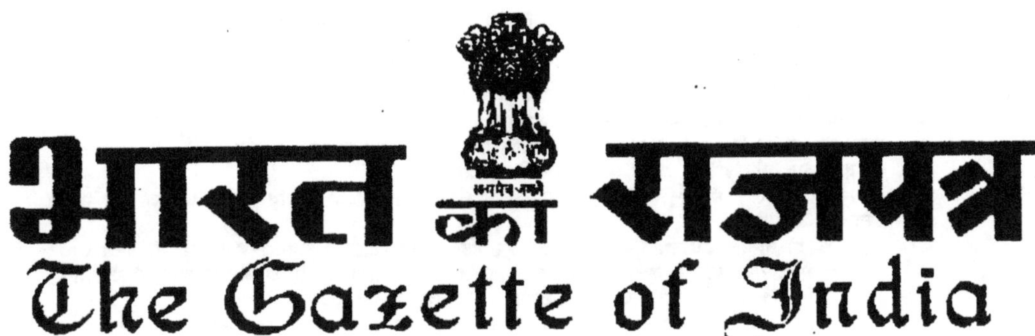

असाधारण

EXTRAORDINARY

भाग II—खण्ड 3—उप-खण्ड (ii)

PART II—Section 3—Sub-section (ii)

प्राधिकार से प्रकाशित

PUBLISHED BY AUTHORITY

सं. 906]	नई दिल्ली, मंगलवार, अप्रैल 23, 2013/वैशाख 3, 1935
No. 906]	**NEW DELHI, TUESDAY, APRIL 23, 2013/VAISAKHA 3, 1935**

वाणिज्य और उद्योग मंत्रालय
(औद्योगिक नीति और संवर्धन विभाग)
अधिसूचना
नई दिल्ली, 23 अप्रैल, 2013

का. आ. 1029(अ).– पेटेंट अधिनियम, 1970 (1970 का 39)की धारा 159 द्वारा प्रदत्त शक्तियों का प्रयोग करते हुए कतिपय प्रारूप नियम, ऐसे व्यक्तियों से, जिनके उनसे प्रभावित होने की संभावना है, उस तारीख से, जिसको अधिसूचना वाले राजपत्र की प्रतियां जनसाधारण को उपलब्ध कराई गई थी, पन्द्रह दिन की अवधि की समाप्ति से पूर्व आक्षेप और सुझाव आमंत्रित करने के लिए भारत के राजपत्र, असाधारण, भाग–II खण्ड 3, उप-खण्ड (ii)में भारत सरकार, उद्योग मंत्रालय (औद्योगिक नीति और संवर्धन विभाग) की अधिसूचना संख्यांक का. आ. 189 (अ), तारीख 17 जनवरी, 2013 द्वारा प्रकाशित किए गए थे।

और उक्त अधिसूचना वाले राजपत्र की प्रतियां तारीख 17 जनवरी, 2013 को जनसाधारण को उपलब्ध करा दी गई थी।

और उक्त प्रारूप नियमों के संबंध में इस विभाग को जनसाधारण से कोई आक्षेप या सुझाव प्राप्त नहीं हुआ है।

अत: अब, केन्द्रीय सरकार, पेटेंट अधिनियम, 1970 (1970 का 39) की धारा 159 द्वारा प्रदत्त शक्तियों का प्रयोग करते हुए, पेटेंट नियम, 2003 का और संशोधन करने के लिए निम्नलिखित नियम बनाती है, अर्थात् –

1   (1) इन नियमों का संक्षिप्त नाम पेटेंट (संशोधन) नियम, 2013 है।

(2) ये उस तारीख को प्रवृत्त होंगे जो केन्द्रीय सरकार राजपत्र में अधिसूचना द्वारा नियत करे।

2.   **पेटेंट नियम, 2003 (जिसे इसमें इसके पश्चात् उक्त नियम कहा गया है) के नियम 4 में उप–नियम (2) में निम्नलिखित उप–नियम अंत: स्थापित किया जाएगा, अर्थात् –**

"(3) उप–नियम (2) में अंतर्विष्ट किसी बात के होते हुए भी, नियंत्रक पेटेंट के लिए इस प्रकार फाइल आवेदन यथास्थिति पेटेंट कार्यालय के प्रधान कार्यालय या शाखा कार्यालय को अंतरित कर सकेगा।

(4) उप—नियम (1) में अंतर्दिष्ट किसी बात के होते हुए भी अधिनियम की धारा 16 में निर्दिष्ट और आवेदन केवल पहले उल्लिखित समुचित कार्यालय में फाइल किया जा सकेगा।

(5)पेटेंट (संशोधन) नियम, 2013 के प्रारंभ के पूर्व पहले उल्लिखित आवेदन के समुचित कार्यालय से भिन्न अधिनियम की धारा 16 में निर्दिष्ट किसी कार्यालय में फाइल सभी और आवेदनों को पहले उल्लिखित आवेदन के समुचित कार्यालय को हस्तांतरित किया जाएगा"।

3. उक्त नियमों के नियम 9 के स्थान पर निम्नलिखित नियम रखा जाएगा, अर्थात् –

"9 दस्तावेज और प्रतियाँ आदि का फाइल किया जाना–

(1) पेटेंट कार्यालय में फाइल किए गए शपथ-पत्र और रेखाचित्रों के सिवाय सभी दस्तावेज और अन्य दस्तावेजों की प्रतियाँ–

(क) न्यूनतम डेढ़ स्थान-अंतराल रखते हुए गहरे अमिट स्याही में कम-से-कम 0.28 सेंटीमीटर उच्च स्पष्ट तथा पठनीय अक्षरों में कागज के केवल एक ही तरफ हिन्दी या अंग्रेजी भाषा में (जब तक नियंत्रक द्वारा अन्यथा निदेश या अनुज्ञात न हो) टंकित अथवा मुद्रित होगी;

(ख) ऐसे किसी कागज पर होगी जो नम्य, सुदृढ, चिकने, अचमकीले तथा टिकाऊ, ए4 आकार के लगभग 29.7 सेंटीमीटर और 21 सेंटीमीटर लम्बाई-चौड़ाई के, जिनके शीर्ष और वाम-हस्त की ओर न्यूनतम 4 सेंटीमीटर तथा नीचे और दाहिनी ओर 3 सेंटीमीटर का हाशिया छोड़ते हुए हो;

(ग) कागज के नीचे केन्द्र में अरेबिक संख्याओं की निरंतर क्रम में संख्यांकित होंगी।

(घ) वर्णन के प्रत्येक पृष्ठ तथा दावों के प्रत्येक पृष्ठ के प्रत्येक पांचवीं पंक्ति पर बाऐं हाशिए के दायें अर्द्ध में संख्या लिखी होगी।

(2) कोई हस्ताक्षर जो पठनीय नहीं है या जो अंग्रेजी या हिन्दी के अतिरिक्त किसी लिपि में लिखित हो, उसके साथ उस नाम का अनुलिपिकरण या तो हिन्दी या अंग्रेजी के बड़े अक्षरों में संलग्न किया जाएगा।

(3) यदि पेटेंट आवेदन न्यूक्लियोटाइड्स की क्रम सूची अथवा अमीनो-अम्ल अनुक्रम प्रकट करता हो, तो वह न्यूक्लियोटाइड्स की क्रम सूची अथवा अमीनो-अम्ल अनुक्रम आवेदन के साथ कम्प्यूटर पठनीय इलेक्ट्रॉनिक प्ररूप में फाइल किया जाएगा और न्यूक्लियोटाइड्स की क्रम सूची अथवा अमीनो-अम्ल अनुक्रम की कोई मुद्रित प्रति देना आवश्यक नहीं होगा।

(4) सभी दस्तावेजों की अतिरिक्त प्रतियाँ समुचित कार्यालय में फाइल किए जाएंगे जो नियंत्रक द्वारा अपेक्षित हो।

(5) आवेदक तथा अन्य व्यक्तियों के नाम और पते, उनकी राष्ट्रीयता और ऐसी अन्य विशिष्टियाँ, यदि हों, जो उनकी पहचान हेतु आवश्यक हो, के साथ पूर्ण रूप में दी जाएगी"।

4. उक्त नियमों के नियम 17 में, खंड (क) के पश्चात् निम्नलिखित खंड अंतःस्थापित किए जाएंगे, अर्थात् :–

(कक) "परीक्षण प्राधिकारी" से नियम 19च के उप-नियम (1) में निर्दिष्ट भारतीय अन्तर राष्ट्रीय प्रारंभिक परीक्षण प्राधिकरण अभिप्रेत है;

(कख) "अन्तरराष्ट्रीय अधिकारी" से विश्व बौद्धिक सम्पदा संगठन का अन्तरराष्ट्रीयखोज प्राधिकारी अभिप्रेत है;

(कग) "खोज अधिकारी" से नियम 19क के उप-नियम (1) में निर्दिष्ट भारतीय अन्तरराष्ट्रीय खोज प्राधिकारी अभिप्रेत है

5. उक्त नियमों के नियम 18 के स्थान पर निम्नलिखित नियम रखा जाएगा, अर्थात् :–

"18 अन्तरराष्ट्रीय आवेदनों के सम्बन्ध में समुचित कार्यालय–

(1)   अन्तरराष्ट्रीय आवेदनों के प्रयोजनों के लिए यथास्थिति प्राप्तकर्ता कार्यालय, अभिहित कार्यालय और चयनित कार्यालय, नियम 4 में निर्दिष्ट समुचित कार्यालय होगा।

(2) उप-नियम (1) में अंतर्विष्ट किसी बात के होते हुए भी, पेटेंट कार्यालय, दिल्ली शाखा अन्तरराष्ट्रीय ब्यूरो तथा किसी अन्य अन्तरराष्ट्रीय खोज प्राधिकारी तथा अन्तरराष्ट्रीय प्रारंभिक परीक्षण प्राधिकारी के साथ कार्य करने हेतु समुचित कार्यालय होगा ।

(3) अन्तरराष्ट्रीय आवेदन, इस अध्याय के उपबन्धों के अनुसार, इस संधि और इस संधि के अधीन स्थापित विनियमों के अनुसार उप-नियम (1) में निर्दिष्ट समुचित कार्यालय में फाइल किया जाएगा और समुचित कार्यालय द्वारा उस पर कार्यवाही की जाएगी।

(4) उप-नियम (1) में उल्लिखित समुचित कार्यालय कोई अन्तरराष्ट्रीय आवेदन प्राप्त होने पर,

(क) उस आवेदन की एक प्रति रख लेगा जिसे "गृह प्रति" कहा जाएगा;

(ख) एक प्रति जिसे "अभिलेख प्रति" कहा जाएगा, अन्तरराष्ट्रीय ब्यूरो को भेजेगा, और

(ग) एक प्रति जिसे "खोज प्रति" कहा जाएगा संधि के अनुच्छेद 16 में निर्दिष्ट अन्तरराष्ट्रीय खोज प्राधिकारी को प्रेषित करेगा और साथ ही ऐसे आवेदन के पूर्ण ब्यौरे पेटेंट कार्यालय दिल्ली को भेजेगा।

6. उक्त नियमों के नियम 19 के स्थान पर निम्नलिखित उप नियम रखा जाएगा, अर्थात् :–

"19 प्राप्तकर्त्ता कार्यालय के रूप में समुचित कार्यालय के साथ फाइल किए गए अन्तरराष्ट्रीय आवेदन–

(1) कोई अन्तरराष्ट्रीय आवेदन या तो अंग्रेजी या हिन्दी में तीन प्रतियों में समुचित कार्यालय के साथ फाइल किया जाएगा।

(2) अन्तरराष्ट्रीय आवेदन की बाबत संदेय फीस, संधि के अधीन विनियमों में विनिर्दिष्ट फीस के अतिरिक्त पहली अनुसूची या पांचवीं अनुसूची में यथा विनिर्दिष्ट फीस होगी।

(3) जहाँ कोई अन्तरराष्ट्रीय आवेदन तीन प्रतियों में फाइल नहीं किए गए हैं वहाँ समुचित कार्यालय प्रथम अनुसूची में विनिर्दिष्ट फीस के संदाय पर अपेक्षित अतिरिक्त प्रतियाँ तैयार करेगा।

(4) आवेदक से अनुरोध प्राप्त होने पर और प्रथम अनुसूची में विनिर्दिष्ट फीस का भुगतान करने के बाद समुचित कार्यालय पूर्विकता दस्तावेज की एक सत्यापित प्रति तैयार करेगा और उसे शीघ्रता से अन्तरराष्ट्रीय ब्यूरो को प्रेषित करते हुए आवेदक और पेटेंट कार्यालय की दिल्ली शाखा को इसकी सूचना देगा।"

३.   क. भारतीय अन्तरराष्ट्रीय खोज प्राधिकारी –

(1)   भारतीय पेटेंट कार्यालय और अन्तरराष्ट्रीय ब्यूरो के बीच हुए समझौते के अनुसरण में संधि के तहत पेटेंट कार्यालय, दिल्ली शाखा भारतीय अन्तरराष्ट्रीय खोज प्राधिकारी के कृत्यों का निष्पादन करेगा।

(2) खोज प्राधिकारी को संदेय फीस, संधि के तहत निर्मित विनियमों में विनिर्दिष्ट फीस के अतिरिक्त, पांचवीं अनुसूची में यथा निर्दिष्ट फीस होगी।

(3)उपनियम (1) में निर्दिष्ट खोज प्राधिकारी, अन्तरराष्ट्रीय आवेदनों के सम्बन्ध में अन्तरराष्ट्रीय खोज रिपोर्ट तैयार करेगा अथवा नियम 19 ख के उपनियम (3) के अनुसार घोषित करेगा, यथास्थिति, जहाँ भारत को सक्षम खोज प्राधिकारी के रूप में इंगित किया गया है।

३.   ख. अन्तरराष्ट्रीय खोज रिपोर्ट–

(1) खोज प्राधिकारी खोज प्रति प्राप्त होने पर, उसके पहचान चिहन 'ISA/IN' के साथ खोज प्रति की अन्तरराष्ट्रीय आवेदन संख्या तथा उसकी क्रम संख्या और प्राप्ति की तारीख देते हुए अन्तरराष्ट्रीय ब्यूरो और उस आवेदक को खोज प्रति की प्राप्ति के सम्बन्ध में अधिसूचित करेगा।

(2) नियम 24ख के उप नियम (2) की मद (i) के परंतुक में अंतर्विष्ट किसी बात के होते हुए भी, खोज प्राधिकारी, खोज प्रति प्राप्त होने पर, उस आदेश में जिसमें खोज प्रति प्राप्त की गई थी, अन्तरराष्ट्रीय आवेदन किसी परीक्षक या अधिनियम की धारा 73 की उप–धारा (2) के तहत नियुक्त किसी अन्य अधिकारी को इस संधि और इसके अंतर्गत स्थापित विनियमों में निहित उपबंधों के अनुसरण में ऐसे संदर्भ की तारीख से सामान्यत: एक महीने की अवधि के भीतर, जो दो महीने से अधिक नहीं होगी, अन्तरराष्ट्रीय खोज रिपोर्ट बनाने के लिए निर्दिष्ट करेगा।

(3) खोज प्राधिकारी का यदि यह विचार है कि –

(क) अन्तरराष्ट्रीय आवेदन उस विषय–वस्तु से संबद्ध है जिस पर खोज प्राधिकारी के लिए खोज करना अपेक्षित नहीं है तथा वह तदनुसार खोज न करने का विनिश्चय करता है; या

(ख) वर्णन, दावे और आरेख विनियमों के अधीन विहित अपेक्षाओं के अनुपालन में उस सीमा तक असफल है कि एक अर्थपूर्ण खोज संचालित नहीं की जा सके,

तो उक्त प्राधिकारी आवेदक तथा अन्तरराष्ट्रीय ब्यूरो को यह घोषणा करेगा तथा अधिसूचित करेगा कि कोई अन्तरराष्ट्रीय खोज रिपोर्ट तैयार नहीं की जाएगी।

(4) ऐसे संदर्भ में जहां उप–नियम (3) के खंड (क) तथा (ख) में निर्दिष्ट कोई स्थिति केवल किसी दावे के सम्बन्ध में विद्यमान पाई गई, तो खोज प्राधिकारी ऐसे दावे की बाबत अन्तरराष्ट्रीय खोज रिपोर्ट में इस तथ्य का उल्लेख करेगा, और अन्य दावे के लिए, वह अन्तरराष्ट्रीय खोज रिपोर्ट तैयार करेगा।

(5) खोज प्राधिकारी का, यदि यह विचार है कि अन्तरराष्ट्रीय आवेदन संधि के तहत विनियमों के नियम 13 में विनिर्दिष्ट उपबंधों के अनुसरण में आविष्कार की एकलता की अपेक्षाओं का अनुपालन नहीं करती है तो वह उन कारणों को विनिर्दिष्ट करते हुए जिसके कारण उस अन्तरराष्ट्रीय आवेदन को आविष्कार की एकलता की अपेक्षाओं का अनुपालन नहीं करने वाला माना गया है एक सूचना भेजेगा और आवेदक को आमंत्रित करेगा:

(क) ऐसे आविष्कार की तारीख से एक मास की अवधि के भीतर संदेय की जाने वाली फीस की रकम उपदर्शित करते हुए पांचवीं अनुसूची में विनिर्दिष्ट फीस का भुगतान करना; और

(ख) ऐसे आविष्कार की तारीख से एक मास की अवधि के लिए संदेय फीस की राशि उपदर्शित करते हुए पांचवीं अनुसूची में विनिर्दिष्ट प्रतिवाद फीस, जहाँ लागू हो, का भुगतान करना।

(6) खोज प्राधिकारी अन्तरराष्ट्रीय आवेदन के उन भागों पर अन्तरराष्ट्रीय खोज रिपोर्ट स्थापित करेगा जो दावे (मुख्य आविष्कार) में सर्वप्रथम उल्लिखित आविष्कार से संबंधित हो जिसके बाबत उक्त फीस का भुगतान किए गया था, के अध्यधीन उप–नियम (5) में विनिर्दिष्ट समयावधि के भीतर अतिरिक्त फीस का भुगतान कर दिया गया हो।

(7) कोई आवेदक विरोध के तहत अतिरिक्त फीस का भुगतान करेगा अर्थात् इस प्रभाव का एक तार्किक कथन-संलग्न करते हुए कि अन्तरराष्ट्रीय आवेदन आविष्कार की एकलता की अपेक्षाओं को पूरा करता है या यह कि अपेक्षित अतिरिक्त फीस की राशि अत्यधिक है।

(8) उप–नियम (7) में निर्दिष्ट प्रतिवाद का परीक्षण नियंत्रक द्वारा गठित एक पुनर्विलोकन समिति द्वारा किया जाएगा।

(9) उप–नियम (8) के अधीन गठित पुनर्विलोकन समिति उस सीमा का परीक्षण करेगी जहाँ तक वह प्रतिवाद युक्तिसंगत है और तदनुसार आवेदक को अतिरिक्त फीस की पूर्ण या आंशिक प्रतिपूर्ति का आदेश देगी।

(10) जहाँ आवेदक ने उप–नियम (5) के उपबंध (ख) के अनुसार प्रतिवाद फीस को सदत्त नहीं किया है, यह मान लिया जाएगा कि विरोध नहीं किया गया है और खोज प्राधिकारी ऐसी घोषणा करेगा।

(11) जहाँ उप–नियम (8) में निर्दिष्ट पुनर्विलोकन समिति यह पाती है कि प्रतिवाद पूर्णतया युक्तिसंगत था तो आवेदक को प्रतिवाद फीस वापस कर दी जाएगी।

(12) जहाँ अन्तरराष्ट्रीय आवेदन में एक या अधिक न्यूक्लियोटाइड या अमीनो अम्ल अनुक्रम अनुसूची का प्रकटीकरण अन्तर्विष्ट है और वह अनुक्रम कम्प्यूटर पठनीय प्ररूप में प्रस्तुत नहीं किया गया है, यहाँ खोज प्राधिकारी उस आवेदक को एक सूचना भेजेगा कि वह उस सूचना की तारीख से एक मास की अवधि के भीतर अनुक्रम अनुसूची को कम्प्यूटर पठनीय प्ररूप में प्रस्तुत करे और पांचवीं अनुसूची में विहित विलम्ब फर्निसिंग फीस का भुगतान करे और यदि आवेदक उस सूचना का अनुपालन करने में असफल रहता है तो खोज प्राधिकारी उस सीमा तक अन्तरराष्ट्रीय खोज संचालित करेगा जहाँ तक कि अनुक्रम अनुसूची किए बिना अर्थपूर्ण खोज संचालित किया जा सके।

19.   ग.   **अन्तरराष्ट्रीय खोज रिपोर्ट स्थापित करने की समय सीमा –**
खोज प्राधिकारी नियम 19 ख के उप–नियम 3 में निर्दिष्ट अन्तरराष्ट्रीय खोज रिपोर्ट तथा, यथास्थिति, लिखित राय या घोषणा उक्त खोज प्राधिकारी द्वारा खोज प्रति प्राप्त होने की तारीख से तीन महीने या प्रायिकता की तारीख से नौ महीने की अवधि के भीतर, जो भी समय सीमा बाद में समाप्त होती हो, स्थापित करेगा।

19.   घ.   **अन्तरराष्ट्रीय खोज रिपोर्ट और लिखित राय आदि का पारेषण –**
अन्तरराष्ट्रीय खोज प्राधिकारी अन्तरराष्ट्रीय खोज रिपोर्ट या इस संधि के अनुच्छेद 17 (2) (क) में निर्दिष्ट उद्घोषणा की एक प्रति और इस संधि के अधीन निर्मित विनियमों के नियम 43 बीआईएस. 1 के अधीन स्थापित लिखित राय की एक प्रति अन्तरराष्ट्रीय ब्यूरो को और एक प्रति आवेदक को उसी दिन पारेषित करेगा।

19.   ङ   **गोपनीय व्यवहार**–अन्तरराष्ट्रीय आवेदन से संबद्ध सभी विषयों को इस संधि और इसके अधीन विनियमों के अनुसार गोपनीय रखा जाएगा।

19.   च.   **भारतीय अन्तरराष्ट्रीय प्रारंभिक परीक्षण प्राधिकारी –**
(1) पेटेंट कार्यालय, दिल्ली शाखा, भारतीय अन्तरराष्ट्रीय प्रारंभिक परीक्षण प्राधिकारी के रूप में कार्य करेगा और भारतीय पेटेंट कार्यालय एवं अन्तरराष्ट्रीय ब्यूरो के बीच हुए समझौते के अनुसार इस संधि के तहत अन्तरराष्ट्रीय प्रारंभिक परीक्षण प्राधिकारी के कृत्यों का निष्पादन करेगा।

(2) उप–नियम (1), में निर्दिष्ट परीक्षण प्राधिकारी निम्नलिखित स्थापित करेगा–

     (क) अन्तरराष्ट्रीय प्रारंभिक परीक्षण प्राधिकारी के रूप में भारत का चयन करने वाले सभी अन्तरराष्ट्रीय आवेदनों के संदर्भ में अन्तरराष्ट्रीय प्रारंभिक परीक्षण रिपोर्ट;

     (ख) अन्य देशों के राष्ट्रीकों अथवा निवासियों द्वारा भारतीय पेटेंट कार्यालय तथा अन्तरराष्ट्रीय ब्यूरो के बीच हुए समझौते के अनुसार फाइल की गई माँगों के सम्बन्ध में, अन्तरराष्ट्रीय ब्यूरो द्वारा अधिसूचित किए जाने के बाद;

     (ग) अन्य देशों के ऐसे राष्ट्रीकों या निवासियों जो इस संधि का भाग नहीं है या इस संधि के अध्याय 2 द्वारा आबद्ध नहीं है, द्वारा की गई माँगों के सम्बन्ध में अन्तरराष्ट्रीय प्रारंभिक परीक्षण, यदि सभा ने इस प्रकार अनुमोदित किया है।

19. छ. **माँग करने की अवधि–**
(1) अन्तरराष्ट्रीय प्रारंभिक परीक्षण की माँग, संधि के अधीन या उस संधि के अधीन बनाए गए विनियमों में विनिर्दिष्ट अवधि के भीतर की जाएगी।

(2) उप–नियम (1) में विनिर्दिष्ट अवधि की समाप्ति के पश्चात् की गई माँग की दशा में, यह समझा जाएगा कि माँग नहीं की गई है और कोई अन्तरराष्ट्रीय प्रारंभिक परीक्षण प्रतिवेदन तैयार नहीं किया जाएगा।

19. ज. **परीक्षणकर्ता प्राधिकारी को संदेय फीस** –परीक्षण प्राधिकारी को संदेय फीस, संधि के अधीन निर्मित विनियमों में निर्दिष्ट फीस के अतिरिक्त पांचवी अनुसूची में यथा निर्दिष्ट फीस होगी।

19. झ. **माँग करने की रीति**–इन नियमों, इस संधि और इसके अधीन विनियमों में निहित उपबंधों के अनुसार माँग की जा सकेगी।

19. ञ. **अन्तरराष्ट्रीय प्रारंभिक परीक्षा हेतु माँगों पर कार्यवाही–**
(1) परीक्षण प्राधिकारी, अन्तरराष्ट्रीय प्रारंभिक परीक्षा हेतु माँग प्राप्त होने पर, यदि परीक्षण प्राधिकारी अन्तरराष्ट्रीय प्रारंभिक परीक्षा संचालित करने में सक्षम है, पहचान चिन्ह 'आईपीईए/आई एन' प्रदान करेगा और आवेदक और अन्तरराष्ट्रीय ब्यूरो को अधिसूचित करेगा।

(2) जहाँ परीक्षण प्राधिकारी अन्तरराष्ट्रीय आवेदन का अन्तरराष्ट्रीय प्रारंभिक परीक्षा संचालित करने में सक्षम नहीं है तो वहाँ प्राधिकारी तुरन्त वह माँग अन्तरराष्ट्रीय ब्यूरो को पारेषित कर देगा।

19. ट. **अन्तरराष्ट्रीय प्रारंभिक परीक्षण प्रतिवेदन** –(1) नियम 24 ख के उप नियम (2) की मद (i) के परंतुक में अंतर्विष्ट किसी बात के होते हुए भी, परीक्षण प्राधिकारी इस संधि और इसके अधीन विनियमों में अंतर्विष्ट उपबंधों के अनुसार अन्तरराष्ट्रीय आवेदन को, भारतीय अन्तरराष्ट्रीय प्रारंभिक परीक्षण प्राधिकारी के समक्ष प्राप्त माँग के क्रमानुसार सामान्यतः तीन महीने किंतु ऐसे संदर्भ की तारीख से चार महीने से कम की अवधि के भीतर एक अन्तरराष्ट्रीय प्रारंभिक परीक्षण प्रतिवेदन तैयार करने के लिए किसी परीक्षक या अधिनियम की धारा 73 की उप–धारा (2) के तहत नियुक्त किसी अन्य अधिकारी के पास भेजेगा।

(2) उस आविष्कार के सम्बन्ध में दावे, जिन पर कोई अन्तरराष्ट्रीय खोज रिपोर्ट तैयार नहीं की गई है वह अन्तरराष्ट्रीय प्रारंभिक परीक्षण का विषय नहीं होगा।

(3) परीक्षण प्राधिकारी यदि यह विचार करता है कि –

(क) वह अन्तरराष्ट्रीय आवेदन उस विषय वस्तु से संबंधित है जिस पर अन्तरराष्ट्रीय प्रारंभिक परीक्षण प्राधिकारी को कोई अन्तरराष्ट्रीय प्रारंभिक परीक्षण संचालित करने की आवश्यकता नहीं है, और उस विशेष मामले में, ऐसा परीक्षण संचालित नहीं करने का विनिश्चय करता है, या

(ख) विवरण, दावे या आरेख इतने अस्पष्ट हैं अथवा दावों के समर्थन में प्रदत्त विवरण इतना अपर्याप्त है कि नवीनता, आविष्कारिक चरण (अभिनव), या औद्योगिक अनुप्रयोग के प्रश्न पर कोई अर्थपूर्ण राय सृजित नहीं की जा सकती, तो परीक्षण प्राधिकारी इन प्रश्नों में नहीं उलझेगा और अपनी राय एवं उसके कारणों की सूचना आवेदक को देगा।

(4) ऐसे किसी मामले में जहाँ उप–नियम (3) के खंड (क) या उपबंध (ख) में निर्दिष्ट कोई स्थिति केवल कतिपय दावे के सम्बन्ध में विद्यमान पायी जाती है तो परीक्षण प्राधिकारी ऐसे दावे की बाबत अन्तरराष्ट्रीय प्रारंभिक परीक्षण रिपोर्ट में इस तथ्य को इंगित करेगा और अन्य दावों के लिए अन्तरराष्ट्रीय प्रारंभिक परीक्षण रिपोर्ट तैयार करेगा।

(5) जहाँ परीक्षण प्राधिकारी यह पाता है कि संधि के अधीन विनियमों के नियम 13 में अंतर्विष्ट उपबंधों के अनुसार अन्तरराष्ट्रीय आवेदन आविष्कार की एकलता की अपेक्षा को पूरा नहीं करता और अपनी राय के अनुसार, आवेदक को दावों का प्रतिबंध अथवा अतिरिक्त फीस का भुगतान करने के लिए आमंत्रित करना चाहता है, वह आवेदक को एक नोटिस जारी करेगा :

    (क) कम से कम एक संभावित निर्वधन विनिर्दिष्ट करेगा जो उस परीक्षण प्राधिकारी की राय में प्रयोज्य अपेक्षा के अनुसरण में हो;

    (ख) उस कारण को निर्दिष्ट करेगा जिसके लिए उस अन्तरराष्ट्रीय आवेदन को आविष्कार की एकलता की अपेक्षा का अनुसरण नहीं करता हुआ पाया गया है;

    (ग) आवेदक को आमंत्रण की तारीख से एक मास के भीतर आमंत्रण का अनुसरण करने के लिए बुलाएगा;

    (घ) अपेक्षित अतिरिक्त फीस की रकम को उपदर्शित करेगा यदि आवेदक ऐसा विकल्प करे; और

    (ड.) आवेदक को आवेदन की तारीख से एक महीने के भीतर प्रतिवाद फीस का भुगतान करने के लिए आमंत्रित करेगा और पांचवीं अनुसूची में यथानिर्दिष्ट भुगतान की जाने वाली रकम का उल्लेख करेगा।

(6) कोई आवेदक अतिरिक्त फीस का भुगतान प्रतिवाद के तहत करेगा अर्थात् इस प्रभाव का एक तार्किक कथन संलग्न करते हुए कि अन्तरराष्ट्रीय आवेदन आविष्कार की एकलता की अपेक्षाओं को पूरा करता है या कि अपेक्षित अतिरिक्त फीस की रकम अत्यधिक है।

(7) उप–नियम (5) में निर्दिष्ट प्रतिवाद का परीक्षण नियंत्रक द्वारा गठित एक पुनर्विलोकन समिति द्वारा किया जाएगा।

(8) उप–नियम (7) के तहत गठित पुनर्विलोकन समिति उस सीमा का परीक्षण करेगी जहाँ तक वह प्रतिवाद युक्तिसंगत है और तदनुसार आवेदक को अतिरिक्त फीस की पूर्ण या आंशिक प्रतिपूर्ति का आदेश देगा।

(9) जहाँ उप–नियम (6) में निर्दिष्ट पुनर्विलोकन समिति यह पाती है कि प्रतिवाद पूर्णतया युक्तिसंगत था तो आवेदक को प्रतिवाद फीस वापस कर दिया जाएगा।

19.   **ठ. अन्तरराष्ट्रीय प्रारंभिक परीक्षण प्रतिवेदन स्थापित करने की समय सीमा और उसका पारेषण** – अन्तरराष्ट्रीय प्रारंभिक परीक्षण प्रतिवेदन स्थापित करने की समयावधि होगी :

i.   पूर्विकता तारीख से अठाईस मास, या

ii.   अन्तरराष्ट्रीय प्रारंभिक परीक्षण प्रारंभ करने के लिए संधि के अधीन विनियमों के नियम 69.1 के अधीन विनिर्दिष्ट अवधि से छः मास; या

iii.   इस संधि के अधीन विनियमों के नियम 55.2 के अधीन परीक्षण प्राधिकारी को उपलब्ध कराए गए अनुवाद की प्राप्ति की तारीख से छः मास, जो भी बाद में समाप्त होता है।

19.   **ड. अन्तरराष्ट्रीय प्रारंभिक परीक्षण प्रतिवेदन का पारेषण** – परीक्षण प्राधिकारी अन्तरराष्ट्रीय प्रारंभिक प्रतिवेदन की एक प्रति और उसके अनुलग्नक, यदि कोई हो, अन्तरराष्ट्रीय ब्यूरो को और एक प्रति आवेदक को उसी दिन पारेषित करेगा।"

19.   **ढ. वापसी की स्थिति और सीमा** – आवेदक द्वारा संदत्त फीस इस संधि में विनिर्दिष्ट शर्तों या संधि के अधीन विनियमों में विहित स्थितियों और भारतीय पेटेंट कार्यालय तथा अन्तरराष्ट्रीय ब्यूरो के बीच हुए समझौते के अनुसार और उस सीमा तक वापस, निरस्त या कम कर दिया जाएगा।"

7.   **उक्त नियमों के नियम 27 में**, "और सार" शब्द के स्थान पर "सार और कोई अन्य दस्तावेज" शब्द रखें जाएंगे;

8.   **उक्त नियमों के नियम 138 के**, उप–नियम (1) में, "नियम 24 ख" शब्द, अंक तथा अक्षर के स्थान पर "इन नियमों के अध्याय 3, नियम 24–ख" शब्द, अंक और अक्षर रखे जाएंगे।

9. उक्त नियमों की चतुर्थ अनुसूची और उससे संबंधित प्रविष्टियों के पश्चात् निम्नलिखित अनुसूची और प्रविष्टियाँ अंतःस्थापित की जाएगी, अर्थात् :–

"पांचवीं अनुसूची
[नियम 19 (2), 19 क (1)(ख), 19 ख(5), 19ख (12), 19ज, 19ट(5) देखें]

क्रम संख्या	किस पर संदेय है (पेटेंट नियम, 2003 के सुसंगत उपबंध, यदि कोई हो)	संधि के अधीन विनियमों से सुसंगत नियम	प्रकृत व्यक्ति के लिए	प्रकृत व्यक्ति से भिन्न या तो अकेले या प्रकृत व्यक्ति के साथ संयुक्त रूप में
(1)	(2)	(3)	(4)	(5)
			(रुपये में)	(रुपये में)
1.	खोज फीस	नियम 16.1 (क)	2500	10000
2.	नियम 19 ख (5) के अधीन अतिरिक्त फीस	नियम 40.2	2500	10000
3.	नियम 19 ख (5) तथा 19 ज (5) के अधीन प्रतिवाद फीस	नियम 40.2 (ड.) और 68.3 (ड़)	1000	4000
4.	प्रारंभिक परीक्षण फीस	नियम 58.1	3000	12000
5.	नियम 19 ज (5) के अधीन अतिरिक्त फीस	नियम 68.3	3000	12000
6.	प्रारंभिक परीक्षण फीस यदि भारतीय अन्तरराष्ट्रीय खोज प्राधिकारी द्वारा अन्तरराष्ट्रीय खोज रिपोर्ट तैयार की जाती है		2500	10000
7.	नियम 19 ज (5) के अधीन यदि भारतीय अन्तरराष्ट्रीय खोज प्राधिकारी द्वारा अन्तरराष्ट्रीय खोज रिपोर्ट तैयार की जाती है		2500	10000
8.	अन्तरराष्ट्रीय ब्यूरो को संदत्त की जाने वाली कार्रवाई फीस	नियम 57	संधि के अधीन बनाए गए विनियमों में संलग्न फीस की अनुसूची में यथा विनिर्दिष्ट	
9.	विलम्ब प्रस्तुति फीस	नियम 13 टीआर. 1(ग) तथा 13 टीईआर.2, 12.3 (ड.), 12.4 (ड.)	1000	4000
10.	विलम्ब भुगतान फीस	नियम 58 बीआईएस. 2, 16 बीआईएस.2	संधि के अधीन बनाए गए विनियमों के अनुसार	
11.	पूर्ववर्ती खोज और पूर्ववर्ती आवेदन के परिणामों की प्रति	12 बीआईएस.1(ग)	1000	4000"

[एफ. सं. 14 / 1 / 2008–आईपीआर–III]

डी. वी. प्रसाद, संयुक्त सचिव

टिप्पण : मूल नियम भारत के राजपत्र, असाधारण में अधिसूचना संख्यांक का. आ. 493 (अ) तारीख 2 मई, 2003 द्वारा प्रकाशित किए गए और निम्नलिखित पश्चातवर्ती अधिसूचना संख्यांकों द्वारा संशोधित किए गए।

i.   का. आ. 1418 (अ), तारीख 28 दिसम्बर, 2004;
ii. का. आ. 657 (अ), तारीख 5 मई, 2006; और
iii. का. आ. 2296 (अ), तारीख 25 सितम्बर, 2012.

MINISTRY OF COMMERCE AND INDUSTRY
(Department of Industrial Policy and Promotion)

NOTIFICATION

New Delhi, the 23rd April, 2013.

S.O.1029 (E).—WHEREAS, certain draft rules were published in exercise of the powers conferred by section 159 of the Patents Act, 1970 (39 of 1970), vide notification of the Government of India in the Ministry of Commerce and Industry (Department of Industrial Policy and Promotion), bearing number S.O. 189 (E) in Part II, Section 3, sub-section (ii) of the Gazette of India, Extraordinary, dated the 17th January, 2013, for inviting objections and suggestions from persons likely to be affected thereby before the expiry of a period of fifteen days from the date on which copies of the Gazette containing the notification were made available to the public;

AND WHEREAS, the copies of the Gazette containing the said notification were made available to the public on the 17th January, 2013;

AND WHEREAS, no objection or suggestion has been received from the public on the said draft rules, by the Central Government;

NOW, THEREFORE, in exercise of the powers conferred by section 159 of the Patents Act, 1970 (39 of 1970), the Central Government hereby makes the following rules further to amend the Patents Rules, 2003, namely:-

1.   (1) These rules may be called the Patents (Amendment) Rules, 2013.
    (2) They shall come into force on such date as the Central Government may, by notification in the Official Gazette, appoint.

2.   In the Patents Rules, 2003 (hereinafter referred to as the said rules), in rule 4, in sub-rule (2), the following sub-rules shall be inserted, namely: -

"(3) Notwithstanding anything contained in sub-rule (2), the Controller may transfer an application for patent so filed, to head office or, as the case may be, branch office of the Patent Office.

(4) Notwithstanding anything contained in sub-rule (1), further application referred to in section 16 of the Act, shall be filed at the appropriate office of the first mentioned application only.

(5) All further applications referred to section 16 of the Act filed in an office other than the appropriate office of the first mentioned application, before the commencement of the Patents (Amendment) Rules, 2013, shall be transferred to the appropriate office of the first mentioned application."

3.   For rule 9 of the said rules, the following rule shall be substituted, namely:-

"**9. Filing of documents and copies, etc.-** (1) All documents and copies of the documents, except affidavits and drawings, filed with patent office, shall -

(a) be typewritten or printed in Hindi or English (unless otherwise directed or allowed by the Controller) in large and legible characters not less than 0.28 centimetre high with deep indelible ink with lines widely spaced not less than one and half spaced only upon one side of the paper;

(b) be on such paper which is flexible, strong, white, smooth, non-shiny, and durable of size A4 of approximately 29.7 centimetre by 21 centimetre with a margin of at least 4 centimetre on the top and left hand part and 3 centimetre on the bottom and right hand part thereof;

(c) be numbered in consecutive Arabic numerals in the centre of the bottom of the sheet; and

(d) contain the numbering to every fifth line of each page of the description and each page of the claims at right half of the left margin.

(2) Any signature which is not legible or which is written in a script other than English or Hindi shall be accompanied by a transcription of the name either in Hindi or English in capital letters.

(3) In case, the application for patent discloses sequence listing of nucleotides or amino acid sequences, the sequence listing of nucleotides or amino acid sequences shall be filed in computer readable text format along with the application, and no print form of the sequence listing of nucleotides or amino acid sequences is required to be given.

(4) Additional copies of all documents shall be filed at the appropriate office as may be required by the Controller.

(5) Names and addresses of applicant and other persons shall be given in full together with their nationality and such other particulars, if any, as are necessary for their identification."

4. **In rule 17 of the said rules, after clause (a), the following clauses shall be inserted, namely:-**

'(aa) "Examining Authority" means the Indian International Preliminary Examining Authority referred to in sub-rule (1) of rule 19F;

(ab) "International Bureau" means the International Bureau of World Intellectual Property Organisation;

(ac) "Searching Authority" means the Indian International Searching Authority referred to in sub-rule (1) of rule 19A;'

5. **For rule 18 of the said rules, the following rule shall be substituted, namely: —**

"**18. Appropriate office in relation to International applications.** —(1) The receiving office, the designated office and the elected office, as the case may be, for the purposes of international applications shall be the appropriate office referred to in rule 4.

(2) Notwithstanding anything contained in sub-rule (1), the Patent Office, Delhi branch shall be the appropriate office for dealing with the International Bureau and any other International Searching Authority and International Preliminary Examining Authority.

(3) An international application shall be filed at and processed by the appropriate office, referred to in sub-rule (1), in accordance with the provisions of this Chapter, the Treaty and the regulations under the Treaty.

(4) The appropriate office referred to in sub-rule (1), shall, on receipt of an international application,

    (a) keep one copy of the application to be called the "home copy" in its office;

    (b) transmit one copy to be called the "record copy" to the International Bureau; and

    (c) transmit one copy to be called "search copy" to the competent International Searching Authority referred to in Article 16 of the Treaty,

And simultaneously furnish complete details of such application to the Patent Office, Delhi branch."

6. **For rule 19 of the said rules, the following rules shall be substituted, namely: —**

"**19. International applications filed with appropriate office as receiving office.** — (1) An international application shall be filed with the appropriate office in triplicate either in English or Hindi language.

(2) The fees payable in respect of an international application shall, in addition to the fees specified in the regulations under the Treaty, be the fees as specified in the First Schedule and the Fifth Schedule.

(3) Where an international application has not been filed in triplicate, the appropriate office shall, upon payment of fees specified in the First Schedule, prepare the required additional copies.

(4) On receipt of a request from the applicant and on payment of the fees specified in the First Schedule, the appropriate office shall prepare a certified copy of the priority document and promptly transmit the same to the International Bureau and intimate the applicant and the Patent Office, Delhi branch."

19A. Indian International Searching Authority.—(1) The Patent Office, Delhi branch shall perform the functions of the Indian International Searching Authority under the treaty in accordance with an agreement between the Indian Patent Office and the International Bureau.

(2) The fees payable to the Searching Authority shall, in addition to the fees specified in the regulations made under the Treaty, be the fees as specified in the Fifth Schedule.

(3) The Searching Authority referred to in sub-rule (1), shall establish international search report in respect of international applications, or, as the case may be, declare in accordance with sub-rule (3) of rule 19B, in cases where India has been indicated as a competent International Searching Authority.

19 B.   International search report.– (1) The Searching Authority shall, on receipt of the search copy, notify the International Bureau and the applicant about the receipt of search copy with identification mark 'ISA/IN' along with the international application number and its serial number and the date of receipt of the search copy.

(2) Notwithstanding anything contained in the proviso to item (i) of sub-rule (2) of rule 24B, the Searching Authority shall, upon receipt of the search copy, refer the international application, in the order in which the search copy was received, to an examiner or any other officer appointed under sub-section (2) of Section 73 of the Act for preparing an international search report, in accordance with the provisions contained in the Treaty and the regulations under the Treaty, ordinarily within a period of one month but not exceeding two months from the date of such reference.

(3)   The Searching Authority, if it considers that-

   (a)   the international application relates to a subject matter which the Searching Authority is not required to search and accordingly decides not to search; or

   (b)   the description, claims or drawings fail to comply with the requirements prescribed under the regulations under the Treaty to such an extent that a meaningful search could not be carried out,

the Authority shall so declare and notify the applicant and the International Bureau that no international search report shall be established.

(4) In a case where any situation referred to in clause (a) or clause (b) of sub-rule (3) is found to exist in connection with certain claims only, the Searching Authority shall indicate this fact in the International Search Report in respect of such claims, and for other claims, it shall establish the International Search Report.

(5) The Searching Authority, if it considers that the international application does not comply with the requirement of unity of invention, in accordance with the provisions contained in Rule 13 of the regulations under the Treaty, shall send a notice specifying the reasons for which the international application is not considered as complying with the requirement of unity of invention and inviting the applicant-

   (a)   to pay the additional fees specified in the Fifth Schedule, indicating the amount of fees to be paid, within a period of one month from the date of such invitation; and

   (b)   to pay, where applicable, the protest fee specified in the Fifth Schedule, indicating the amount of fee to be paid, within a period of one month from the date of such invitation.

(6) The Searching Authority shall establish the International Search Report on those parts of the international application which relate to the invention first mentioned in the claims ("main invention") and subject to payment of additional fee within the period specified in sub-rule (5), on those parts of the international application which relate to inventions in respect of which such additional fees were paid.

(7) Any applicant may pay the additional fees under protest, that is, accompanied by a reasoned statement to the effect that the international application complies with the requirement of unity of invention or that the amount of the required additional fees is excessive.

(8) The examination of the protest referred to in sub-rule (7) shall be carried out by a Review Committee constituted by the Controller.

(9) The Review Committee constituted under sub-rule (8) shall examine the extent to which the protest is justified and shall accordingly order for the total or partial reimbursement of the additional fee to the applicant.

(10) Where the applicant has not paid the fees for the protest in accordance with clause (b) of sub-rule (5),the protest shall be considered not to have been made and the Searching Authority shall so declare.

(11) The protest fee shall be refunded to the applicant where the Review Committee referred to in sub-rule (8) finds that the protest was entirely justified.

(12) Where the international application contains the disclosure of one or more nucleotide or amino acid sequences and the sequences are not furnished in computer-readable text format, the Searching Authority shall send a notice to the applicant to submit the sequence listing in computer-readable text format and pay the late furnishing fee specified in the Fifth Schedule, within a period of one month from the date of such notice and if the applicant fails to comply with the notice, the Searching Authority shall search the international application to the extent that a meaningful search can be carried out without the sequence listing.

19 C. Time limit for establishing international search report. – The Searching Authority shall establish the International Search Report and written opinion or, as the case may be, the declaration referred to in sub-rule (3) of rule 19B within a period of three months from the date of receipt of the search copy by the Searching Authority, or within a period of nine months from the date of priority, whichever expires later.

19D. Transmittal of the International Search Report and written opinion,–
The Searching Authority shall transmit one copy of the International Search Report or of the declaration referred to in Article 17(2)(a) of the Treaty, and one copy of the written opinion established under Rule 43*bis*.1 of the regulations under the Treaty, to the International Bureau and one copy to the applicant, on the same day.

19E. Confidential treatment.–All matters pertaining to international applications shall be kept confidential in accordance with the treaty and the regulations under the Treaty.

19F.   Indian International Preliminary Examining Authority. - (1) The Patent Office, Delhi branch shall perform the functions of the International Preliminary Examining Authority under the Treaty in accordance with an agreement between the Indian Patent Office and the International Bureau.

(2) The Examining Authority referred to in sub-rule (1), shall establish—

    (a) the International Preliminary Examination Report in respect of all international applications electing India as an International Preliminary Examining Authority;

    (b) the International Preliminary Examination Report in respect of the demands filed by the nationals or residents of other countries in accordance with an agreement between Indian Patent Office and the International Bureau, upon being notified by the International Bureau;

    (c) the International Preliminary Examination in respect of demands made by the nationals or residents of other countries not party to the Treaty or not bound by Chapter II of the Treaty, if the Assembly has so approves.

19G.   Period for making a demand. – (1) The demand for international preliminary examination shall be made within the period specified in the Treaty or regulations under the Treaty.

(2)   In case the demand is made after the expiry of the period specified in sub-rule (1), it shall be considered to have not been made and no International Preliminary Examination Report shall be prepared.

19H.   Fees payable to Examining Authority. –The fees payable to the Examining Authority shall, in addition to the fees specified in the regulations under the Treaty, be the fees specified in the Fifth Schedule.

19I.   Manner of making a demand.–A demand shall be made in accordance with the provisions contained in these rules, the Treaty and the regulations under the Treaty.

19J.   Processing of demands for international preliminary examination.– (1) The Examining Authority, on receipt of the demand for international preliminary examination, if the Examining Authority is competent to conduct an international preliminary examination, shall assign the identification mark 'IPEA/IN' and shall notify the Applicant and the International Bureau.

(2)   In case where the Examining Authority is not competent to conduct the international preliminary examination of the international application, it shall transmit the demand promptly to the International Bureau.

19K. International Preliminary Examination Report. – (1)Notwithstanding anything contained in the proviso to item (i) of sub-rule (2) of rule 24B, the Examining Authority shall refer the international application, in accordance with the provisions contained in the Treaty and the regulations under the Treaty, in the order in which the demand was received in the Examining Authority to an examiner or any other officer appointed under sub-section (2) of section 73 of the Act for preparing an International Preliminary Examination Report ordinarily within a period of three months but not exceeding four months from the date of such reference.

(2)   Claims relating to inventions in respect of which no International Search Report has been established shall not be the subject of international preliminary examination.

(3)   The Examining Authority, if considers that –
  (a)   the international application relates to a subject matter on which the Examining Authority is not required to carry out an international preliminary examination, and, decides not to carry out such examination; or
  (b)   that the description, the claims, or the drawings, are so unclear, or the claims are so inadequately supported by the description, that no meaningful opinion can be formed on the questions of novelty, inventive step (non-obviousness), or industrial applicability, the Examining Authority shall not go into these questions and shall inform the applicant of this opinion and the reasons therefor.

(4) In a case where any situation referred to in clause (a) or clause (b) of sub-rule (3) is found to exist in connection with certain claims only, the Examining Authority shall indicate this fact in the International Preliminary Examination Report in respect of such claims, and for other claims, it shall establish the International Preliminary Examination Report.

(5) Where the Examining Authority finds that the international application does not comply with the requirement of unity of invention, in accordance with the provisions contained in Rule 13 of the regulations under the Treaty and chooses to invite the applicant, at his option, to restrict the claims or to pay additional fees, it shall issue a notice to the applicant:

  (a) specifying at least one possibility of restriction which, in the opinion of the Examining Authority, would be in compliance with the applicable requirement;

(b) specifying the reasons for which the international application is not considered as complying with the requirement of unity of invention;

(c) inviting the applicant to comply with the invitation within one month from the date of such notice;

(d) indicating the amount of the required additional fees to be paid in case the applicant so chooses; and

(e) inviting the applicant to pay, the protest fee within one month from the date of such notice, and indicate the amount to be paid, as specified in the Fifth Schedule.

(6) Any applicant may pay the additional fees under protest, that is, accompanied by a reasoned statement to the effect that the international application complies with the requirement of unity of invention or that the amount of the required additional fees is excessive.

(7) The examination of the protest referred to in sub-rule (5) shall be carried out by a Review Committee constituted by the Controller.

(8) The Review Committee constituted under sub-rule (7) shall examine the extent to which the protest is justified and shall accordingly order for the total or partial reimbursement to the applicant of the additional fee.

(9) The protest fee shall be refunded to the applicant where the Review Committee referred to in sub-rule (6) finds that the protest was entirely justified.

19 L. Period for establishing international preliminary examination report and its transmission. – The period for establishing the International Preliminary Examination Report shall be:

(i)   twenty eight months from the priority date; or

(ii)   six months from the period specified under Rule 69.1 of the regulations under the Treaty for the start of the international preliminary examination; or

(iii)   six months from the date of receipt by the Examining Authority of the translation furnished under Rule 55.2 of the regulations under the Treaty,

whichever expires last.

19M.Transmittal of the International Preliminary Examination Report.-The Examining Authority shall transmit one copy of the International Preliminary Examination Report and its annexures, if any, to the International Bureau, and one copy to the applicant, on the same day.

19N. Conditions for and extent of refund. – The fee paid by the applicant may be refunded, waived or reduced to the extent and in accordance with the conditions specified in the Treaty or the regulations under the Treaty and the agreement entered between the Indian Patent Office and the International Bureau."

7. In rule 27 of the said rules, for the words "and the abstract", the words "the abstract and any other document" shall be substituted.

8. In rule 138 of the said rules, in sub-rule (1), for the word, figures and letter "rules 24B", the words, figures and letters "Chapter III of these rules, rule 24B," shall be substituted.

9. After the FOURTH SCHEDULE to the said rules and the entries relating thereto, the following SCHEDULE and entries shall be inserted, namely:-

"THE FIFTH SCHEDULE

[See rules 19(2), 19A(1)(b), 19B(5),19B(12), 19H, 19K(5)]

Sl. No.	On what payable (Relevant provision of Patents Rules, 2003, if any)	Relevant Rule of regulations under the Treaty	For Natural Person	Other than natural person either alone or jointly with natural person
(1)	(2)	(3)	(4)	(5)
			(In Rupees)	(In Rupees)
1.	Search fee	Rule 16.1(a)	2500	10000
2.	Additional fee under rule 19B (5)	Rule 40.2	2500	10000
3.	Protest fee under rules 19B (5) and 19J(5)	Rules 40.2(e) and 68.3(e)	1000	4000
4.	Preliminary examination fee	Rule 58.1	3000	12000
5.	Additional fee under rule 19J(5)	Rule 68.3	3000	12000
6.	Preliminary examination fee, if the International Search Report was prepared by the Indian International Searching Authority		2500	10000
7.	Additional fee under rule 19J(5), if the International Search Report was prepared by the Indian International Searching Authority		2500	10000
8.	Handling fee to be paid to be IB	Rule 57	As specified in the schedule of fee annexed to the regulations made under the Treaty	
9.	Late furnishing fee	Rule 13ter.1(c),13ter.2, 12.3(e), 12.4(e)	1000	4000
10.	Late payment fee	Rule 58bis.2, 16bis.2	In accordance with the regulations made under the Treaty	
11.	Copy of Results of Earlier Search and of Earlier Application	12bis.1(c)	1000	4000"

Note. – The principal rules were published in the Gazette of India, Extraordinary, vide notification number S.O. 493 (E), dated the 2nd May, 2003 and subsequently amended vide notification numbers –

(i) S.O. 1418(E), dated the 28th December, 2004;

(ii) S.O. 657 (E), dated the 5th May, 2006; and

(iii)S.O. 2296 (E), dated the 25th September, 2012.

ANNEXURE 15

IPO AS RECEIVING OFFICE

<table>
<tr><td>C</td><td align="center">Receiving Offices</td><td align="right">C</td></tr>
<tr><td>IN</td><td align="center">INDIAN PATENT OFFICE</td><td align="right">IN</td></tr>
</table>

Competent receiving Office for nationals and residents of:	India
Language in which international applications may be filed:	English or Hindi[1]
Language in which the request may be filed:	English
Number of copies on paper required by the receiving Office:	3
Does the receiving Office accept the filing of international applications with requests in PCT-EASY format?[2]	Yes
Does the receiving Office accept requests for restoration of the right of priority (PCT Rule 26bis.3)?	No
Competent International Searching Authority:	Australian Patent Office, Austrian Patent Office, European Patent Office, Indian Patent Office, State Intellectual Property Office of the People's Republic of China, Swedish Patent and Registration Office or United States Patent and Trademark Office
Competent International Preliminary Examining Authority:	Australian Patent Office, Austrian Patent Office, European Patent Office,[3] Indian Patent Office, State Intellectual Property Office of the People's Republic of China, Swedish Patent and Registration Office or United States Patent and Trademark Office[4]

[Continued on next page]

---

[1] If the language in which the international application is filed is not accepted by the International Searching Authority (see Annex D), the applicant will have to furnish a translation (PCT Rule 12.3).

[2] Where the request is filed in PCT-EASY format together with the electronic file on a physical medium and the receiving Office accepts such filings, the total amount of the international filing fee is reduced (see "Fees payable to the receiving Office").

[3] The European Patent Office is competent only if the international search is or has been carried out by that Office, by the Austrian Patent Office or by the Swedish Patent and Registration Office.

[4] The United States Patent and Trademark Office is competent only if the international search is or has been carried out by that Office.

(9 January 2014)

PCT Applicant's Guide – International Phase – Annex C

| C
IN | **Receiving Offices**

INDIAN PATENT OFFICE | C
IN |

[Continued]

Fees payable to the receiving Office:	Currency: Indian rupee (INR) and US dollar (USD)
Transmittal fee:	INR 8,000 (2,000)[5]
International filing fee:[6]	USD 1,471
Fee per sheet in excess of 30:[6]	USD 17
Additional component:[6]	Where applicable
Reductions (under Schedule of Fees, item 4):	
PCT-EASY:[7]	USD 111
Search fee:	See Annex D(AT), (AU), (CN), (EP), (IN), (SE) or (US)
Fee for priority document:	INR 4,000 (1,000)[5]
Late payment fee:	INR 8,000 (2,000)[5]

Is an agent required by the receiving Office?	No, but an address for service in India is required

Who can act as agent?	Any patent agent registered to practice before the Office[8]

---

[5]   The amount in parentheses is applicable in case of filing by an individual.

[6]   This fee is reduced by 90% if certain conditions apply (see Annex C(IB)).

[7]   See footnote 2.

[8]   The list of registered patent agents is available on the website of the Office at:
http://ipindia.nic.in/ipr/patent/patent_agent/List_PatentAgent_01April2010.pdf

(9 January 2014)

ANNEXURE 16

PCT APPLICATION

PCT

REQUEST

The undersigned requests that the present
international application be processed
according to the Patent Cooperation Treaty.

<table>
<tr><td colspan="2">For receiving Office use only</td></tr>
<tr><td colspan="2">International Application No.</td></tr>
<tr><td colspan="2">International Filing Date</td></tr>
<tr><td colspan="2">Name of receiving Office and "PCT International Application"</td></tr>
<tr><td>Applicant's or agent's file reference
(if desired) (12 characters maximum)</td><td>CHOCO 95549</td></tr>
</table>

Box No. I	TITLE OF INVENTION

PROCESS FOR FOLDING WRAPPING PAPER FOR CHOCOLATES

Box No. II	APPLICANT	☐ This person is also inventor

Name and address: *(Family name followed by given name; for a legal entity, full official designation. The address must include postal code and name of country. The country of the address indicated in this Box is the applicant's State (that is, country) of residence if no State of residence is indicated below.)*

CANDY WRAP UNLIMITED, INC.
300 Colorado Street
Baltimore, Maryland 21201-4307
United States of America

Telephone No.
(+1-301) 876-5432

Facsimile No.
(+1-301) 876-5555

Applicant's registration No. with the Office

E-mail authorization: Marking one of the check-boxes below authorizes the receiving Office, the International Searching Authority, the International Bureau and the International Preliminary Examining Authority to use the e-mail address indicated in this Box to send, notifications issued in respect of this international application to that e-mail address if those offices are willing to do so.
☐ as advance copies followed by paper notifications; or   ☒ exclusively in electronic form (no paper notifications will be sent).
   E-mail address: candy@anumma.com

State *(that is, country)* of nationality: US	State *(that is, country)* of residence: US

This person is applicant for the purposes of: ☒ all designated States   ☐ the States indicated in the Supplemental Box

Box No. III	FURTHER APPLICANT(S) AND/OR (FURTHER) INVENTOR(S)

☒ Further applicants and/or (further) inventors are indicated on a continuation sheet.

Box No. IV	AGENT OR COMMON REPRESENTATIVE; OR ADDRESS FOR CORRESPONDENCE

The person identified below is hereby/has been appointed to act on behalf of the applicant(s) before the competent International Authorities as: ☒ agent   ☐ common representative

Name and address: *(Family name followed by given name; for a legal entity, full official designation. The address must include postal code and name of country.)*

DAVIS, Catherine
2500 Virginia Avenue, N.W.
Washington, D.C. 20037-1902
United States of America

Telephone No.
(+1-301) 557-3054

Facsimile No.
(+1-301) 557-3060

Agent's registration No. with the Office
44,111

E-mail authorization: Marking one of the check-boxes below authorizes the receiving Office, the International Searching Authority, the International Bureau and the International Preliminary Examining Authority to use the e-mail address indicated in this Box to send, notifications issued in respect of this international application to that e-mail address if those offices are willing to do so.

☐ as advance copies followed by paper notifications; or   ☒ exclusively in electronic form (no paper notifications will be sent).
   E-mail address: davispatents@anumma.com

☐ **Address for correspondence:** Mark this check-box where no agent or common representative is/has been appointed and the space above is used instead to indicate a special address to which correspondence should be sent.

Sheet No. ...2...

Box No. III   FURTHER APPLICANT(S) AND/OR (FURTHER) INVENTOR(S)

If none of the following sub-boxes is used, this sheet should not be included in the request.

Name and address: *(Family name followed by given name; for a legal entity, full official designation. The address must include postal code and name of country. The country of the address indicated in this Box is the applicant's State (that is, country) of residence if no State of residence is indicated below.)*

JONES, Mary
1600 South Eads Street
Arlington, Virginia 22202-2913
United States of America

This person is:

☐ applicant only

☐ applicant and inventor

☒ inventor only *(If this check-box is marked, do not fill in below.)*

Applicant's registration No. with the Office

State *(that is, country)* of nationality:

State *(that is, country)* of residence:

This person is applicant for the purposes of: ☐ all designated States ☐ the States indicated in the Supplemental Box

---

Name and address: *(Family name followed by given name; for a legal entity, full official designation. The address must include postal code and name of country. The country of the address indicated in this Box is the applicant's State (that is, country) of residence if no State of residence is indicated below.)*

This person is:

☐ applicant only

☐ applicant and inventor

☐ inventor only *(If this check-box is marked, do not fill in below.)*

Applicant's registration No. with the Office

State *(that is, country)* of nationality:

State *(that is, country)* of residence:

This person is applicant for the purposes of: ☐ all designated States ☐ the States indicated in the Supplemental Box

---

Name and address: *(Family name followed by given name; for a legal entity, full official designation. The address must include postal code and name of country. The country of the address indicated in this Box is the applicant's State (that is, country) of residence if no State of residence is indicated below.)*

This person is:

☐ applicant only

☐ applicant and inventor

☐ inventor only *(If this check-box is marked, do not fill in below.)*

Applicant's registration No. with the Office

State *(that is, country)* of nationality:

State *(that is, country)* of residence:

This person is applicant for the purposes of: ☐ all designated States ☐ the States indicated in the Supplemental Box

---

Name and address: *(Family name followed by given name; for a legal entity, full official designation. The address must include postal code and name of country. The country of the address indicated in this Box is the applicant's State (that is, country) of residence if no State of residence is indicated below.)*

This person is:

☐ applicant only

☒ applicant and inventor

☐ inventor only *(If this check-box is marked, do not fill in below.)*

Applicant's registration No. with the Office

State *(that is, country)* of nationality:

State *(that is, country)* of residence:

This person is applicant for the purposes of: ☐ all designated States ☐ the States indicated in the Supplemental Box

---

☐ Further applicants and/or (further) inventors are indicated on another continuation sheet.

Form PCT/RO/101 (continuation sheet) (16 September 2012)   *See Notes to the request form*

Sheet No. . . . .

Supplemental Box	*If the Supplemental Box is not used, this sheet should not be included in the request.*

1.   *If, in any of the Boxes, except Boxes Nos. VIII(i) to (v) for which a special continuation box is provided, **the space is insufficient** to furnish all the information: in such case, write "Continuation of Box No...." (indicate the number of the Box) and furnish the information in the same manner as required according to the captions of the Box in which the space was insufficient, in particular:*

(i)   ***if more than one person is to be indicated as applicant and/or inventor** and no "continuation sheet" is available: in such case, write "Continuation of Box No. III" and indicate for each additional person the same type of information as required in Box No. III. The country of the address indicated in this Box is the applicant's State (that is, country) of residence if no State of residence is indicated below;*

(ii)   *if, in Box No. II or in any of the sub-boxes of Box No. III, the indication **"the States indicated in the Supplemental Box"** is checked: in such case, write "Continuation of Box No. II" or "Continuation of Box No. III" or "Continuation of Boxes No. II and No. III" (as the case may be), indicate the name of the applicant(s) involved and, next to (each) such name, the State(s) (and/or, where applicable, ARIPO, Eurasian, European or OAPI patent) for the purposes of which the named person is applicant;*

(iii)   *if, in Box No. II or in any of the sub-boxes of Box No. III, **the inventor or the inventor/applicant is not inventor for the purposes of all designated States**: in such case, write "Continuation of Box No. II" or "Continuation of Box No. III" or "Continuation of Boxes No. II and No. III" (as the case may be), indicate the name of the inventor(s) and, next to (each) such name, the State(s) (and/or, where applicable, ARIPO, Eurasian, European or OAPI patent) for the purposes of which the named person is inventor;*

(iv)   *if, in addition to the agent(s) indicated in Box No. IV, there are **further agents**: in such case, write "Continuation of Box No. IV" and indicate for each further agent the same type of information as required in Box No. IV;*

(v)   *if, in Box No. VI, there are **more than three earlier applications whose priority is claimed**: in such case, write "Continuation of Box No. VI" and indicate for each additional earlier application the same type of information as required in Box No. VI.*

2.   *If the applicant intends to make an indication of the wish that the international application be treated, in certain designated States, as an application for a patent of addition, certificate of addition, inventor's certificate of addition or utility certificate of addition: in such case, write the name or two-letter code of each designated State concerned and the indication **"patent of addition," "certificate of addition," "inventor's certificate of addition"** or **"utility certificate of addition,"** the number of the parent application or parent patent or other parent grant and the date of grant of the parent patent or other parent grant or the date of filing of the parent application (Rules 4.11(a)(i) and 49bis.1(a) or (b)).*

3.   *If the applicant intends to make an indication of the wish that the international application be treated, in the United States of America, as a continuation or continuation-in-part of an earlier application: in such case, write "United States of America" or "US" and the indication **"continuation"** or **"continuation-in-part"** and the number and the filing date of the parent application (Rules 4.11(a)(ii) and 49bis.1(d)).*

Form PCT/RO/101 (supplemental sheet) (16 September 2012)   *See Notes to the request form*

Sheet No. ...3...

<table>
<tr><td colspan="2">Box No. V   DESIGNATIONS</td></tr>
</table>

The filing of this request **constitutes under Rule 4.9(a) the designation** of all Contracting States bound by the PCT on the international filing date, for the grant of every kind of protection available and, where applicable, for the grant of both regional and national patents.

However,

☐   DE Germany **is not designated** for any kind of national protection

☐   JP Japan **is not designated** for any kind of national protection

☐   KR Republic of Korea **is not designated** for any kind of national protection

(The check-boxes above may only be used to exclude (irrevocably) the designations concerned if, at the time of filing or subsequently under Rule 26bis.1, the international application contains in Box No. VI a priority claim to an earlier national application filed in the particular State concerned, in order to avoid the ceasing of the effect, under the national law, of this earlier national application.)

Box No. VI   PRIORITY CLAIM AND DOCUMENT

The priority of the following earlier application(s) is hereby claimed:

Filing date of earlier application *(day/month/year)*	Number of earlier application	Where earlier application is:		
		national application: country or Member of WTO	regional application: regional Office	international application: receiving Office
item (1) 26 October 2011 (26.10.2011)	61/274,654	US		
item (2) 13 December 2011 (13.12.2011)	11187654.4		EP	
item (3)				

☐ Further priority claims are indicated in the Supplemental Box.

Furnishing the priority document(s):

☒ The **receiving Office** is requested to prepare and transmit to the International Bureau a certified copy of the earlier application(s) *(only if the earlier application(s) was filed with the receiving Office which, for the purposes of this international application, is the receiving Office)* identified above as:

    ☐ all items   ☒ item (1)   ☐ item (2)   ☐ item (3)   ☐ other, see Supplemental Box

☐ The **International Bureau** is requested to obtain from a digital library a certified copy of the earlier application(s) identified above, using, where applicable, the access code(s) indicated below *(if the earlier application(s) is available to it from a digital library)*:

    ☐ item (1)   ☐ item (2)   ☐ item (3)   ☐ other, see Supplemental Box
    access code _______   access code _______   access code _______

Restore the right of priority: the receiving Office is requested to restore the right of priority for the earlier application(s) identified above or in the Supplemental Box as item(s) (_______________________). *(See also the Notes to Box No. VI; further information **must** be provided to support a request to restore the right of priority.)*

Incorporation by reference: where an element of the international application referred to in Article 11(1)(iii)(d) or (e) or a part of the description, claims or drawings referred to in Rule 20.5(a) is not otherwise contained in this international application but is completely contained in an earlier application whose priority is claimed on the date on which one or more elements referred to in Article 11(1)(iii) were first received by the receiving Office, that element or part is, subject to confirmation under Rule 20.6, incorporated by reference in this international application for the purposes of Rule 20.6.

Box No. VII INTERNATIONAL SEARCHING AUTHORITY

Choice of International Searching Authority (ISA) *(if more than one International Searching Authority is competent to carry out the international search, indicate the Authority chosen; the two-letter code may be used)*:

ISA/ EP

Form PCT/RO/101 (second sheet) (16 September 2012)   *See Notes to the request form*

Sheet No. ...4...

Continuation of Box No. VII	USE OF RESULTS OF EARLIER SEARCH, REFERENCE TO THAT SEARCH

☒ The ISA indicated in Box No. VII is requested to take into account the results of the earlier search(es) indicated below (*see also Notes to Box VII; use of results of more than one earlier search*).

Filing date *(day/month/year)*	Application Number	Country *(or regional Office)*
13 December 2011 (13.12.2011)	11187654.4	EP

☐ **Statement (Rule 4.12(ii))**: this international application is the same, or substantially the same, as the application in respect of which the earlier search was carried out except, where applicable, that it is filed in a different language.

☒ **Availability of documents**: the following documents are available to the ISA in a form and manner acceptable to it and therefore do not need to be submitted by the applicant to the ISA (Rule 12*bis*.1(f)):

☒ a copy of the results of the earlier search,*
☒ a copy of the earlier application,
☐ a translation of the earlier application into a language which is accepted by the ISA,
☐ a translation of the results of the earlier search into a language which is accepted by the ISA,
☒ a copy of any document cited in the results of the earlier search. (*If known, please indicate below the document(s) available to the ISA):*

☐ **Transmit copy of results of earlier search and other documents** (*where the earlier search was not carried out by the ISA indicated above but by the same Office as that which is acting as the receiving Office*): the **receiving Office** is requested to prepare and transmit to the ISA (Rule 12*bis*.1(c)):

☐ a copy of the results of the earlier search,*
☐ a copy of the earlier application,
☐ a copy of any document cited in the results of the earlier search.

* Where the results of the earlier search are neither available from a digital library nor transmitted by the receiving Office, the applicant is required to submit them to the receiving Office (Rule 12*bis*.1(a)) (*See item 11. in the check-list and also Notes to Box No. VII*).

Filing date *(day/month/year)*	Application Number	Country *(or regional Office)*

☐ **Statement (Rule 4.12(ii))**: this international application is the same, or substantially the same, as the application in respect of which the earlier search was carried out except, where applicable, that it is filed in a different language.

☐ **Availability of documents**: the following documents are available to the ISA in a form and manner acceptable to it and therefore do not need to be submitted by the applicant to the ISA (Rule 12*bis*.1(f)):

☐ a copy of the results of the earlier search,*
☐ a copy of the earlier application,
☐ a translation of the earlier application into a language which is accepted by the ISA,
☐ a translation of the results of the earlier search into a language which is accepted by the ISA,
☐ a copy of any document cited in the results of the earlier search. (*If known, please indicate below the document(s) available to the ISA):*

☐ **Transmit copy of results of earlier search and other documents** (*where the earlier search was not carried out by the ISA indicated above but by the same Office as that which is acting as the receiving Office*): the **receiving Office** is requested to prepare and transmit to the ISA (Rule 12*bis*.1(c)):

☐ a copy of the results of the earlier search,*
☐ a copy of the earlier application,
☐ a copy of any document cited in the results of the earlier search.

* Where the results of the earlier search are neither available from a digital library nor transmitted by the receiving Office, the applicant is required to submit them to the receiving Office (Rule 12*bis*.1(a)) (*See item 11. in the check-list and also Notes to Box No. VII*).

☐ Further earlier searches are indicated on a continuation sheet.

Box No. VIII DECLARATIONS	

The following **declarations** are contained in Boxes Nos. VIII (i) to (v) *(mark the applicable check-boxes below and indicate in the right column the number of each type of declaration)*:

Number of declarations

☐	Box No. VIII (i)	Declaration as to the identity of the inventor	:
☒	Box No. VIII (ii)	Declaration as to the applicant's entitlement, as at the international filing date, to apply for and be granted a patent	: 1
☐	Box No. VIII (iii)	Declaration as to the applicant's entitlement, as at the international filing date, to claim the priority of the earlier application	:
☒	Box No. VIII (iv)	Declaration of inventorship (only for the purposes of the designation of the United States of America)	: 1
☐	Box No. VIII (v)	Declaration as to non-prejudicial disclosures or exceptions to lack of novelty	:

Form PCT/RO/101 (third sheet) (16 September 2012)   *See Notes to the request form*

Sheet No. . . . .

Box No. VIII (i)   DECLARATION: IDENTITY OF THE INVENTOR
The declaration must conform to the standardized wording provided for in Section 211; see Notes to Boxes Nos. VIII, VIII (i) to (v) (in general) and the specific Notes to Box No. VIII (i). If this Box is not used, this sheet should not be included in the request.

Declaration as to the identity of the inventor (Rules 4.17(i) and 51*bis*.1(a)(i)):

NOT INCLUDED

(not needed since the inventor is named in Box No. III)

☐ This declaration is continued on the following sheet, "Continuation of Box No. VIII (i)".

Form PCT/RO/101 (declaration sheet (i)) (16 September 2012)   *See Notes to the request form*

Sheet No.   5

Box No. VIII (ii)   DECLARATION: ENTITLEMENT TO APPLY FOR AND BE GRANTED A PATENT

The declaration must conform to the standardized wording provided for in Section 212; see Notes to Boxes Nos. VIII, VIII (i) to (v) (in general) and the specific Notes to Box No.VIII (ii). If this Box is not used, this sheet should not be included in the request.

Declaration as to the applicant's entitlement, as at the international filing date, to apply for and be granted a patent (Rules 4.17(ii) and 51*bis*.1(a)(ii)), in a case where the declaration under Rule 4.17(iv) is not appropriate:

in relation to this international application,

CANDY WRAP UNLIMITED, INC., is entitled to apply for and be granted a patent by virtue of the following:

an assignment from JONES, Mary, to CANDY WRAP UNLIMITED, INC.,
dated 10 April 2012 (10.04.2012).

☐ This declaration is continued on the following sheet, "Continuation of Box No. VIII (ii)".

Form PCT/RO/101 (declaration sheet (ii)) (16 September 2012)   *See Notes to the request form*

Sheet No. . . . .

Box No. VIII (iii)   DECLARATION: ENTITLEMENT TO CLAIM PRIORITY
The declaration must conform to the standardized wording provided for in Section 213; see Notes to Boxes Nos. VIII, VIII (i) to (v) (in general) and the specific Notes to Box No.VIII (iii). If this Box is not used, this sheet should not be included in the request.

Declaration as to the applicant's entitlement, as at the international filing date, to claim the priority of the earlier application specified below, where the applicant is not the applicant who filed the earlier application or where the applicant's name has changed since the filing of the earlier application (Rules 4.17(iii) and 51*bis*.1(a)(iii)):

TO BE INCLUDED
ONLY IF NECESSARY

☐ This declaration is continued on the following sheet, "Continuation of Box No. VIII (iii)".

Form PCT/RO/101 (declaration sheet (iii)) (16 September 2012)   *See Notes to the request form*

Sheet No. ..6....

Box No. VIII (iv)   DECLARATION: INVENTORSHIP (only for the purposes of the designation of the United States of America)

The declaration must conform to the following standardized wording provided for in Section 214; see Notes to Boxes Nos. VIII, VIII (i) to (v) (in general) and the specific Notes to Box No.VIII (iv). If this Box is not used, this sheet should not be included in the request.

**Declaration of inventorship (Rules 4.17(iv) and 51*bis*.1(a)(iv))
for the purposes of the designation of the United States of America:**

I hereby declare that I believe I am the original inventor or an original joint inventor of a claimed invention in the application.

This declaration is directed to the international application of which it forms a part (if filing declaration with application).

This declaration is directed to international application No. PCT/............................ (if furnishing declaration pursuant to Rule 26*ter*).

I hereby declare that the above-identified international application was made or authorized to be made by me.

I hereby acknowledge that any willful false statement made in this declaration is punishable under 18 U.S.C. 1001 by fine or imprisonment of not more than five (5) years, or both.

Name: JONES, Mary

Residence: Arlington, Virginia
(city and either US state, if applicable, or country)

Mailing Address: 1600 South Eads Street
Arlington, Virginia 22202-2913
United States of America

Inventor's Signature: *Mary Jones*　　　Date: 18 September 2012 (18.09.2012)
(The signature must be that of the inventor, not that of the agent)

Name: ....

Residence: ....
(city and either US state, if applicable, or country)

Mailing Address: ....

Inventor's Signature: ....　Date: ....
(The signature must be that of the inventor, not that of the agent)

Name: ....

Residence: ....
(city and either US state, if applicable, or country)

Mailing Address: ....

Inventor's Signature: ....　Date: ....
(The signature must be that of the inventor, not that of the agent)

☐ This declaration is continued on the following sheet, "Continuation of Box No. VIII (iv)".

Form PCT/RO/101 (declaration sheet (iv)) (16 September 2012)　　　*See Notes to the request form*

Sheet No. . . . .

Box No. VIII (v)   DECLARATION: NON-PREJUDICIAL DISCLOSURES OR EXCEPTIONS TO LACK OF NOVELTY

The declaration must conform to the standardized wording provided for in Section 215; see Notes to Boxes Nos. VIII, VIII (i) to (v) (in general) and the specific Notes to Box No.VIII (v). If this Box is not used, this sheet should not be included in the request.

Declaration as to non-prejudicial disclosures or exceptions to lack of novelty (Rules 4.17(v) and 51*bis*.1(a)(v)):

☐ This declaration is continued on the following sheet, "Continuation of Box No. VIII (v)".

Form PCT/RO/101 (declaration sheet (v)) (16 September 2012)   *See Notes to the request form*

Sheet No. . . . .

Continuation of Box No. VIII (i) to (v)   DECLARATION

*If the space is insufficient in any of Boxes Nos. VIII (i) to (v) to furnish all the information, including in the case where **more than two inventors are to be named** in Box No. VIII (iv), in such case, write "Continuation of Box No. VIII ..." (indicate the item number of the Box) and furnish the information in the same manner as required for the purposes of the Box in which the space was insufficient. If additional space is needed in respect of two or more declarations, a separate continuation box must be used for each such declaration. If this Box is not used, this sheet should not be included in the request.*

Sheet No. ....7....

| Box No. IX | CHECK LIST for PAPER filings – this sheet is only to be used when filing an international application on **PAPER** |

This international application **contains the following**:	Number of sheets	This international application is **accompanied by** the following item(s) *(mark the applicable check-boxes below and indicate in right column the number of each item)*:	Number of items
(a) request form PCT/RO/101 (including any declarations and supplemental sheets) . . . . :	7	1. ☒ fee calculation sheet . . . . :	1
		2. ☒ original separate power of attorney . . . . :	1
		3. ☐ original general power of attorney . . . . :	
(b) description (excluding any sequence listing part of the description, see (f), below) . . . . :	24	4. ☐ copy of general power of attorney; reference number: . . . . :	
		5. ☒ priority document(s) identified in Box No. VI as item(s) .2 . . . . :	1
		6. ☐ Translation of international application into *(language)*: . . . . :	
(c) claims . . . . :	3	7. ☐ separate indications concerning deposited microorganism or other biological material . . . . :	
(d) abstract . . . . :	1	8. ☐ copy in electronic form (Annex C/ST.25 text file) on physical data carrier(s) of the sequence listing, not forming part of the international application, which is **furnished only for the purposes of international search** under Rule 13*ter* *(type and number of physical data carriers)*	
(e) drawings (if any) . . . . :	4		
(f) sequence listing part of the description (if any) . . . . :			
		9. ☐ a statement confirming that "the information recorded in electronic form submitted under Rule 13*ter* is identical to the sequence listing as contained in the international application" as filed on paper	
Total number of sheets :	39		
		10. ☐ copy of results of earlier search(es) (Rule 12*bis*.1(a)) . . . :	
		11. ☐ other *(specify)*: . . . . :	

| **Figure of the drawings** which should accompany the abstract: | 3 | **Language of filing** of the international application: | English |

| Box No. X | SIGNATURE OF APPLICANT, AGENT OR COMMON REPRESENTATIVE |

Next to each signature, indicate the name of the person signing and the capacity in which the person signs (if such capacity is not obvious from reading the request).

Catherine Davis

Catherine Davis

═══════════════════ For receiving Office use only ═══════════════════

1. Date of actual receipt of the purported international application:		2. Drawings:
3. Corrected date of actual receipt due to later but timely received papers or drawings completing the purported international application:		☐ received:
4. Date of timely receipt of the required corrections under PCT Article 11(2):		☐ not received:
5. International Searching Authority (if two or more are competent): ISA /	6. ☐ Transmittal of search copy delayed until search fee is paid	

═══════════════════ For International Bureau use only ═══════════════════

Date of receipt of the record copy by the International Bureau:

Form PCT/RO/101 (last sheet – paper) (16 September 2012) *See Notes to the request form*

Sheet No. . . . .

Box No. IX   CHECK LIST for EFS-Web filings - this sheet is only to be used when filing an international application with RO/US via **EFS-Web**

This international application **contains** the following:	Number of sheets
(a) request form PCT/RO/101 (including any declarations and supplemental sheets) . . . . :	
(b) description (excluding any sequence listing part of the description, see (f), below) . . . . . :	
(c) claims . . . . :	
(d) abstract . . . . :	
(e) drawings (if any) . . . . :	
(f) sequence listing part of the description in the form of an **image file** (e.g. PDF) . . . . :	

Total number of sheets (including the sequence listing part of the description if **filed as an image file**) . . . . :

(g) sequence listing part of the description

☐ filed in the form of an **Annex C/ST.25 text file**

☐ WILL BE filed separately on physical data carrier(s), on the same day and in the form of an **Annex C/ST.25 text file**

Indicate type and number of physical data carrier(s) . . . . :

This international application is **accompanied by** the following item(s) *(mark the applicable check-boxes below and indicate in right column the number of each item)*:

Number of items

1. ☐ fee calculation sheet . . . . :
2. ☐ original separate power of attorney . . . . :
3. ☐ original general power of attorney . . . . :
4. ☐ copy of general power of attorney; reference number: . . . . :
5. ☐ priority document(s) identified in Box No. VI as item(s) . . . . :
6. ☐ Translation of international application into *(language)*: . . . . :
7. ☐ separate indications concerning deposited microorganism or other biological material . . . . :
8. ☐ *(only where item (f) is marked in the left column)* copy of the sequence listing in electronic form (Annex C/ST.25 text file) not forming part of the international application but **furnished only for the purposes of international search** under Rule 13*ter* . . . . :
9. ☐ *(only where item (f) is marked in the left column)* a statement confirming that "the information recorded in electronic form submitted under Rule 13*ter* is identical to the sequence listing contained in the international application" as filed via EFS-Web: . . . . :
10. ☐ copy of results of earlier search(es) (Rule 12*bis*.1(a)) . . :
11. ☐ other *(specify)*: . . . . :

Figure of the drawings which should accompany the abstract:	**Language of filing** of the international application:

Box No. X   SIGNATURE OF APPLICANT, AGENT OR COMMON REPRESENTATIVE
Next to each signature, indicate the name of the person signing and the capacity in which the person signs (if such capacity is not obvious from reading the request).

═══ For receiving Office use only ═══

1. Date of actual receipt of the purported international application:	2. Drawings:
3. Corrected date of actual receipt due to later but timely received papers or drawings completing the purported international application:	☐ received:
4. Date of timely receipt of the required corrections under PCT Article 11(2):	☐ not received:
5. International Searching Authority (if two or more are competent): **ISA /**	6. ☐ Transmittal of search copy delayed until search fee is paid

═══ For International Bureau use only ═══

Date of receipt of the record copy by the International Bureau:

Form PCT/RO/101 (last sheet – EFS) (16 September 2012)   *See Notes to the request form*

This sheet is not part of and does not count as a sheet of the international application.

PCT

FEE CALCULATION SHEET

Annex to the Request

For receiving Office use only

International Application No.

Applicant's or agent's file reference **CHOCO 95549**

Date stamp of the receiving Office

Applicant

CANDY WRAP UNLIMITED, INC., et al.

CALCULATION OF PRESCRIBED FEES

1. TRANSMITTAL FEE . . . . USD 240 [T]

2. SEARCH FEE . . . . USD 2,426 [S]

   International search to be carried out by ______ **EP** ______

   (If two or more International Searching Authorities are competent to carry out the international search, indicate the name of the Authority which is chosen to carry out the international search.)

3. INTERNATIONAL FILING FEE

   Enter total number of sheets indicated in Box No IX: ______ **39** ______

   [i1] first 30 sheets . . . . 1,453 [i1]

   [i2] ___ **9** ___ x ___ **16** ___ = 144 [i2]
   number of sheets in excess of 30   fee per sheet

   Add amounts entered at i1 and i2 and enter total at I . . . . 1,597 [I]

   (Applicants from certain States are entitled to a reduction of 90% of the international filing fee. Where the applicant is (or all applicants are) so entitled, the total to be entered at I is 10% of the international filing fee.)

4. FEE FOR PRIORITY DOCUMENT *(if applicable)* . . . . [P]

5. FEE FOR RESTORATION OF THE RIGHT OF PRIORITY *(if applicable)* . [RP]

6. FEE FOR EARLIER SEARCH DOCUMENTS *(if applicable)* . . . . . . [ES]

7. TOTAL FEES PAYABLE . . . . **USD 4,263**

   Add amounts entered at T, S, I, P, RP and ES, and enter total in the TOTAL box

   TOTAL

MODE OF PAYMENT *(Not all modes of payment may be available at all receiving Offices)*

- [X] authorization to charge deposit or current account (see below)
- [ ] postal money order
- [ ] credit card *(details should be furnished separately and not included on this sheet)*
- [ ] cash
- [ ] check
- [ ] bank transfer
- [ ] revenue stamps
- [ ] other *(specify):*

AUTHORIZATION TO CHARGE (OR CREDIT) DEPOSIT OR CURRENT ACCOUNT

(This mode of payment may not be available at all receiving Offices)

- [X] Authorization to charge the total fees indicated above.
- [X] *(This check-box may be marked only if the conditions for deposit or current accounts of the receiving Office so permit)* Authorization to charge any deficiency or credit any overpayment in the total fees indicated above.
- [ ] Authorization to charge the fee for priority document.

Receiving Office: RO/ **US**

Deposit or Current Account No.: **12-3456**

Date: **20 September 2012 (20.09.2012)**

Name: **Catherine Davis**

Signature: *Catherine Davis*

ANNEXURE 17

IPO AS INTERNATIONAL SEARCH AUTHORITY

D International Searching Authorities D

IN INDIAN PATENT OFFICE IN

Search fee (PCT Rule 16):[1]	Indian rupee (INR)	10,000	(2,500)[2]
	Euro (EUR)	119	(30)[2]
	Swiss franc (CHF)	147	(27)[2]
	US dollar (USD)	162	(41)[2]

Additional search fee (PCT Rule 40.2):[3]   INR   10,000   (2,500)[2]

Fee for copies of documents
cited in the international search report
(PCT Rule 44.3):   INR   4 per page

Conditions for refund and amount of refund of the search fee:

Money paid by mistake, without cause, or in excess, will be refunded.

Where the international application is withdrawn or is considered withdrawn, under PCT Article 14(1), (3) or (4), before the start of the international search: refund of 100%

Where the Authority benefits from an earlier search already made by the Authority on an application whose priority is claimed in the international application: refund of 25% to 50%, depending upon the extent of the benefit

Protest fee
(PCT Rule 40.2(e)):   INR   4,000   (1,000)[2]

Late furnishing fee
(PCT Rule 13*ter*.1(c)):   INR   4,000   (1,000)[2]

Languages accepted for international search: English

Does the Authority require that nucleotide and/or amino acid sequence listings be furnished in electronic form (PCT Rule 13*ter*.1)?   Yes

Types of electronic carrier required: The entire printable copy of the sequence listing and identifying data should be contained within one text file on a single diskette, CD-ROM, CD-R, DVD, DVD-R.

Subject matter that will not be searched: The subject matter specified in items (i) to (vi) of PCT Rule 39.1 with the exception of subject matter which is searched under the Patents Act, 1970 administered by the Indian Patent Office

Waiver of power of attorney:

Has the Authority waived the requirement that a separate power of attorney be submitted?   No

Has the Authority waived the requirement that a copy of a general power of attorney be submitted?   No

---

[1]   This fee is payable to the receiving Office in the currency or one of the currencies accepted by it (see Annex C).

[2]   The amount in parentheses is applicable in case of filing by an individual.

[3]   This fee is payable to the International Searching Authority and only in particular circumstances.

ANNEXURE 18

**ISA REPORT
CASE STUDY**

PATENT COOPERATION TREATY

<table>
<tr>
<td>

To:

HETERO DRUGS LIMITED
Hetero House, 8-3-166/7/1, Erragadda,
Hyderabad,
Andhrapradesh.
500 018 Hyderabad
India

</td>
<td>

PCT

**WRITTEN OPINION OF THE
INTERNATIONAL SEARCHING AUTHORITY**

(PCT Rule 43bis.1)

</td>
</tr>
</table>

	Date of mailing *(day/month/year)* 14 December 2009 (14.12.2009)

Applicant's or agent's file reference **HDL-PCT-63**	**FOR FURTHER ACTION** See paragraph 2 below

International application No. PCT/IN 2007/000466	International filing date *(day/month/year)* 8 October 2007 (08.10.2007)	Priority Date *(day/month/year)* ----------

International Patent Classification (IPC) or both national classification and IPC
C07D 401/12 (2006.01); **A61K 31/44** (2006.01)

Applicant
HETERO DRUGS LIMITED

1. This opinion contains indications relating to the following items:

- ☒ Cont. No. I — Basis of the opinion
- ☐ Cont. No. II — Priority
- ☐ Cont. No. III — Non-establishment of opinion with regard to novelty, inventive step and industrial applicability
- ☒ Cont. No. IV — Lack of unity of invention
- ☒ Cont. No. V — Reasoned statement under Rule 43bis.1(a)(i) with regard to novelty, inventive step or industrial applicability; citations and explanations supporting such statement
- ☐ Cont. No. VI — Certain documents cited
- ☐ Cont. No. VII — Certain defects in the international application
- ☒ Cont. No. VIII — Certain observations on the international application

2. FURTHER ACTION

If a demand for international preliminary examination is made, this opinion will be considered to be a written opinion of the International Preliminary Examining Authority ("IPEA") except that this does not apply where the applicant chooses an Authority other than this one to be the IPEA and the chosen IPEA has notified the International Bureau under Rule 66.1bis(b) that written opinions of this International Searching Authority will not be so considered.

If this opinion is, as provided above, considered to be a written opinion of the IPEA, the applicant is invited to submit to the IPEA a written reply together, where appropriate, with amendments, before the expiration of 3 months from the date of mailing of Form PCT/ISA/220 or before the expiration of 22 months from the priority date, whichever expires later.

For further options, see Form PCT/ISA/220.

3. For further details, see notes to Form PCT/ISA/220.

Name and mailing address of the ISA/ AT **Austrian Patent Office** Dresdner Straße 87, A-1200 Vienna	Authorized officer HOFBAUER P.
Facsimile No. **+43 / 1 / 534 24 / 535**	Telephone No. **+43 / 1 / 534 24 / 225**

Form PCT/ISA/237 (cover sheet) (January 2004)

**WRITTEN OPINION OF THE
INTERNATIONAL SEARCHING AUTHORITY**

International application No.
PCT/IN 2007/000466

Continuation No. I

Basis of the opinion

1. With regard to the **language**, this opinion has been established on the basis of the international application in the language in which it was filed.

Continuation No. IV:

Lack of unity of invention

In response to the invitation (Form PCT/ISA/206) to pay additional fees the applicant has paid additional fees.

4. Consequently, this opinion has been established in respect of the following parts of the international application: all parts.

Continuation No. V

Reasoned statement under Rule 43bis.1(a)(i) with regard to novelty, inventive step or industrial applicability; citations and explanations supporting such statement

1. Statement

Novelty (N)	Claims **1-27, 35-101**	**YES**
	Claims **28-34**	**NO**
Inventive step (IS)	Claims **64, 73, 85-86**	**YES**
	Claims **1-63, 65-72, 74-84, 87-101**	**NO**
Industrial applicability (IA)	Claims **1-101**	**YES**
	Claims **----**	**NO**

2. Citations and explanations:

EP 2000468 A1 (DR. REDDY'S LAB. LTD) 09.05.2008
E whole document, 1-101
WO 2007/140608 A1 (APOTEX PHARMA. INC.) 13.12.2007
E whole document, 1-101

International application No.
PCT/IN 2007/000466

The following documents cited in the Search Report are considered for the purpose of this report.

D1: WO 1998/54171 A1 (ASTRA AKTIEBOLAG) 25.05.1998
D2: WO 2005/105786 A1 (HETERO DRUGS LIM) 10.11.2005
D3: WO 2004/020436 A1 (REDDY'S LABORATORIES LIM.) 11.03.2004
D4: www.sigmaaldrich.com/catalog/
D5: WO 2008/102145 A2 (CIPLA LIM) 28.08.2008
D6: US 2008/0076929 A1 (HETERO DRUGS LIM) 27.03.2008
D7: WO 2004/002982 A2 (REDDY'S LABORATORIES LIM.) 08.01.2004
D8: WO 2005/082888 A1 (MILEN MERKEZ ILAC ENDUSTRISI A.S.) 09.09.2005
D9: WO 2004/037253 A1 (RANBAXY LAB. LIM.) 06.05.2004
D10: US 5693818 A (VON UNGE) 02.12.1997
D11: WO 2007/054951 A1 (HETERO DRUGS LIM) 18.05.2007
D12: WO 98/28294 A1 (ASTRA AKTIEBOLAG) 02.07.1998
D13: US 2004/0235903 A1 (KHANNA et al) 25.11.2004
D14: WO 97/41114 A1 (ASTRA AKTIEBOLAG) 06.11.1997
D15: WO 03/089408 A2 (SUN PHARMA IND LIM) 30.10.2003
D16: US 2008/0119654 A1 (KHANNA et al) 22.05.2008
D17: EP 2000468 A1 (DR. REDDY'S LAB. LTD) 09.05.2008
D18: WO 2007/140608 A1 (APOTEX PHARMA. INC.) 13.12.2007

D1 discloses a process in which esomeprazole magnesium dihydrate was synthesized.
esomeprazole magnesium salt in methanol was concentrated by evaporation,
a mixture of water and acetone was added
the solution was allowed to crystallize at room temperature,
the crystals were filtered off and dried (D1: Example 5-6, Figure 3., Table 4.)

D2 relates to a process for preparing substituted sulfoxides either as a single enantiomer or in an
enantionerically enriched form.
Potassium salt of esomeprazole was dissolved in water,
Magnesium chloride was added,
Stirring the mass obtained in the previous step
The solid precipitated was filtered,
Washed with water and dried (D2: Example 5-6).

D3 discloses a process in which esomeprazole magnesium was synthesized, in which magnesium metal was
suspended in an alcohol-containing solvent in the presence of a haloalkene and esomeprasole base was
added to the mixture. The preferred haloalkenes were dichloromethane and chloroform (D3: page 9 lines 29-
35).

D4 provides for purchase esomeprazole magnesium dihydrate (assay≥98%).

D7 discloses a process in which optically pure esomeprazole and salts such as esomeprazole magnesium was
synthesized. Re-precipitating the residue of esomeprazole from a mixture of water and acetone to
obtain a solid which is an amorphous form of free species of (S)-omeprazole. Reacting the free
species of omeprazole with a magnesium metal in the presence of dichloromethane in an alcoholic
solvent (preferably methanol) obtaining a residue of magnesium salt of (S)-omeprazole, and dissolving
the residue of magnesium salt of (S)-omeprazole in acetone and lowering the temperature of the
acetone solution to precipitate the magnesium salt of (S)-omeprazole (D7: page 15 lines 28- page 16 line
25; Claims 47, 57).

D8 provides the preparation of magnesium or calcium salt of esomeprazole, where the calcium hydroxide and
alcohol (particularly ethanol) is used instead of magnesium hydroxide in calcium salt preparation. The method
involves:(i) treating esomeprazole in a solution with magnesium or calcium hydroxide as magnesium source (ii)

<table>
<tr><td>WRITTEN OPINION OF THE
INTERNATIONAL SEARCHING AUTHORITY</td><td>International application No.
PCT/IN 2007/000466</td></tr>
</table>

removing unreacted magnesium hydroxide from the reaction mixture;(iii) crystallization of magnesium or calcium esomeprazole; and(iv) purifying by washing with ethyl acetate.

The esomeprazole and magnesium hydroxide are reacted at 15-30C. The magnesium hydroxide is reacted in solid form or as aqueous solution. The esomeprazole and magnesium hydroxide are reacted and followed by crystallization where hydrocarbon and seeds are used during the crystallization of magnesium esomeprazole, which also contains magnesium hydroxide. The crystallization temperature is 15-30 C. Crystallization is followed by distillation at 30-45C under vacuum until no solvent remains, followed by separation of magnesium hydroxide from magnesium esomeprazole using methanol and active carbon at 20-35C. The separation step is followed by removing magnesium hydroxide by filtration, then water addition to the magnesium esomeprazole crystals and distillation under vacuum (preferably 60-90% of initial volume evaporated by distillation). The amount of added water is equal or less amount of methanol, preferably half of it. The crystallization starts by distillation where 60-90% of the initial volume evaporates. The solution temperature during the crystallization is 0-30C. The separation of the magnesium esomeprazole is performed by centrifuge or filtration and the crystals then washed with water and dried at 50-75C. Purification of the crystals is performed by washing the crystals with ethyl acetate and drying at 40-50C (D8: page 5 line 5- page 6 line 8; Claims 36-39).

D9 describes processes for preparing amorphous salts such as Na, Mg, Ca of esomeprazole. In general, the solution of esomeprazole salt in a suitable solvent for example a mixture of dichloromethane and methanol. The solvent may be removed from the solution by a technique which includes distillation, distillation under vacuum, evaporation, spray drying (D9: whole document).

D10 provides optically pure (+)- and (-)-omeprazole (5-methoxy 2-(4-methoxy-3,5-dimethyl-pyridinyl)methyl)sulphinyl)-1H- benzimidazole) (I) and (II), and their Na, Mg, Li, K, Ca, and tetra-(1-4C alkyl) ammonium salts. To obtain the optically pure Mg salts of the invention, optically pure Na salts are treated with an aqueous solution of an inorganic magnesium salt such as MgCl2, whereupon the Mg salts are precipitated. The optically pure Mg salts may also be prepared by treating single enantiomers of omeprazole with a base, in a non-aqueous solvent such as alcohol (only for alcoholates). In an analogous way, also alkaline salts wherein the cation is Ca can be prepared, using an aqueous solution of an inorganic calcium salt such as CaCl2 (D10: whole document).

D11 provides a process for amorphous esomeprazole. Esomeprazole (50 g) was suspended in water (100 ml) at 25C and stirred at the same temperature for 3 hours. Then, the water was removed from the reaction mixture by lyophilization at 70C and isolated to give amorphous esomeprazole (49.7 g) (99.89% of purity) (D11: whole document).

D12 provides esomeprazole in a neutral form in a solid state. Also claimed are methods for obtaining both crystalline form A and form B of esomeprazole. The method comprising evaporation of a solution of esomeprazole in one or more organic solvents to give a concentrate, addition of a further solvent and evaporation to afford solid amorphous neutral esomeprazole. The solution may be obtained by dissolution of an alkaline salt of esomeprazole in water, extracting with an organic solvent while decreasing the pH in the water phase with a water soluble acid to provide the neutral esomeprazole in solution in the organic phase; (2) crystallisation from a solution of neutral esomeprazole in one or more organic solvents and optionally water, when (a) the solution is obtained by dissolving isolated esomeprazole in ethyl acetate or acetonitrile or (b) the solution is obtained from a reaction solution or from the extraction phase in e.g. methylene chloride or toluene. Optionally an anti-solvent such as ethyl acetate or isooctane is added and (3) precipitation from a solution of an alkaline salt of esomeprazole in water with a suitable acid (to give a final pH of 7-10), optionally in the presence of one or more organic solvents (D12: whole document).

D13 describes the preparation of the amorphous form of esomeprazole salt. Preparation of the amorphous form of esomeprazole salt involves preparing a solution of an esomeprazole salt in at least one solvent and recovering the esomeprazole salt in the amorphous form from its solution by removal of the solvent. The solvent is removed by distillation, distillation under vacuum, evaporation, spray drying and/or freeze-drying. The salt of esomeprazole in an amorphous form is recovered from the solution. The cation is selected from Na, Mg, Li, K, Ca, or N(R) (D13: whole document).

WRITTEN OPINION OF THE
INTERNATIONAL SEARCHING AUTHORITY

International application No.
PCT/IN 2007/000466

D14-15 are interesting examples of the state of the art.

<u>Novelty/Inventive step</u>

Group I. (Claims 1-32)
Group I. of the present application refers to a high assayed esomeprazole magnesium dihydrate substantially free of its trihydrate form and an improved and commercially viable process for preparation of the same. The process comprises the following steps:
Adding magnesium chloride or magnesium sulfate to the solution of an alkali metal salt of esomeprazole in an alcoholic solvent; or adding esomeprazole to a solution of magnesium alkoxide in an alcoholic solvent
Stirring the mass obtained in the previous step
Distilling off the solvent
Dissolving the residue in a chlorinated solvent
Filtering the solution
Distilling off the solvent
Dissolving the residue in methanol and water
Precipitating the product
Adding acetone

The subject matter of claims 1-27 appears to be new over the state of the art.
Esomeprazole magnesium dihydrate substantially free of its trihydrate form was synthesized in D1-D2, D4 and it is the state of the art.
Therefore the subject matter of claims 28-32 is considered to lack novelty and inventive step over D1-D2 and D4.

Nevertheless, claims 1-27 of the present application are not considered to involve an inventive step in view of documents D1-D3, D8 because it is considered to be obvious to skilled personnel to combine and optimize the features of document D1-D3, D8 arriving at the improved process for the preparation of esomeprazole magnesium dihydrate according to the present application.
Claims 1-27 differ from D1, D2 and D8 by using chlorinated solvent to dissolve the residue, which missing feature is well described in D3. Therefore the subject matter of claims 1-27 is considered to lack inventive step over D1-D3 and D8.

Group II. (Claims 33-34)
Group II. of the present application refers to an improved process for preparation of pure amorphous esomeprazole magnesium. The process comprises the following steps:
Reacting an alkali metal salt of esomeprazole with magnesium chloride in aqueous medium.
Filtering or centrifuging the reaction mass.

A process for preparation of amorphous esomeprazole magnesium is known from D2, D7, D9 and it is the state of the art.
Therefore the subject matter of claims 33-34 is considered to lack novelty and inventive step over D2, D7 and D9.

Nevertheless, claims 33-34 of the present application are not considered to involve an inventive step in view of documents D1-D3 and D9-D13 because it is considered to be obvious to skilled personnel to combine and optimize the features of document D1-D3, D9-D13 arriving at the improved process for the preparation of amorphous esomeprazole magnesium according to the present application.
Therefore the subject matter of claims 33-34 is considered to lack inventive step over D1-D3 and D9-D13.

Group III. (Claims 35-60)
Group III. of the present application refers to an improved and commercially viable process for preparation of substantially enantiomerically pure esomeprazole in neutral form or as a

<table>
<tr><td style="text-align:center">WRITTEN OPINION OF THE
INTERNATIONAL SEARCHING AUTHORITY</td><td>International application No.
PCT/IN 2007/000466</td></tr>
</table>

pharmaceutically acceptable salt or as its solvates including hydrates from enantiomerically impure esomeprazole calcium salt. The process comprises the following steps:
Dissolving enantiomerically impure esomeprazole calcium salt in an alcoholic solvent.
Isolating the product.
Neutralizing with an acid.
Moreover, the present application refers to an enantiomerically pure esomeprazole calcium salt.

The subject matter of claims 35-60 appears to be new over the state of the art.
Nevertheless, claims 35-60 of the present application are not considered to involve an inventive step in view of documents D3, D7-D10 and D12 because it is considered to be obvious to skilled personnel to combine and optimize the features of document D3, D7-D10 and D12 arriving at the process for preparation of substantially enantiomerically pure esomeprazole in neutral form or as a pharmaceutically acceptable salt or as its solvates including hydrates from enantiomerically impure esomeprazole calcium salt according to the present application.
Therefore the subject matter of claims 35-60 is considered to lack inventive step over D3, D7-D10 and D12.

Group IV. (Claims 61-63)
Group IV. of the present application refers to a solid form of esomeprazole calcium salt.

The subject matter of claims 61-63 appears to be new over the state of the art.
Nevertheless, claims 61-63 of the present application are not considered to involve an inventive step in view of documents D1-D3, D7-D13 because it is considered to be obvious to skilled personnel to combine and optimize the features of document D1-D3, D7-D13 arriving at the solid form of esomeprazole calcium salt according to the present application.
Therefore the subject matter of claims 61-63 is considered to lack inventive step over D1-D3, D7-D13.

Group V. (Claims 64-72)
Group V. of the present application refers to stable and novel crystalline form 1 of esomeprazole calcium salt and a process for preparing them and pharmaceutical compositions comprising them.

The subject matter of claim 64 appears to be new and inventive over the state of the art.
The subject matter of claims 65-72 appears to be new over the state of the art.
Nevertheless, claims 65-72 of the present application are not considered to involve an inventive step in view of documents D1-D3, D7-D13 because it is considered to be obvious to skilled personnel to combine and optimize the features of document D1-D3, D7-D13 arriving at process for the preparation of crystalline form 1 of esomeprazole calcium salt according to the present application.
Therefore the subject matter of claims 65-72 is considered to lack inventive step over D1-D3, D7-D13.

Group VI. (Claims 73-84)
Group VI. of the present application refers to stable and novel crystalline form 2 of esomeprazole calcium salt and a process for preparing them and pharmaceutical compositions comprising them.

The subject matter of claim 73 appears to be new and inventive over the state of the art.
The subject matter of claims 74-84 appears to be new over the state of the art.
Nevertheless, claims 74-84 of the present application are not considered to involve an inventive step in view of documents D1-D3, D7-D13 because it is considered to be obvious to skilled personnel to combine and optimize the features of document D1-D3, D7-D13 arriving at process for the preparation of crystalline form 2 of esomeprazole calcium salt according to the present application.
Therefore the subject matter of claims 74-84 is considered to lack inventive step over D1-D3, D7-D13.

Group VII. (Claims 85-101)
Group VII. of the present application refers to stable and novel amorphous form of esomeprazole calcium salt and a process for preparation of the same and a pharmaceutical composition comprising it.

<table>
<tr><td>WRITTEN OPINION OF THE
INTERNATIONAL SEARCHING AUTHORITY</td><td>International application No.
PCT/IN 2007/000466</td></tr>
</table>

The subject matter of claim 85-86 appears to be new and inventive over the state of the art.
The subject matter of claims 87-101 appears to be new over the state of the art.
Nevertheless, claims 87-101 of the present application are not considered to involve an inventive step
in view of documents D1-D3, D7-D13 because it is considered to be obvious to skilled personnel to
combine and optimize the features of document D1-D3, D7-D13 arriving at process for the preparation
of amorphous form of esomeprazole calcium salt according to the present application.
Therefore the subject matter of claims 87-101 is considered to lack inventive step over D1-D3, D7-
D13.

Industrial applicability

Claims 1-101 are industrially applicable.

———————

Continuation No. VIII:

Certain observations on the international application

The following observations on the clarity of the claims, description, and drawings or on the
question whether the claims are fully supported by the description, are made:

In claims 28-32 the subject matter is not clear, it is not suitably characterized. The claim must
define the matter for which protection is sought and be clear and concise. The subject matter
could be characterized by technical features, which give the claim a precise meaning, and
allows the skilled person to repeat the process or repeat the product as claimed in the
application.

———————

ANNEXURE 19

IPO AS INTERNATIONAL PRELIMINARY EXAMINATION AUTHORITY

E	**International Preliminary Examining Authorities**	**E**
IN	**INDIAN PATENT OFFICE**	**IN**

Preliminary examination fee (PCT Rule 58):[1]	Indian rupee (INR) $12,000^2$ $(3,000)^3$
Additional preliminary examination fee (PCT Rule 68.3):[4]	INR $12,000^2$ $(3,000)^3$
Handling fee (PCT Rule 57.1):[5]	USD 221
Fee for copies of documents cited in the international preliminary examination report (PCT Rule 71.2):	INR 4 per page
Fee for copies of documents contained in the file of the international application (PCT Rule 94.2):	INR 4 per page
Conditions for refund and amount of refund of the preliminary examination fee:	Money paid by mistake, without cause, or in excess, will be refunded. In the cases provided for under PCT Rule 58.3: refund of 100% If the international application or the demand is withdrawn before the start of the international preliminary examination: refund of 100%[6]
Protest fee (PCT Rule 68.3(e)):	INR 4,000 $(1,000)^7$
Late furnishing fee (PCT Rule 13*ter*.2):	INR 4,000 $(1,000)^7$
Languages accepted for international preliminary examination:	English
Subject matter that will not be examined:	The subject matter specified in items (i) to (vi) of PCT Rule 67.1 with the exception of subject matter which is examined under the Patents Act, 1970 administered by the Indian Patent Office
Waiver of power of attorney:	
Has the Authority waived the requirement that a separate power of attorney be submitted?	No
Has the Authority waived the requirement that a copy of a general power of attorney be submitted?	No

---

[1]   This fee is payable to the International Preliminary Examining Authority.

[2]   This fee is reduced to INR 10,000 when the international search report was prepared by the Indian Patent Office.

[3]   The amount in parentheses is applicable in case of filing by an individual. It is reduced to INR 2,500 when the international search report was prepared by the Indian Patent Office.

[4]   This fee is payable to the International Preliminary Examining Authority and only in particular circumstances.

[5]   This fee is payable to the International Preliminary Examining Authority. It is reduced by 90% if certain conditions apply (see Annex C(IB)).

[6]   A processing fee equivalent to the amount of the transmittal fee (see Annex C(IN)) will be deducted from this refund.

[7]   The amount in parentheses is applicable in case of filing by an individual.

PATENT COOPERATION TREATY

PCT

INTERNATIONAL PRELIMINARY REPORT ON PATENTABILITY
(Chapter I of the Patent Cooperation Treaty)

(PCT Rule 44*bis*)

Applicant's or agent's file reference HDL-PCT-63	FOR FURTHER ACTION	See item 4 below
International application No. PCT/IN2007/000466	International filing date *(day/month/year)* 08 October 2007 (08.10.2007)	Priority date *(day/month/year)*

International Patent Classification (8th edition unless older edition indicated) See relevant information in Form PCT/ISA/237

Applicant HETERO DRUGS LIMITED

1. This international preliminary report on patentability (Chapter I) is issued by the International Bureau on behalf of the International Searching Authority under Rule 44 *bis*.1(a).

2. This REPORT consists of a total of 8 sheets, including this cover sheet.

   In the attached sheets, any reference to the written opinion of the International Searching Authority should be read as a reference to the international preliminary report on patentability (Chapter I) instead.

3. This report contains indications relating to the following items:

   ☒ Box No. I   Basis of the report

   ☐ Box No. II   Priority

   ☐ Box No. III   Non-establishment of opinion with regard to novelty, inventive step and industrial applicability

   ☒ Box No. IV   Lack of unity of invention

   ☒ Box No. V   Reasoned statement under Article 35(2) with regard to novelty, inventive step or industrial applicability; citations and explanations supporting such statement

   ☐ Box No. VI   Certain documents cited

   ☐ Box No. VII   Certain defects in the international application

   ☒ Box No. VIII   Certain observations on the international application

4. The International Bureau will communicate this report to designated Offices in accordance with Rules 44*bis*.3(c) and 93*bis*.1 but not, except where the applicant makes an express request under Article 23(2), before the expiration of 30 months from the priority date (Rule 44*bis* .2).

	Date of issuance of this report 13 April 2010 (13.04.2010)
The International Bureau of WIPO 34, chemin des Colombettes 1211 Geneva 20, Switzerland	Authorized officer Dorothée Mülhausen
Facsimile No. +41 22 338 82 70	e-mail: pt01.pct@wipo.int

Form PCT/IB/373 (January 2004)

PATENT COOPERATION TREATY

<table>
<tr>
<td>
To:

HETERO DRUGS LIMITED
Hetero House, 8-3-166/7/1, Erragadda,
Hyderabad,
Andhrapradesh.
500 018 Hyderabad
India
</td>
<td>

PCT

**WRITTEN OPINION OF THE
INTERNATIONAL SEARCHING AUTHORITY**

(PCT Rule 43bis.1)
</td>
</tr>
</table>

Date of mailing *(day/month/year)*	14 December 2009 (14.12.2009)

Applicant's or agent's file reference HDL-PCT-63	**FOR FURTHER ACTION** See paragraph 2 below

International application No. PCT/IN 2007/000466	International filing date *(day/month/year)* 8 October 2007 (08.10.2007)	Priority Date *(day/month/year)* ----------

International Patent Classification (IPC) or both national classification and IPC
C07D 401/12 (2006.01); **A61K 31/44** (2006.01)

Applicant

HETERO DRUGS LIMITED

1. This opinion contains indications relating to the following items:

☒ Cont. No. I   Basis of the opinion

☐ Cont. No. II   Priority

☐ Cont. No. III   Non-establishment of opinion with regard to novelty, inventive step and industrial applicability

☒ Cont. No. IV   Lack of unity of invention

☒ Cont. No. V   Reasoned statement under Rule 43bis.1(a)(i) with regard to novelty, inventive step or industrial applicability; citations and explanations supporting such statement

☐ Cont. No. VI   Certain documents cited

☐ Cont. No. VII   Certain defects in the international application

☒ Cont. No. VIII   Certain observations on the international application

2. FURTHER ACTION

If a demand for international preliminary examination is made, this opinion will be considered to be a written opinion of the International Preliminary Examining Authority ("IPEA") except that this does not apply where the applicant chooses an Authority other than this one to be the IPEA and the chosen IPEA has notified the International Bureau under Rule 66.1bis(b) that written opinions of this International Searching Authority will not be so considered.

If this opinion is, as provided above, considered to be a written opinion of the IPEA, the applicant is invited to submit to the IPEA a written reply together, where appropriate, with amendments, before the expiration of 3 months from the date of mailing of Form PCT/ISA/220 or before the expiration of 22 months from the priority date, whichever expires later.

For further options, see Form PCT/ISA/220.

3. For further details, see notes to Form PCT/ISA/220.

Name and mailing address of the ISA/ AT **Austrian Patent Office** Dresdner Straße 87, A-1200 Vienna	Authorized officer HOFBAUER P.
Facsimile No. **+43 / 1 / 534 24 / 535**	Telephone No. **+43 / 1 / 534 24 / 225**

Form PCT/ISA/237 (cover sheet) (January 2004)

<table>
<tr><td>WRITTEN OPINION OF THE
INTERNATIONAL SEARCHING AUTHORITY</td><td>International application No.
PCT/IN 2007/000466</td></tr>
</table>

Continuation No. I

Basis of the opinion

1. With regard to the **language**, this opinion has been established on the basis of the international application in the language in which it was filed.

———————

Continuation No. IV:

Lack of unity of invention

In response to the invitation (Form PCT/ISA/206) to pay additional fees the applicant has paid additional fees.

4. Consequently, this opinion has been established in respect of the following parts of the international application: all parts.

———————

Continuation No. V

Reasoned statement under Rule 43bis.1(a)(i) with regard to novelty, inventive step or industrial applicability; citations and explanations supporting such statement

1. Statement

Novelty (N)	Claims **1-27, 35-101**	**YES**
	Claims **28-34**	**NO**
Inventive step (IS)	Claims **64, 73, 85-86**	**YES**
	Claims **1-63, 65-72, 74-84, 87-101**	**NO**
Industrial applicability (IA)	Claims **1-101**	**YES**
	Claims **----**	**NO**

2. Citations and explanations:

EP 2000468 A1 (DR. REDDY'S LAB. LTD) 09.05.2008
E whole document, 1-101
WO 2007/140608 A1 (APOTEX PHARMA. INC.) 13.12.2007
E whole document, 1-101

<table>
<tr><td align="center">WRITTEN OPINION OF THE
INTERNATIONAL SEARCHING AUTHORITY</td><td>International application No.
PCT/IN 2007/000466</td></tr>
</table>

The following documents cited in the Search Report are considered for the purpose of this report.

D1: WO 1998/54171 A1 (ASTRA AKTIEBOLAG) 25.05.1998
D2: WO 2005/105786 A1 (HETERO DRUGS LIM) 10.11.2005
D3: WO 2004/020436 A1 (REDDY'S LABORATORIES LIM.) 11.03.2004
D4: www.sigmaaldrich.com/catalog/
D5: WO 2008/102145 A2 (CIPLA LIM) 28.08.2008
D6: US 2008/0076929 A1 (HETERO DRUGS LIM) 27.03.2008
D7: WO 2004/002982 A2 (REDDY'S LABORATORIES LIM.) 08.01.2004
D8: WO 2005/082888 A1 (MILEN MERKEZ ILAC ENDUSTRISI A.S.) 09.09.2005
D9: WO 2004/037253 A1 (RANBAXY LAB. LIM.) 06.05.2004
D10: US 5693818 A (VON UNGE) 02.12.1997
D11: WO 2007/054951 A1 (HETERO DRUGS LIM) 18.05.2007
D12: WO 98/28294 A1 (ASTRA AKTIEBOLAG) 02.07.1998
D13: US 2004/0235903 A1 (KHANNA et al) 25.11.2004
D14: WO 97/41114 A1 (ASTRA AKTIEBOLAG) 06.11.1997
D15: WO 03/089408 A2 (SUN PHARMA IND LIM) 30.10.2003
D16: US 2008/0119654 A1 (KHANNA et al) 22.05.2008
D17: EP 2000468 A1 (DR. REDDY'S LAB. LTD) 09.05.2008
D18: WO 2007/140608 A1 (APOTEX PHARMA. INC.) 13.12.2007

D1 discloses a process in which esomeprazole magnesium dihydrate was synthesized.
esomeprazole magnesium salt in methanol was concentrated by evaporation,
a mixture of water and acetone was added
the solution was allowed to crystallize at room temperature,
the crystals were filtered off and dried (D1: Example 5-6, Figure 3., Table 4.)

D2 relates to a process for preparing substituted sulfoxides either as a single enantiomer or in an enantionerically enriched form.
Potassium salt of esomeprazole was dissolved in water,
Magnesium chloride was added,
Stirring the mass obtained in the previous step
The solid precipitated was filtered,
Washed with water and dried (D2: Example 5-6).

D3 discloses a process in which esomeprazole magnesium was synthesized, in which magnesium metal was suspended in an alcohol-containing solvent in the presence of a haloalkene and esomeprasole base was added to the mixture. The preferred haloalkenes were dichloromethane and chloroform (D3: page 9 lines 29-35).

D4 provides for purchase esomeprazole magnesium dihydrate (assay≥98%).

D7 discloses a process in which optically pure esomeprazole and salts such as esomeprazole magnesium was synthesized. Re-precipitating the residue of esomeprazole from a mixture of water and acetone to obtain a solid which is an amorphous form of free species of (S)-omeprazole. Reacting the free species of omeprazole with a magnesium metal in the presence of dichloromethane in an alcoholic solvent (preferably methanol) obtaining a residue of magnesium salt of (S)-omeprazole, and dissolving the residue of magnesium salt of (S)-omeprazole in acetone and lowering the temperature of the acetone solution to precipitate the magnesium salt of (S)-omeprazole (D7: page 15 lines 28- page 16 line 25; Claims 47, 57).

D8 provides the preparation of magnesium or calcium salt of esomeprazole, where the calcium hydroxide and alcohol (particularly ethanol) is used instead of magnesium hydroxide in calcium salt preparation. The method involves:(i) treating esomeprazole in a solution with magnesium or calcium hydroxide as magnesium source (ii)

<table>
<tr><td>WRITTEN OPINION OF THE
INTERNATIONAL SEARCHING AUTHORITY</td><td>International application No.
PCT/IN 2007/000466</td></tr>
</table>

removing unreacted magnesium hydroxide from the reaction mixture;(iii) crystallization of magnesium or calcium esomeprazole; and(iv) purifying by washing with ethyl acetate.

The esomeprazole and magnesium hydroxide are reacted at 15-30C. The magnesium hydroxide is reacted in solid form or as aqueous solution. The esomeprazole and magnesium hydroxide are reacted and followed by crystallization where hydrocarbon and seeds are used during the crystallization of magnesium esomeprazole, which also contains magnesium hydroxide. The crystallization temperature is 15-30 C. Crystallization is followed by distillation at 30-45C under vacuum until no solvent remains, followed by separation of magnesium hydroxide from magnesium esomeprazole using methanol and active carbon at 20-35C. The separation step is followed by removing magnesium hydroxide by filtration, then water addition to the magnesium esomeprazole crystals and distillation under vacuum (preferably 60-90% of initial volume evaporated by distillation). The amount of added water is equal or less amount of methanol, preferably half of it. The crystallization starts by distillation where 60-90% of the initial volume evaporates. The solution temperature during the crystallization is 0-30C. The separation of the magnesium esomeprazole is performed by centrifuge or filtration and the crystals then washed with water and dried at 50-75C. Purification of the crystals is performed by washing the crystals with ethyl acetate and drying at 40-50C (D8: page 5 line 5- page 6 line 8; Claims 36-39).

D9 describes processes for preparing amorphous salts such as Na, Mg, Ca of esomeprazole. In general, the solution of esomeprazole salt in a suitable solvent for example a mixture of dichloromethane and methanol. The solvent may be removed from the solution by a technique which includes distillation, distillation under vacuum, evaporation, spray drying (D9: whole document).

D10 provides optically pure (+)- and (-)-omeprazole (5-methoxy 2-(4-methoxy-3,5-dimethyl-pyridinyl)methyl)sulphinyl)-1H- benzimidazole) (I) and (II), and their Na, Mg, Li, K, Ca, and tetra-(1-4C alkyl) ammonium salts. To obtain the optically pure Mg salts of the invention, optically pure Na salts are treated with an aqueous solution of an inorganic magnesium salt such as MgCl2, whereupon the Mg salts are precipitated. The optically pure Mg salts may also be prepared by treating single enantiomers of omeprazole with a base, in a non-aqueous solvent such as alcohol (only for alcoholates). In an analogous way, also alkaline salts wherein the cation is Ca can be prepared, using an aqueous solution of an inorganic calcium salt such as CaCl2 (D10: whole document).

D11 provides a process for amorphous esomeprazole. Esomeprazole (50 g) was suspended in water (100 ml) at 25C and stirred at the same temperature for 3 hours. Then, the water was removed from the reaction mixture by lyophilization at 70C and isolated to give amorphous esomeprazole (49.7 g) (99.89% of purity) (D11: whole document).

D12 provides esomeprazole in a neutral form in a solid state. Also claimed are methods for obtaining both crystalline form A and form B of esomeprazole. The method comprising evaporation of a solution of esomeprazole in one or more organic solvents to give a concentrate, addition of a further solvent and evaporation to afford solid amorphous neutral esomeprazole. The solution may be obtained by dissolution of an alkaline salt of esomeprazole in water, extracting with an organic solvent while decreasing the pH in the water phase with a water soluble acid to provide the neutral esomeprazole in solution in the organic phase; (2) crystallisation from a solution of neutral esomeprazole in one or more organic solvents and optionally water, when (a) the solution is obtained by dissolving isolated esomeprazole in ethyl acetate or acetonitrile or (b) the solution is obtained from a reaction solution or from the extraction phase in e.g. methylene chloride or toluene. Optionally an anti-solvent such as ethyl acetate or isooctane is added and (3) precipitation from a solution of an alkaline salt of esomeprazole in water with a suitable acid (to give a final pH of 7-10), optionally in the presence of one or more organic solvents (D12: whole document).

D13 describes the preparation of the amorphous form of esomeprazole salt. Preparation of the amorphous form of esomeprazole salt involves preparing a solution of an esomeprazole salt in at least one solvent and recovering the esomeprazole salt in the amorphous form from its solution by removal of the solvent. The solvent is removed by distillation, distillation under vacuum, evaporation, spray drying and/or freeze-drying. The salt of esomeprazole in an amorphous form is recovered from the solution. The cation is selected from Na, Mg, Li, K, Ca, or N(R) (D13: whole document).

**WRITTEN OPINION OF THE
INTERNATIONAL SEARCHING AUTHORITY**

International application No.
PCT/IN 2007/000466

D14-15 are interesting examples of the state of the art.

<u>Novelty/Inventive step</u>

Group I. (Claims 1-32)
Group I. of the present application refers to a high assayed esomeprazole magnesium dihydrate substantially free of its trihydrate form and an improved and commercially viable process for preparation of the same. The process comprises the following steps:
Adding magnesium chloride or magnesium sulfate to the solution of an alkali metal salt of esomeprazole in an alcoholic solvent; or adding esomeprazole to a solution of magnesium alkoxide in an alcoholic solvent
Stirring the mass obtained in the previous step
Distilling off the solvent
Dissolving the residue in a chlorinated solvent
Filtering the solution
Distilling off the solvent
Dissolving the residue in methanol and water
Precipitating the product
Adding acetone

The subject matter of claims 1-27 appears to be new over the state of the art.
Esomeprazole magnesium dihydrate substantially free of its trihydrate form was synthesized in D1-D2, D4 and it is the state of the art.
Therefore the subject matter of claims 28-32 is considered to lack novelty and inventive step over D1-D2 and D4.

Nevertheless, claims 1-27 of the present application are not considered to involve an inventive step in view of documents D1-D3, D8 because it is considered to be obvious to skilled personnel to combine and optimize the features of document D1-D3, D8 arriving at the improved process for the preparation of esomeprazole magnesium dihydrate according to the present application.
Claims 1-27 differ from D1, D2 and D8 by using chlorinated solvent to dissolve the residue, which missing feature is well described in D3. Therefore the subject matter of claims 1-27 is considered to lack inventive step over D1-D3 and D8.

Group II. (Claims 33-34)
Group II. of the present application refers to an improved process for preparation of pure amorphous esomeprazole magnesium. The process comprises the following steps:
Reacting an alkali metal salt of esomeprazole with magnesium chloride in aqueous medium.
Filtering or centrifuging the reaction mass.

A process for preparation of amorphous esomeprazole magnesium is known from D2, D7, D9 and it is the state of the art.
Therefore the subject matter of claims 33-34 is considered to lack novelty and inventive step over D2, D7 and D9.

Nevertheless, claims 33-34 of the present application are not considered to involve an inventive step in view of documents D1-D3 and D9-D13 because it is considered to be obvious to skilled personnel to combine and optimize the features of document D1-D3, D9-D13 arriving at the improved process for the preparation of amorphous esomeprazole magnesium according to the present application.
Therefore the subject matter of claims 33-34 is considered to lack inventive step over D1-D3 and D9-D13.

Group III. (Claims 35-60)
Group III. of the present application refers to an improved and commercially viable process for preparation of substantially enantiomerically pure esomeprazole in neutral form or as a

WRITTEN OPINION OF THE
INTERNATIONAL SEARCHING AUTHORITY

International application No.
PCT/IN 2007/000466

pharmaceutically acceptable salt or as its solvates including hydrates from enantiomerically impure esomeprazole calcium salt. The process comprises the following steps:
Dissolving enantiomerically impure esomeprazole calcium salt in an alcoholic solvent.
Isolating the product.
Neutralizing with an acid.
Moreover, the present application refers to an enantiomerically pure esomeprazole calcium salt.

The subject matter of claims 35-60 appears to be new over the state of the art.
Nevertheless, claims 35-60 of the present application are not considered to involve an inventive step in view of documents D3, D7-D10 and D12 because it is considered to be obvious to skilled personnel to combine and optimize the features of document D3, D7-D10 and D12 arriving at the process for preparation of substantially enantiomerically pure esomeprazole in neutral form or as a pharmaceutically acceptable salt or as its solvates including hydrates from enantiomerically impure esomeprazole calcium salt according to the present application.
Therefore the subject matter of claims 35-60 is considered to lack inventive step over D3, D7-D10 and D12.

Group IV. (Claims 61-63)
Group IV. of the present application refers to a solid form of esomeprazole calcium salt.

The subject matter of claims 61-63 appears to be new over the state of the art.
Nevertheless, claims 61-63 of the present application are not considered to involve an inventive step in view of documents D1-D3, D7-D13 because it is considered to be obvious to skilled personnel to combine and optimize the features of document D1-D3, D7-D13 arriving at the solid form of esomeprazole calcium salt according to the present application.
Therefore the subject matter of claims 61-63 is considered to lack inventive step over D1-D3, D7-D13.

Group V. (Claims 64-72)
Group V. of the present application refers to stable and novel crystalline form 1 of esomeprazole calcium salt and a process for preparing them and pharmaceutical compositions comprising them.

The subject matter of claim 64 appears to be new and inventive over the state of the art.
The subject matter of claims 65-72 appears to be new over the state of the art.
Nevertheless, claims 65-72 of the present application are not considered to involve an inventive step in view of documents D1-D3, D7-D13 because it is considered to be obvious to skilled personnel to combine and optimize the features of document D1-D3, D7-D13 arriving at process for the preparation of crystalline form 1 of esomeprazole calcium salt according to the present application.
Therefore the subject matter of claims 65-72 is considered to lack inventive step over D1-D3, D7-D13.

Group VI. (Claims 73-84)
Group VI. of the present application refers to stable and novel crystalline form 2 of esomeprazole calcium salt and a process for preparing them and pharmaceutical compositions comprising them.

The subject matter of claim 73 appears to be new and inventive over the state of the art.
The subject matter of claims 74-84 appears to be new over the state of the art.
Nevertheless, claims 74-84 of the present application are not considered to involve an inventive step in view of documents D1-D3, D7-D13 because it is considered to be obvious to skilled personnel to combine and optimize the features of document D1-D3, D7-D13 arriving at process for the preparation of crystalline form 2 of esomeprazole calcium salt according to the present application.
Therefore the subject matter of claims 74-84 is considered to lack inventive step over D1-D3, D7-D13.

Group VII. (Claims 85-101)
Group VII. of the present application refers to stable and novel amorphous form of esomeprazole calcium salt and a process for preparation of the same and a pharmaceutical composition comprising it.

<table>
<tr><td align="center">WRITTEN OPINION OF THE
INTERNATIONAL SEARCHING AUTHORITY</td><td>International application No.
PCT/IN 2007/000466</td></tr>
</table>

The subject matter of claim 85-86 appears to be new and inventive over the state of the art.
The subject matter of claims 87-101 appears to be new over the state of the art.
Nevertheless, claims 87-101 of the present application are not considered to involve an inventive step in view of documents D1-D3, D7-D13 because it is considered to be obvious to skilled personnel to combine and optimize the features of document D1-D3, D7-D13 arriving at process for the preparation of amorphous form of esomeprazole calcium salt according to the present application.
Therefore the subject matter of claims 87-101 is considered to lack inventive step over D1-D3, D7-D13.

Industrial applicability

Claims 1-101 are industrially applicable.

Continuation No. VIII:

Certain observations on the international application

The following observations on the clarity of the claims, description, and drawings or on the question whether the claims are fully supported by the description, are made:

In claims 28-32 the subject matter is not clear, it is not suitably characterized. The claim must define the matter for which protection is sought and be clear and concise. The subject matter could be characterized by technical features, which give the claim a precise meaning, and allows the skilled person to repeat the process or repeat the product as claimed in the application.

ANNEXURE 21

JAPANESE GUIDELINE ON TECHNOLOGY TRANSFER

Guideline for Technology Transfer

1.   Preface

1.1   Background

According to the revised Japanese Pharmaceutical Affairs Law in July 2003, the manufacturing approval system has been replaced with the manufacturing and marketing approval system in April 2005, resulting in a big change in the Japanese pharmaceutical system and regulations. Under these circumstances, it is highly desired to improve a quality assurance system of drugs at all stages through research and development (R&D), manufacturing and marketing in line with the trends by reviewing the current quality assurance system and its methods including existing Good Manufacturing Practice (GMP) to comply with the new system and adopting achievements of technological progress and international harmonization of pharmaceutical regulations.

In recent years, there is a growing awareness that an appropriate transfer of manufacturing technologies (technology transfer) is important to upgrade drug quality as designed during R&D to be a final product during manufacture as well as assure stable quality transferred for many reasons between contract giver and contract acceptor during manufacture. Also, to assure the drug quality, it is desired to make sure 5 W's and 1 H, that is what, when and why information should be transferred to where and by whom and how to transfer, then share knowledge and information of the technology transfer each other between stake holders related to drug manufacturing. Fur that purpose, it is necessary to establish an appropriate guideline for the technology transfer and upgrade the quality assurance system. This guideline categorizes information generated in the processes through pharmaceutical R&D and manufacturing as well as the information flows, discusses information necessary for the technology transfer and communication route, and proposes ideal technological transfer.

1.2   Objective

The objectives of this guideline are:
1) To elucidate necessary information to transfer technology from R&D to actual manufacturing by sorting out various information obtained during R&D;
2) To elucidate necessary information to transfer technology of existing products between various manufacturing places; and
3) To exemplify specific procedures and points of concern for the two types of technology transfer in the above to contribute to smooth technology transfer.

1.3   Scope

This guideline applies to the technology transfer through R&D and production of drugs (chemically synthesized drug substances and drug products) and the technology transfer related to post-marketing changes in manufacturing places. The both technologies include those of manufacturing and quality control (manufacturing methods and tests).

1.4   Organization

This guideline consists of the followings:
- Explanation of technology transfer process
- Explanation of procedures and necessary documents for technology transfer
- Examples of technical information to be transferred
- Points of concern for documenting technology transfer

2. Technology Transfer Process

The drug quality is designed based on basic data concerning efficacy and safety obtained from various studies in preclinical phases and data concerning efficacy, safety and stability of drug products obtained from clinical studies. The quality of design will be almost completed in Phase II clinical study. Various standards for manufacturing and tests will be established in process of reviewing factory production and Phase III study to realize the quality of design, and the quality of design will be verified in various validation studies, and will be upgraded to be the quality of product, and the actual production will be started. The technology transfer consists of actions taken in these flows of development to realize the quality as designed during the manufacture. Even if the production starts, the technology transfer will take place in processes such as changes in manufacturing places. The processes are classified broadly into the following five categories.

2.1 Quality Design (Research Phase)

The quality design is to design properties and functions of drugs, and often performed in phases from late preclinical studies to Phase II study. For drug products, the quality design corresponds to so-called pharmaceutical design to design properties and functions such as elimination of adverse reactions, improvement of efficacy, assurance of stability during distribution, and adding usefulness based on various data such as chemical and physical properties, efficacy, safety and stability obtained from preclinical studies. For drug substances, the quality design is to determine starting materials and their reaction paths, and basic specifications of the drug substances.

2.2 Scale-up and Detection of Quality Variability Factors (Development Phase)

2.2.1 Research for Factory Production

To manufacture drugs with qualities as designed, it is required to establish appropriate quality control method and manufacturing method, after detecting variability factors to secure stable quality in the scale-up validation that is performed to realize factory production of drugs designed on the basis of results from small-scale experiments. In general, this process is called the research for factory production where the quality of design will be upgraded to be the quality of product.

2.2.2 Consistency between Quality and Specification

When the product specification is established on the basis of the quality of product determined in the above, it is required to verify that the specification adequately specifies the product quality. (Consistency between quality and specification)

In short, the consistency between quality and specification is to ensure in the product specification that the quality predetermined in the quality design is assured as the manufacturing quality, and the product satisfies the quality of design.

In reviewing factory production, since manufacturing methods are established with limited amount of lots and limited resources of raw materials, the product specification should be established based on data from study results with limited lots; however, relations between upper and lower limits of manufacturing formula (compositions and manufacturing methods) and upper and lower of control limits of the product specification should be fully understood, and the consistency between the product quality and specification should be maintained.

Also, since initial manufacturing formula and specification are established based on limited information, the consistency between the quality and specification should be fully verified after the start of manufacturing, and the consistency should be revised through appropriate change controls, if necessary.

2.2.3 Assurance of consistency through development and manufacturing

To make developed product have indications as predetermined in clinical phases, the quality of design should be reproducible as the quality of product (assurance of consistency). For this purpose, the transferring party in charge of development should fully understand what kind of technical information is required by the transferred party in charge of manufacturing, and should establish an appropriate evaluation method to determine whether a drug to be manufactured meets the quality of design.

It should be recognized that technical information of developed product are generated from data of a limited amount of batches, various standards have been established from the limited data, and quality evaluation method established in development phase is not always sufficient for factory production. For stable production of consistent products, it is fundamental to fully refer to information of similar products of the past maintained by the manufacturer when research for factory production is implemented, and this is a key to successful technology transfer.

2.3   Technology Transfer from R&D to Production

Transfer of technical information is necessary to realize manufacturing formula established in the above in the actual production facility. In the past, the technology transfer was mainly seen as standard transfer or as technology instruction from technology department to production department within the same company. In future, since contract manufacturing is expected to increase under the revised Pharmaceutical Affairs Law, the technology transfer between companies will increase. In principle, how accurately transfer technical information (know-how) from transferring party to transferred party is important, and it is essential to establish responsibility system and prepare documents clarifying 5 W's and 1 H, and have adequate technology exchange between the both parties for successful transfer.

When transfer technology of new products from research and development department to production department, technical information to be transferred should be complied as research and development report (development report and recommend to use the development report as a part of technology transfer documentations).

2.4   Validation and Production (Production Phase)

Production is implemented after various validation studies verify that it is able to stably produce based on transferred manufacturing formula. While the manufacturing facility accepting technology is responsible for validation, the research and development department transferring technology should take responsibility for validations such as performance qualification (PQ), cleaning validation, and process validation (PV) unique to subject drugs. For validations such as installation qualification (IQ) and operational qualification (OQ), which are not unique to the subject drugs, it is possible to effectively use data of already implemented validations.

2.5   Feedback of Information Generated from Production Phase and Technology Transfer of Marketed Products

As a result of technology transfer, products are manufactured and brought to the hands of consumers. Since the technical information of developed products are obtained from data of a limited amount of batches, various standards have been established from the limited data, and quality evaluation method established in development phase is not always sufficient for factory production, it is highly desired to feed back and accumulate technical information obtained from repeated production, if necessary. Also, it is important to appropriately modify various standards established before on the basis of these information, and accountability (responsibility for giving sufficient explanation) and responsibility (responsibility for outcomes of actions) for design and manufacturing should be executed. For this purpose, appropriate feedback system for technical information and documentation management of technology transfer should be established. For drugs as they have long product shelf life, documentation management should be performed assuming that the technology transfer would occur several decades after the completion of development. Also since product improvements and changes of specifications and methods are often implemented, the initial technical information should be reviewed and updated at regular intervals.

For this kind of documentation management and information updating, it is desirable to establish product specification describing entire characteristics of the product in addition to the development report, which is to be revised and updated regularly.

Since manufacturing places of marketed drugs are often changed for many reasons, already standardized test methods and manufacturing methods are sometimes transferred to other offices or other companies. In this case, subject drug should contain rigorous equivalency including bioequivalency rather than consistency needed for newly developed drugs. Although there are no significant differences between existing drugs and development drugs in terms of technology transfer, it is desirable that subject technical information of the existing drugs should be compiled in forms such as product specification. Also as in the case of technology transfer from research and development to production, responsibilities for the technology transfer should be clearly defined, documentation of technology transfer should be prepared, and the technology transfer should be implemented through adequate exchanges of technical information.

3.   Procedures and Documentation of Technology Transfer

To properly transfer technology according to the above processes, documentation of technology transfer including appropriate procedures and technical documents is necessary. Procedures and documentation of technology transfer are indicated as follows. Items to be specified in the documentation will be referred in detail in the 5th chapter.

3.1   Organization for Technology Transfer

One of the most significant elements for successful technology transfer is close communication between transferring and transferred parties. Therefore, organization for technology transfer should be established and composed of both party members, roles and scope of responsibilities of each party should be clarified, and adequate communication and feedback of information should be ensured.

It is desirable that this organization complies with GMP.

3.2   Research and Development Report

To realize quality assurance at all stages from drug development to manufacturing, transfer of technical documents concerning product development or corresponding documents should be considered. The research and development report (development report) is a file of technical information necessary for drug manufacturing, which is obtained from pharmaceutical development, and the research and development department is in charge of its documentation. This report is an important file to indicate rationale for the quality design of drug substances and drug products including information such as raw materials, components, manufacturing methods, specifications and test methods. The development report should also include the above rationales, and it is desirable to document the report before the approval inspection. Although the development report is not prerequisite for the application for approval, it can be used at the pre-approval inspection as valid document for the quality design of new drug. Also, this report can be used as raw data in case of post-marketing technology transfer. The following exemplifies information to be contained in the development report.

Historical data of pharmaceutical development of new drug substances and drug products at stages from early development phase to final application of approval

Raw materials and components

Synthetic route

Rationale for dosage form and formula designs

Rationale for design of manufacturing methods

Rational and change histories of important processes and control parameters

Quality profiles of manufacturing batches (including stability data)

Specifications and test methods of drug substances, intermediates, drug products, raw materials, and components, and their rationale (validity of specification range of important tests such as contents, impurities and dissolution, rationale for selection of test methods, regents, and columns, and traceability of raw data of those information)

3.3   Technology Transfer Documentation

Technology transfer documentation are generally interpreted as documents indicating contents of technology transfer for transferring and transferred parties. The raw data of the documents (such as development report) should be prepared and compiled according to purposes, and should be always readily available and traceable. For successful technology transfer, task assignments and responsibilities should be clarified, and acceptance criteria for the completion of technology transfer concerning individual technology to be transferred. In principle, it is desirable to prepare product specification with detailed information of product (drug substances or drug products) subject to transfer, then proceed with the technology transfer according to the technology transfer plan established on the basis of this specification, and document the results as the technology transfer report.

3.3.1   Product Specification (Product Specification File)

The product specification is to compile information which enable the manufacture of the product, and to define specification, manufacturing and evaluation methods of the product and its quality, and the transferring party is responsible for documenting the file.
For new products, the development report can be used as a part of product specification file.
The product specification file should be reviewed at regular intervals, and incorporate various information obtained after the start of production of the product, and be revised as appropriate.
The product specification file should contain the following.

- Information necessary for the start and continuation of product manufactuirng} Development Report
- Information necessary for quality assurance of the product
- Information necessary for assurance of operation safety
- Information necessary for environmental impact assessment
- Information of costs
- Other specific information of the product

3.3.2   Technology Transfer Plan

The technology transfer plan is to describe items and contents of technology to be transferred and detailed procedures of individual transfer and transfer schedule, and establish judgment criteria for the completion of the transfer. The transferring party should prepare the plan before the implementation of the transfer, and reach an agreement on its contents with the transferred party.

3.3.3   Technology Transfer Report

The technology transfer report is to report the completion of technology transfer after data of actions taken according to the technology plan is evaluated and the data is confirmed pursuant to the predetermined judgment criteria. Both transferring and transferred parties can document the technology transfer report; however, they should reach an agreement on its contents.

3.3.4   Check and Approval by Quality Assurance Department

It is desirable that the quality assurance department should establish confirmation process for all kinds of technology transfer documentation, and should check and approve the documentation.

3.4   For Implementation of Technology Transfer

Avoid as much as possible the technology transfer from transferring to transferred party only by handing over the technology transfer documentation.
It is recommended that the both parties should cooperate to implement technology education, training and validations at facilities where the transferred technology is actually used.

3.5 Manufacturing Related Documents Including Drug Product Standards

The transferred party should compile documents such as drug product standards necessary for manufacturing, various standards and validation plans/reports after the completion of technology transfer. While the transferred party is responsible for compiling these documents, the transferring party should make necessary confirmation for these documents.

3.6 Verification of Results of Technology Transfer

After the completion of technology transfer and before the start of manufacturing of the product, the transferring party should verify with appropriate methods such as product testing and audit that the product manufactured after the technology transfer meets the predetermined quality, and should maintain records of the results.

3.7 Points of Concern for Post-Marketing Technology Transfer

While there are no fundamental differences in technology transfer between new development product and marketed product, some marketed products do not have development report which can be used as raw data. In this case, a development report needs not to be newly documented; however, it is strongly recommended that the file should be prepared including information of specified items. This file can be used as reference file in case of regular inspection.

4. Examples of Technical Information to be Contained in Technology Transfer Documentation

The1st to 3rd chapters indicate technology transfer processes and procedures. This chapter describes practical concept and contents of technical information to be included in the technology transfer documentation.

4.1 Technical Information of Facilities and Equipments

For technology transfer, technical information of products as well as those of manufacturing facilities and equipments are important. To establish facilities and equipments conforming to GMP, it is essential to obtain and understand information from R&D process so that quality assurance of subject drugs can be secured and the facilities and equipments can comply with required conditions for manufacturing. For that purpose, the following technical information should be transferred.

> ➤ The R&D department should clarify considerations of GMP compliance specific to subject drugs and manufacturing methods (manufacturing processes), and present them to a facility and equipment department.
> ➤ The facility and equipment department should establish facilities and equipments reflecting the above considerations, clearly details of the establishment and operational considerations of those facilities and equipments, and present them to a drug manufacturing department.
> ➤ The drug manufacturing department should fully understand the above information, implement validations, perform appropriate operations and controls in conformity to the established facilities and equipments, and records results of operations and controls.

4.1.1 Technical Information to Establish New Facilities and Equipments

To establish new facilities and equipments in conformity to manufacture of subject drugs, the facility and equipment department should set up required specifications (so called objectives) based on considerations presented by the R&D department, and realize functions in view of considerations specific to the facilities and equipments. In this regard, some functions may be combined, and it is required to prepare definite rationale for establishing functions. To comply with GMP, it is prerequisite to prepare documents of processes through specification decision and realization of functions as well as qualifications, which can be explained to the third party (so called design qualification (DQ)) as technical information.

Information Necessary for the Establishment of Facilities and Equipments (Input Information)

Information necessary for the establishment of facilities and equipments in conformity to GMP are classified into the following three categories.

1) Required Functions of facilities and equipments necessary for quality assurance of subject drugs
2) Required functions of facilities and equipments specific to manufacturing methods (manufacturing processes)
3) Basic required functions necessary for GMP compliance such as prevention of contamination, and human failures, etc.

Regarding 1) and 2), the drug manufacturing department should extract information affecting facilities and equipments from results of quality design during drug development (information on composition, manufacturing and specification), review results of scale-up and quality variability factors during possible factory production, fully understand them and present documents containing

clarified considerations of GMP compliance specific to subject drugs and manufacturing methods (manufacturing processes) to the facility and equipment department.
The facility and equipment department should document interpretations of the above information in forms such as "quality requirement specification" and present the documentation to the R&D department to confirm each other. The both departments should clarify differences of each thought by conforming documents prepared from their own perspectives, and establish certain input data of facility and equipment establishment by obtaining necessary or unnecessary evidence data, extracting unnecessary data, and feeding back them to the R&D department.
Concerning 3), information can be collected by sorting out and reviewing GMP requirements for properties of subject drugs and manufacturing methods and organization of facilities and equipments. Degree of contamination and acceptable contamination level of the subject drugs and acceptable limit of residues are important to determine prevention level of contamination and cleaning methods at the facilities and equipments. Since policies on facilities and equipments such as multi-item production level and automatic production level may have a great impact on granting levels to facilities and equipments regarding prevention for human failures such as cross-contamination or mix-up, measures should be taken in view of all properties of drugs and manufacturing methods which are to be used at the facilities and equipments to be established.

Information of Results of the Establishment of Facilities and Equipments (Output Information)

Establishing facilities and equipments includes actions to upgrade facilities and equipments to be functions for achieving established objectives (required specifications), plan and design details while reflecting considerations specific to the facilities and equipments, construct them in time for the start of manufacturing, and perform qualifications upon the trial operation, while it is important to transfer results of the establishment of facilities and equipments to the drug manufacturing department so that the department can implement validations and production.
It is important for GMP compliance to prepare documents including series of activities from initial stages of establishment (plan and design), the trial operation through qualifications and present them to the third party. In short, output information should be documented by extracting facility and equipment related information from documents compiled during the establishment of facilities and equipments (design, procurement, construction, and trial operation, etc.) to assure the quality of the subject drugs. Cross checking of input and output information are equal to series of qualifications such as DQ, IQ and OQ, while results of qualifications are integrations of output information.

4.1.2 Technical Information When Applied to Established Facilities and Equipments
Subject drugs are often manufactured in existing facilities and equipments. Although there are limitations attributable to the characteristics of the existing facilities and equipments, technical documents should be prepared to demonstrate that those facilities and equipments meet required specifications (so called objectives) for quality assurance of drugs, and this kind of preparation can be equal to the establishment of facilities and equipments in conformity to the subject drug manufacturing. Basic contents of necessary technical documents are similar to those of new facilities and equipments, while only difference is documentation method.

Information necessary for the establishment of existing facilities and equipments are classified into the following three categories as in the case of the new facilities and equipments.

1) Required Functions of facilities and equipments necessary for quality assurance of subject drugs
2) Required functions of facilities and equipments specific to manufacturing methods (manufacturing processes)
3) Basic required functions necessary for GMP compliance such as prevention of contamination, and human failures, etc.

Concerning considerations of applications to existing facilities and equipments in 1) and 2), existing functions should be clarified, and it should be verified that the functions are maintained by maintenance and inspection including routine monitoring. Then, activities are required to compare documents such as "quality requirement specification" prepared as in the case of input information of new facilities and equipments with existing functions and maintenance conditions in the existing facilities and equipments, and identify differences between them. If there are any differences, input information should be realigned by feedback of necessary and unnecessary evidence data and other required information to the R&D department.

Regarding 3), activities are required to compare properties of facilities and equipments such as multi-item production level and automatic production level of the existing facilities and equipments as well as granting levels to facilities and equipments regarding prevention for human failures such as cross-contamination or mix-up with conditions for quality assurance attributable to properties of subject drugs and manufacturing methods, and to clarify differences between them. If there are any differences, measures should be taken as in the cases of 1) and 2).

4.2   Technology Transfer of Test Methods

This chapter exemplifies items to be included in the development report and the technology transfer plan both of which are important to technology transfer of test methods, and describe general concepts.

4.2.1   Development Report of Test Methods

The main objective of documenting development report of test methods is to make quality assurance of drugs more secured one by appropriately transferring technical information accumulated at each stage from design of test methods through those implementation between various departments (organizations).

Therefore, it is desirable that the development report should include details of test methods, information related to drug properties such as physicochemical properties, biological properties, and safety information, background of development of the test methods and rationale for the establishment, and validity and rationale for specifications from early research and development phase to production.

Specifications and Test Methods

Test methods subject to technology transfer include the following.

- Test methods for drug substances
- Test methods for drug products
- Test methods for raw materials and components
- Test methods for in-process tests
- Test methods for drug residue tests
- Test methods for environmental tests

Rational for Specifications and Background

Especially for historic records of specifications of contents, impurities, and degradation products, rationales for their establishment and changes should be included.

Results of Validations

Results of analytical validations for established test methods should be described.

Development History of Important Test Methods (Development Report on Test Methods)

Concerning test methods necessary for the evaluation of product quality and important attributes, development and change histories including their rationales should be described. The test methods include the followings.

> Test methods to measure contents and organic impurities
> Test methods to measure residual solvents and volatile compounds
> Dissolution tests for oral solid drug products
> Test methods to measure residual minerals in drug substances such as metals
> Test methods to evaluate physicochemical properties of drug substances and drug products such as polymorphism and hygroscopicity

It is especially important to describe in detail significant operating conditions (including test equipments, reagents and test solutions, and items concerning reference standards) in relation to developmental history of tests so that transferred party can effectively understand transferred information and attain its technology as well as the description may contribute to future modification of test methods. Also, failure mode factors for the test methods identified during reviewing process may be a part of important information.

Developmental history of already established test methods specified in pharmacopoeia, etc. need not to be described; however, the applicability of such pharmacopoeia method and rationale for adopting the test methods should be described.

Summary of Test Results (Summary of Batch Analysis)

Summary of test results of batches used to develop test methods described in the development report should be described as tables including references to raw data.

Reference Standards

Reference standards to be used in tests of subject substances and impurities should be described. The description should include methods of manufacturing, purification, evaluation for the purity and quality, and storage.

Other information

Items other than the above such as information of drug substances and drug products (properties, stability, manufacturing methods, and formula, background of drug development, containers, etc.) should be described if necessary. If those information are described in the Common Technical Document (CTD), references to raw data should be included.

4.2.2   Technology Transfer Plan

For technology transfer of test methods, it is required to clarify validation range and acceptance criteria of conformity of technology transfer regarding individual test methods to be transferred. The validation range (e.g. full validations, reproducibility, etc.) should be judged on the basis of results of evaluation of technologies, facilities and equipments of transferred party, and the range may be influenced by information to be contained in the technology transfer documentation.

To compare test results, samples (including dose range, number of batches, etc.), specific test methods and evaluation methods to be used in the transferring and transferred parties should be specified.

Acceptance criteria should be established for each test method of subject items on the basis of accumulated test results of the past and analytical validation data, and rationales for the acceptance criteria should be clearly described.

Technical information to be described in or attached to the technology transfer plan (including references to the development report) are shown as follows.

Information of Raw Materials
- Summary including physical and chemical properties and stability
  - Name and structural formula
  - Stability data
- Specifications and test methods
  - Specific test methods and specifications
  - Change history of specifications and test methods and its rationale
  - Results of analytical validation
- List of reference standards (Test results should be attached.)
- Information of toxicity and stability for laboratory use
- List of subject samples for comparative evaluation and their test results

Information of Drug Substances
- Summary including physicochemical properties and stability
  - Name and structural formula
  - Elucidation of chemical structure
  - Possible isomers
  - Physical and chemical properties (including physicochemical properties)
  - Stability data (including severe test data)
- Batch records
  - Chemical synthesis methods of subject batches
  - Analytical data of batches
  - Impurity profile of representative batch
- Specifications and test methods
  - Specific test methods and specifications (including items related to efficacy such as particle size distribution, polymorphism, crystallinity, and hygroscopicity)
  - Change history of specifications and test methods and their rationales
  - Results of analytical method validation
- List of reference standards (Test results should be attached.)
- Development report on test methods (Interim report is acceptable depending on development phases.)
- Information of toxicity and stability for laboratory use
- List of subject samples for comparative evaluation and their test results

Information of Drug Products
- Summary including formula and stability
  - Formula and contents
  - Elucidation of dissolution profile
  - Stability data (including severe test data)
  - Storage conditions and expiry date (if established)
- Analytical data of batches
- Specifications and test methods
  - Specific test methods and specifications (including items related to efficacy such as particle size distribution and hygroscopicity)
  - Change history of specifications and test methods and its rationale
  - Results of analytical method validation
- List of reference standards (Test results should be attached.)

- Development report on test methods (Interim report is acceptable depending on development phases.)
- Information of toxicity and stability for laboratory use
- List of subject samples for comparative evaluation and their test results

Information on Implementation of Technology Transfer
- Persons in charge of planning, checking and settlement of technology transfer
- Test methods (test method number
- Objectives
- Persons in charge of transferring and transferred parties
- Training plan (including explanation of test methods and demonstration)
- Plan of comparative evaluation study
  - Samples: Lot No. (including rationale for the number of lots), storage condition during test, and handling after the completion of the test (disposal or return to the transferred party, etc.)
  - Test period
  - Number of repeated tests
  - Handling of data (Handling method)
  - Retest and handling of outlier
  - Acceptance criteria
  - Storage of raw data (storage department, storage place, and duration, etc.)
  - Judge (person in charge of judgment in the transferring party)

4.3 Technology Transfer of Drug Substances

During R&D processes prior to technology transfer of drug substances, information indicated in 4.3.1 to 4.3.3 should be collected, and based on these information, technology transfer documentation including those indicated from 4.3.4 onward should be prepared.

4.3.1 Information to be Collected During Quality Design (Research Phase)
Items Concerning Raw Materials, Intermediates and Drug Substances
- Impurity profile and information on residual solvents (structure of impurities and route of synthesis)
- Information on descriptions of crystals of drug substances (crystallization, salt and properties of powders)
- Information on stability and description (raw materials, drug substances (including packaged drug substances), intermediates, solutions, crystal slurry, and humid crystals)
- Information on safety of drug substances, intermediates, and raw materials (Material Safety Data Sheet (MSDS))
- Information on animal origins of raw materials, etc.
- Information on packaging materials and storage methods (quality of packaging materials, storage temperature, and humidity)
- Information on reference standards and seed crystals (method of dispensing, specifications and test methods, and storage methods)

Items Concerning Manufacturing Methods
- Information on manufacturing methods (synthetic routes and purification methods)
- Information on operating conditions (control parameters and acceptable range)
- Information on important processes and parameters (identification of processes and parameters which will affect quality)
- Information on in-process control
- Information on reprocess and rework (places and methods)

> Basic data concerning manufacture (properties, heat release rate, reaction rate, and solubility, etc.)
> Data concerning environment and safety (environmental load and process safety)

Items Concerning Facilities and Equipments
> Information on equipment cleaning (cleaning methods, cleaning solvents, and sampling methods)
> Information on facilities (selection of materials, capacity, and equipment types, and necessity of special equipments)

Items Concerning Test Methods and Specifications
> Information on specifications and test methods of drug substances, intermediates, and raw materials (physical and chemical, microbiological, endotoxin and physicochemical properties, etc.)
> Validations for test methods of drug substances and intermediates

4.3.2   Items to be Checked in the Review of Scale-up
Manufacturing processes of drug substances often involve handling of unstable chemical substances, and they are unsteady processes accompanied with chemical changes. Therefore, scale-up should be considered with much attention to prediction of handling period for each operational unit and stability of subject compounds during operation, and conditions of scale-up should be established.
Also, since factors of equipments may have significant influence on qualities regarding scale dependent parameters of operational parameters, considerations should be given in this regard.
Items to be confirmed in reviewing scale-up of reaction and crystallization processes are shown as follows:

Items to be Confirmed in Reviewing Scale-Up of Reaction Processes
> Reproducibility of temperature pattern and its effects (effects of delay in temperature up and down on quality)
> Effects of churning in heterogeneous and semi-batch reactions (formations of concentration distribution and diffusion-controlled zone)
> Prediction and effect of operation period of consecutive reaction or exothermic reaction in semi-batch reactors (extension of operation period due to insufficient capacity of facilities and its effects on quality)
> Balance between heat release rate and heat dissipation capacity (temperature pattern of exothermic reaction and its effects)
> Effects of facilities (validity of required capacity of utility, and effects from temperature distribution, dead volume, and overheating of laminar film)
> Confirmation of fluctuations due to scale-up (phenomenon which did not appear at flask levels)

Items to be Confirmed in Reviewing Scale-up of Crystallization Processes
> Effects of churning (effects on particle size and polymorphism, and selection of scale-up factors)
> Reproducibility of temperature pattern (reproducibility of established temperature pattern and effects on quality)
> Effects on facilities (temperature pattern, changes in flow pattern, effects of local concentration distribution and temperature distribution, supercooling of laminar film, and scaling)
> Prediction of time for solid-liquid separation and its effects (stability of slurry waiting for filtration)

> Confirmation of ease of operation (problems at actual equipment levels such as slurry emission, transfer, and churn load)

4.3.3 Elucidation of Quality Variability Factors

To elucidate quality variability factors, the following items should be reviewed during quality design through scale-up review.

Processes Affecting Quality

To identify processes which may affect quality of final drug substances, such as processes to generate final substances, structures with pharmacological activities, and impurities that cannot be eliminated in purification.

Establishment of Critical Parameters Affecting Quality

To search parameters among those controlling the above processes which may affect quality of final drug substances, such as generation and elimination of impurities, and physicochemical properties of final drug substances, and establish range of control.

Establishment of Other Parameters

Parameters not affecting quality of final drug substances are not subject to validations; however, they are subject to change control and change histories should be recorded.

4.3.4 Development Report on Synthetic Drug Substances

Items concerning drug substances and intermediates to be described are as follows:

> Development history including different synthetic methods used to manufacture investigational drugs
> Finally determined chemical synthetic route
> Change history of processes
> Quality profile of manufactured batches
> Specifications and test methods of intermediates and final drug substances
> Rationale for establishment of critical processes
> Critical parameters and control range
> References to existing reports and literatures, etc.

4.3.5 Technology Transfer of Synthetic Drug Substances from R&D Department to Manufacturing Department

Technology transfer information which transferring party should compile are shown as follows.

- **Information on Manufacturing Methods**
  > Development report on synthetic drug substances or those corresponding to the development report
  > Master batch records of manufacturing of investigational drugs or samples (format of manufacturing records)
  > Manufacturing records of investigational drugs or samples (batches for establishment of specifications for application, validation batches, etc.)
  > Plan and report of process validations
  > Items of in-process control: IPC (test methods and specifications)
  > Investigation report on causes of abnormalities (if occurred)

- **Information on Cleaning Procedures**
  > Master batch record of cleaning
  > Record of cleaning
  > Plan and report of cleaning validation

> Test methods and specifications
> Validation report on analytical methods used for cleaning validation

- **Information on Analytical Methods**
  > Development report on analytical methods or those corresponding to the development report
  > Test methods and specifications (raw materials, intermediates, final drug substances, and container/closure)
  > Validation report on release test methods
  > Stability test (validation report on analytical method, plan/report of stability test, container form, reference standard, and relevant reports)
  > Investigation report on causes of OOS (out of specification)
- **Information on Methods of Storage/Transportation**
  > Container/closure system
  > Date of retest/expiry date
  > Conditions of transportation
  > Information on sensitivity to temperature, humidity, light, and oxygen
  > Instructions of temperature monitoring for drug substances which need cold storage

- **Information on Facilities**
  > Structural materials
  > Category and type of main facility
  > <u>Critical</u> facilities for final processing that may affect physicochemical properties (particle size and surface conditions, etc.)

- **Information on Environmental Management (Drug Substances for Injection and Highly Potent Substances, etc.)**
  > Cleaning area (temperature, humidity, microorganism monitoring, airborne particles, and control of differential pressure)
  > Information on safety
    - ✧ Safety information of hazardous raw materials, intermediates, and final drug substances
    - ✧ Information on degradability
    - ✧ Information on dust explosion
    - ✧ Information on deflagration

- **Information on Industrial Hygiene/Occupational Health**
  > Protection for operators
  > Protection for products

4.4   Technology Transfer of Drug Products

During R&D processes prior to technology transfer of drug products, information indicated in 4.4.1 to 4.4.3 should be collected, and based on these information, technology transfer documentation including those indicated from 4.4.4 onward should be prepared.

4.4.1   Information to be Collected During Quality Design (Research Phase)
(Solid form)
Items Concerning Compositions
> Physicochemical properties of drug substances (crystal form, melting point, solubility, distribution coefficient, hygroscopicity, degradation products, impurities, particle size, particle size distribution, wetness, moisture, and handling, etc.)
> Biopharmaceutical properties of drug substances (hygroscopicity and dose dependency,

etc.)
- Stability of drug substances (temperature, humidity, and light)
- Incompatibility of drub substances with raw materials of drug products
- Initial formula design of drug products (absorbability and dose dependency, etc.)
- Formula design of prototype drug products
- Formula design of final drug products (reasons for combining individual inactive ingredients and validities)
- Change histories of formula during development and rationales for assurance of equivalence
- Packaging design
- Stability of drug products (temperature, humidity, and light)
- Information on drug substances, raw materials of drug products, and packaging materials (such as specifications, packaging manufacturers, Drug Master File (DMF) and MSDS)
- Information on origins of drug substances and raw materials of drug products (raw materials of animal origins, etc.)

Items Concerning Manufacturing Methods
- Information on selection of dosage forms (direct compressed tablets, dry and wet granulation, agitation fluidized bed granulation, uncoated tablets, and coated tablets)
- Manufacturing methods of initial drug products (manufacturing flows, manufacturing conditions, and in-process control)
- Manufacturing methods of prototype drug products (manufacturing flows, manufacturing conditions, and in-process control)
- Manufacturing methods of final prescribed drug products (manufacturing flows, manufacturing conditions, in-process control, scale-up, and validation)
- Information on other important processes and manufacturing procedures (information on determination of granulation end-point, determination of mixing time with lubricants, cleaning methods, and cleaning validation, etc.)

Items Concerning Facilities and Equipments
- Information on equipment cleaning (cleaning methods, cleaning solvents and sampling methods)
- Information on equipments (selection of materials, capacity and equipment types, and necessity of special equipments)

Items Concerning Test Methods and Specifications
- Specifications and test methods of drug substances (physical and chemical, and microorganism)
- Specifications and test methods of raw materials of drug products (grade, physical and chemical, and microorganism)
- Specifications and test methods of packaging materials (specifications, physical and chemical, and microorganism)
- Acceptance criteria for product assessment (internal control criteria based on stability, etc.) and specifications for application (specifications for approval to ensure expiry date)
- Validation for test methods of drug substances and products

(Injectable Solutions (sterile drug products))

Items Concerning Compositions
- Information on formula design (reasons for combining individual inactive ingredients and validities; pH, relations between inactive ingredients and stability, and overages, etc.)
- Information on stability of drug substances (heat, light and gas)
- Information on safety of drug substances and raw materials (MSDS)
- Information on origins of drug substances and raw materials (raw materials of animal origins, etc.)
- Disparities in quality between different lots of drug substances and raw materials, stability of lots of raw materials, and effects on impurities
- Basic documents to ensure sterilization and cleaning in view of composition
- Information on stability of drug products (heat, light, oscillation, and gas)

Items Concerning Manufacturing Methods
- Information on selection of dosage forms (solution, freeze dry or powder preparations; relations between those dosage forms and stability)
- Information on determination of container/closure system and its validity (eluting materials from containers or closures, interactions between drug products and containers (absorbability), etc.)
- Information on initial design of manufacturing methods (aseptic manipulation or final sterilization method; effects of heat sterilization on stability)
- Information on selection of process filters (absorbability, etc.)
- Process design and important processes (test items in important processes and specifications)
- Rationale for design to ensure sterilization and cleaning in view of manufacturing methods

Items Concerning Facilities and Equipments
- Information on equipment cleaning (cleaning methods, cleaning solvents, and sampling methods)
- Information on facilities (selection of materials, capacity, and equipment types, and necessity of special equipments)

Items Concerning Test Methods and Specifications
- Specifications and test methods of drug substances (physical and chemical, microbiological, and endotoxin, etc.)
- Specifications and test methods of raw materials of drug products (physical and chemical, microbiological, and endotoxin, etc.)
- Specifications and test methods of containers and closures (physical and chemical, microbiological, and endotoxin, etc.)
- Specifications and test methods of packaging materials (specifications, etc.)
- Specifications and test methods of products (physical and chemical, microbiological, and endotoxin, etc.)
- Specifications of shipment (internal control specifications in view of stability, etc.) and specifications of products (approval specifications to ensure expiry date)
- Validation of test methods of drug substances and products
- Reference standard and reference substance (dispensing methods, specifications and test methods, and storage methods and stability, etc.)

4.4.2 Scale-up Validation and Detection of Quality Variability Factors (Development Phase)

(Solid Form)
- Mixing conditions in mixing process of raw materials (uniformity of contents)

> Granulation conditions in granulation process (determination of granulation end-point, tablet hardness, and elution)
> Drying end-point in drying process (tablet hardness, compression problems, and stability)
> Mixing conditions in granulation mixing process (uniformity of contents)
> Mixing conditions in lubricant mixing process (tablet hardness and elution)
> Time series fluctuations in tablet compressing process or filling process (tablet weight, tablet hardness, and uniformity of contents)
> Fluctuations due to raw materials (processes in manufacturers of raw materials and changes in material qualities, etc.)
> Fluctuations due to facilities (exchange of consumable parts, changes of equipments, and changes in manufacturing processes including automated processes, etc.)

(Injectable Solutions (Sterile Drug Products))
> Dispersion of final moisture and contents between different shelves and/or within the same shelf in freeze drying process
> Changes and dispersion in water content in rubber closures of vials
> Dispersion of contents and impurities, etc. after the final sterilization
> Concerning fluctuations of raw materials, dispersion in particle size which may affect solubility, peroxide which affect stability, and viable cell counts which affect abacterial situations should be evaluated.
> Concerning facilities, effects of temperature distribution within facilities and effects of changes in important parameters on product quality should be evaluated. Especially for drugs or minor constitutes such as protein which are highly sensitive to oxygen, water and light, relations between conditions of facility operations and stability should be fully understood.
> Validity of solution preparation process (uniformity of contents of all raw materials and stability in solution conditions, etc.)
> Validity of sterile filtration processes (completeness, conformity of filtration process and drug solution, stability of filtrated drug solution, and initial disposal rate, etc.)
> Microorganism capture efficiency of barrier filter (validation data)
> Validity of cleaning of containers and closures (cleaning validation, drying and residual moisture, etc.)
> Validity of sterilization of containers and closures (validations of sterilization and removal of ethyl, and drying and residual moisture of closures, etc.)
> Validity of filling processes (accuracy of filling, conformity of filling system and drug solution, stability of filled drug solution, and initial disposal rate, etc.)
> Validity of freeze drying process (cycle conditions, uniformity of inside of freeze-dry equipment, water contents, and stability, etc.)
> Validity of capping and metal sealing (replacement rate of inactive gas in a head space and stability of the inactive gas)
> Validity of final sterilization process (validation of sterilization)
> Validity of test process (development of test process, types of foreign substances, and accuracy of test)
> Development of cleaning methods of facilities and validation of cleaning
> Development of sterilization methods of facilities and validation of sterilization
> Validity of in-process control of sterile operation (culture media filling test, etc.)
> Methods of environmental management and monitoring data (methods of sterilization)
> Control parameters of important processes and process test data
> Data of all batches of preclinical lots and investigational drug lots, etc.

4.4.3   Development Report
The development report should contain the following elements.

- Rationale for selection of dosage forms
- Explanation of formula design
- Development history including different manufacturing methods used for manufacturing investigational drugs
- Consideration of scale-up
- Finally determined manufacturing methods
- Change history of processes
- Quality profile of manufactured batches
- Specifications and test methods of final drug products
- Rationale for establishment of important processes
- Control range of process parameters
- References to existing reports and literatures, etc.

4.4.4   Information of Technology Transfer of Drug Products
Information of technology transfer are shown as follows.

Information on Manufacturing Methods
- Development report on drug products or those corresponding to the development report
- Master batch records of manufacture (format of manufacturing records)
- Manufacturing records (batches for establishment of specifications for approval and validation batches, etc.)
- Plan and report of process validations
- Items of in-process control: IPC (test methods and specifications)
- Investigation report on causes of abnormalities (if occurred)

Information on Test and Packaging
- Inspection procedures (precision of inspection and limit of defects)
- Container closure system
- Specifications of primary packaging (moisture proof and light blocking, etc.) and conformity to primary packaging materials

Information on Cleaning Procedures
- Master batch records of cleaning
- Records of cleaning
- Plan and report of cleaning validations
- Test methods and specifications
- Validation report on analytical methods used for cleaning validations

Information on Analytical Methods
- Development report on analytical methods or those corresponding to the development report
- Test methods and specifications (raw materials, drug substances, final drug products, container/closure, and packaging materials)
- Validation report on release test methods
- Stability tests (validation report on analytical methods, plan and report of stability tests, packaging conditions, reference standards, and relevant reports)
- Investigation report on causes of OOS (out of specification)

Information on Storage and Transportation Methods
- Specifications of secondary packaging
- Expiry date
- Transportation conditions and tests

- ➢ Information on sensitivity to temperature, humidity, and light
- ➢ Instructions of temperature monitoring for drug products which need cold storage

Information on Facilities
- ➢ Structural materials
- ➢ Category and type of main facility

Information on Environmental Management
- ➢ Cleaning area (temperature and humidity, microorganism monitoring, airborne particles, and control of differential pressure)
- ➢ Information on safety
  - ✧ Safety information of hazardous raw materials, drug substances, and final drug products

Information on Industrial Hygiene/Occupational Health
- ➢ Protection for operators
- ➢ Protection for products

5.   Points of Concern For Preparing Technology Transfer Documentation

For smooth technology transfer, transferring and transferred parties should establish organizations in conformity to GMP, and appropriately document and record necessary information relevant to the technology transfer. In this regard, summaries are already described in the above; however, it is recommended to prepare the following documents.

1) Documents to clarify applicable technologies, burden shares, responsibilities, and approval systems, etc. concerning the technology transfer (written agreements and memorandums, etc.)
2) Organizations of technology transfer (at both of transferring and transferred parties)
3) Development report
4) Product specifications
5) Technology transfer Plan
6) Technology transfer Report

Concerning 1), 3) and 4) which need comments on descriptions, this chapter will show details of items to describe, and points of concern for description.

5.1   Documents To Clarify Applicable Technologies, Burden Shares and Responsibility System, etc. Concerning Technology Transfer

The following chart shows details of items to be described in documents clarifying applicable technologies, burden shares, responsibilities, and approval system, etc. concerning technology transfer, and points of concern for description. Any types and forms of the documents are acceptable if they include the items in the following chart, and no duplications of the items stipulated or described in detail in other technology transfer documents are required.

Items		Details	Remarks
1	GMP compliance		
1.1	Organizations	Organizational framework, organization chart, department (person) in charge, and separation between manufacturing and quality departments	
1.2	Supervisor	Clarify supervisor of technology transfer (manufacturing supervisor is acceptable) and his/her responsibilities.	
1.3	Responsibility system	Clarify organization and its responsibilities, document control system, persons in charge of manufacturing department and quality control department.	
1.4	Structure and equipments	Maintenance, inspection and calibration of manufacturing facilities and equipments, and antipollution measurements, etc.	
1.5	Documentation and records	Clarify all technology transfer documentations. Describe control methods of documentation and records, and storage period.	SOP list may substitute the documentation and records, if under the control of GMP; however, "cleaning categories" and "cleaning methods of facilities and equipments" should be described in detail.

Table *Contd…*

1.6	Manufacturing control	Standard manufacturing procedure, and manufacturing instructions and records Industrial hygiene control methods of buildings and facilities Industrial hygiene control methods of operators Report on manufacturing control and quality control Control methods of raw materials, intermediates, and products	For existing products, existing GMP documents can be used.
1.7	Quality control	Determination of test results and report methods Control method of reference samples Maintenance and inspection of pilot facilities and equipments Control methods of test results Control methods of reference standards, reagents, and test solutions, etc. Handling of retest	
1.8	Product release	Control methods of release (procedures and judge)	
1.9	Validation	Organization for validation Describe communication and confirmation methods, discussion, and approval, etc. concerning validations. Facility qualification	
1.10	Change control	Specify handling of change controls in advance.	
1.11	Deviations	Clarify handling of abnormalities, deviations, and OOS.	
4	Other necessary items		
4.1	Persons in charge	Describe persons in charge at both parties.	
4.2	Periodic report	Describe formats of periodic reports, such as annual report.	
4.3	Changes in technology transfer documentation such as required specifications and product specifications	Describe communication and confirmation methods and necessary formats for changes.	
4.4	Retention of technology transfer documentation such as required specifications and product specifications	Specify retention period and disposal time.	
4.5	Revision history	Documents should be replaced according to revisions.	
4.6	Others	Handling of not specified items	

Table _Contd..._

5.2   Technical information to be Described in the Development Report, and Product Specification, etc.

The following chart shows technical information and points of concern to be described in documents such as the development report, and product specification, etc. of drug substances.

Items	Details	Remarks
Report on design of drug substances		
1 Change history of process design and manufacturing methods during development	• History of manufacturing methods of drug substance used in Phase I, II and III studies, etc., bioequivalence of drug substance quality, and justification for starting materials and manufacturing methods, etc.	
2 Information on final product		
2.1 Product name	• Scheduled brand name in the certificate of approval	• Not necessary, if not yet determined.
2.2 Specifications and test methods	• Describe all of specifications and test methods described in the certificate of approval.	• Describe agreed specifications as well, if any.
2.2.1 Raw materials	• Specifications and test methods of raw materials to be used	• Clarify suppliers. • Test results
2.2.2 Container and closure	• Specifications and test methods of container and closure to be used	• Clarify suppliers. • Test results
2.2.3 Packaging and labeling materials	• Specifications and test methods of packaging and labeling materials to be used	• Clarify suppliers. • Test results
2.2.4 Intermediates	• Sampling procedures, specifications and test methods of intermediates	• For intermediates not to be isolated, description can be omitted, provided that the rationale should be described in the development report. • Describe added specifications for trading (such as acceptance criteria for product assessment), if any.
2.2.5 Drug substance	• Sampling procedures, specifications and test methods of drug substance	• Describe added specifications for trading (such as acceptance criteria for product assessment), if any.
2.2.6 Form of test results	• Attach sample form of manufacturer.	
2.3 Manufacturing methods and procedures, etc.	• Describe manufacturing flows, manufacturing procedures, in-process control, and required facility capacity, etc. as detail as possible.	• Describe scientific evidence based data (including stability data to determine unit operating conditions) in the development report. • Confirm important parameters at the time of predictive validation and change validation.
2.4 Packaging methods and procedures, etc.	• Describe packaging methods and procedures.	
2.5 Storage conditions	• Describe storage conditions of raw materials, intermediates, and drug substances.	• Temperature and humidity ranges, light, and container in use • Describe evidence data in the development report.

Table *Contd...*

2.6	Expiry date	• Expiry dates of raw materials, intermediates, and drug substances	• Describe evidence data in the development report. • Describe stability data as much as possible.
2.7	Transportation conditions	• Describe transportation conditions and cautions for transportation of raw materials, intermediates and drug substances.	
2.8	Information on safety	• Describe information on safety of raw materials, intermediates, and drug substances. • Describe information on safety of each unit operation (reaction and post-treatment, etc.).	• Attach MSDS as much as possible. • Attach safety data of processes as much as possible.
3	Stability		
3.1	Raw materials		• Describe physicochemical safety (temperature, humidity, and light).
3.2	Intermediates		
3.3	Drug substances		• Describe microbiological safety.
4	Environmental assessment	• Describe influence on environment.	• Describe waste disposal methods as well.

The following chart shows technical information and points of concern of drug products to be described in documents such as the development report, and product specification, etc.

	Items	Details	Remarks
Report on drug product design			
1	Properties of drug substances	• Physicochemical and pharmaceutical properties necessary for drug product design (such as dissolution, particle size, hygroscopicity, incompatibility, absorbability and stability, etc.)	
2	Change history of formula design and manufacturing methods during development *	• History of formula and manufacturing methods of drug product used for exploratory pharmacokinetic study, Phase I study, proof of concept (POC) study, Phase II and Phase III studies, bioequivalence between different drug products, formula of final drug product, and rational for the manufacturing methods, etc.	
3	Information on final drug product		
3.1	Product name	• Scheduled brand name in the certificate of approval	• Not necessary, if not yet determined.
3.2	Indications and dosage and administration	• Indications in the certificate of approval	• Not necessary, if not yet determined.
3.3	Ingredients/contents	• Ingredients/contents in the certificate of approval	• In case of revision of contents, its rationale should be included.
3.4	Specifications and test methods	• Describe all specifications and test methods in the certificate of approval.	• Describe agreed specifications, if any.
3.4.1	Drug substances	• Specifications and test methods of drug substances to be used	• Clarify suppliers. • DMF No., if any, and letter of authorization (LOA)

Table *Contd...*

3.4.2	Drug substance raw materials	• Specifications and test methods of drug substance raw materials to be used	• Clarify suppliers. • DMF No., if any, and letter of authorization (LOA)
3.4.3	Primary packaging materials	• Specifications and test methods of primary packaging materials	• Clarify suppliers. • DMF No., if any, and letter of authorization (LOA)
3.4.4	Secondary packaging materials	• Specifications and test methods of secondary packaging materials	
3.4.5	Intermediates	• Specifications and test methods of intermediates	
3.4.6	Final products	• Specifications and test methods of final products	• Describe applied specifications for application and/or specifications before shipment, if any.
3.4.7	Forms of test results	• Attach sample form of an manufacturer.	
3.5	Manufacturing methods and manufacturing procedures, etc.	• Describe manufacturing flows, manufacturing procedures, and in-process control as detail as possible.	
3.6	Packaging methods and packaging procedures, etc.	• Describe packaging flows, packaging procedures, and in-process control as detail as possible.	
3.7	Storage conditions	• Storage conditions of drug substances, drug product raw materials, primary packaging materials, secondary packaging materials, intermediates, and final products	Temperature and humidity ranges, light and container in use
3.8	Expiry date	• Expiry dates of drug substances, drug product raw materials, primary packaging materials, secondary packaging materials, intermediates, and final products	• Describe rationale for expiry dates. • Describe stability data as much as possible.
3.9	Transportation conditions	• Describe transportation conditions of drug substances, drug product raw materials, primary packaging materials, secondary packaging materials, intermediates, and final products, and cautions for their transportation.	
3.10	Information on safety	• Describe information on safety of drug substances, drug product raw materials, primary packaging materials, secondary packaging materials, intermediates and final products.	• Attach MSDS as much as possible.
4	Stability		
4.1	Drug substance		• Describe physicochemical stability (temperature, humidity, and light).
4.2	Intermediates		
4.3	Final products		• Describe microbiological stability as well.
5	Environmental assessment	• Describe influence on environment.	• Describe waste disposal methods as well.

ANNEXURE 22

STATISTICS AND RELAVANT PUBLICATIONS

An Overview of Patent System

Ravali. A & Rau. B. S

Abstract: Creations of brain are called intellect. Since these creations have commercial value are called as property. As these creations are rights of an individual, the term was coined as intellectual property rights. It is believed that intellectual property rights increase the economy of the country due to industrial applicability leading to business within the country as well as exports. There is a necessity of still the basics since many of the creators of intellectual property are prone for research paper journal publications instead for patent protection and emphasis is made on Indian perspective.

Introduction

Now a day the numbers of pharmacy colleges are increasing throughout the country. It can be interpreted that as the intellectuals increases, creations increases leading to industrial applicability and hence increasing the economy of the country either through business within the country or as exports. The Indian government has brought out a tremendous change in protecting the intellectual property especially over the last one and a half decade. Currently, Indian patent office takes the role of international search authority as well as international preliminary examination authority for patent applications, indicating the in house established facility for making decisions on patentability of inventions made by the creator at the international level. Several professionals involved in academics, industry are contributing extensively in research in pharmaceuticals but finally leading to journal publications (especially in case of academicians) without any intellectual property protections. During the last one and a half decade the number of patent applications, patent grants increased exponentially. There is a need to review such applications, grants by the innovators at the academic level so that the inventions made to be confirmed for patentability criteria. Only if the invention meets the patentability criteria, the invention can be considered as patentable. With the increase in the patent grants, it has become crucial for the intellectuals to brain storm so that the outcome of the research is really patentable. There is a misconception that intellectual property rights belong to law discipline, but it is necessary to understand that framing the Act mainly deals with law where as technical people should understand the law and based on the provisions, intellectual property can be protected. The objective of this article is to bring awareness, increase patent filings, increase individual/ independent patent filings at academic level at least by some professionals who can afford the patent filing and maintenance fees which may bring out good business after patent grants.

Components of Intellectual Property Rights

Intellectual property rights (IPR) are governed by Intellectual property law. Intellectual property rights are classified into two i.e., industrial property rights, copyrights. Industry property rights comprises of patents, trademarks, designs, integrated circuits, geographical indicators, protection of plant varieties, trade secrets, traditional knowledge, biodiversity. Copyrights comprise of author rights, artistic rights, film rights, broadcasting rights, performers rights etc. In India, there is no protection relating to trade secrets (like data exclusivity).

Term of Intellectual Property Rights

In case of Industrial property rights, the duration of patent is for 20 years from date of first filing, while for the other property the duration ranges from 10 to 15 years and extendable for some selected property. In case of copyrights especially author rights,

Associate Professor, RBVRR Women's College of Pharmacy, Barkatpura, Hyderabad, A.P.

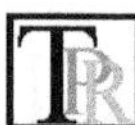 **ARTICLE**

the duration of protection is life time of author plus 60 years. In several other cases especially copyright in government works, works of public undertaking, works of international organisations etc., the term is for 60 years.

Objective and Role of International and National Governing bodies

General Agreement on Tariffs and Trade (GATT) converted to World Trade Organisation (WTO) with additional inclusion of safeguarding rights of individuals as intellectual property rights. The main objective was to provide stable and predictable international trade system while monitoring and settling disputes among countries. Trade related aspects of intellectual property rights (TRIPS) came into existence with origin of WTO and India became a signatory since 1995 fulfilling the up gradation of The Patents Act, 1970, infrastructure within the stipulated transition period.

World Intellectual Property Organisation (WIPO) is an international body that promote international co-operation with respect to creation, dissemination, use and protection of works of the human mind for economic, social, cultural progress of all mankind.

In India, Department of Industrial Policy and Promotion (DIPP), Department of Pharmaceuticals, Department of Commerce of the respective ministries play a critical role in the implementation of intellectual property rights (especially relating to patents) in India.

Indian patent office (IPO) located at Mumbai, Kolkata, Chennai, New Delhi accepts and grants applications for a patent.

Conventions and Treaties

Among the different conventions and treaties relating to intellectual property rights, Paris convention (PC) and Patent Co-operation Treaty (PCT) play a critical role relating to patents. Paris Convention provides a provision to claim priority of the invention among the countries who are members of the convention. In other words, the convention has brought national treatment i.e., a foreign national is treated as a national of India provided the foreign national's country and India are members of Paris Convention. Patent Co-operation Treaty has brought a single patent filing procedure for the member countries of the PCT. The treaty is beneficial with single filing, examination procedures avoiding translations and repetition of patent office procedures. Moreover, the provision provides economic benefit during filings as well as saving time.

What is a Patent?

A patent is a document issued by the government to the inventor granting him exclusive rights to sell, make, use, import the invention for a stipulated period upon disclosure of the invention.

Criteria for Patentability

A subject matter (invention) is said to be a patentable subject matter provided it is novel, non-obvious, useful (industrial application) and enabled. It is necessary that the subject matter of the invention fulfill all the patentability criteria.

Term of Patent

A term of a patent is 20 years from the date of filing.

Types of Patent Applications

Patent applications are filed as provisional, complete, additional and divisional. In a provisional application, the inventor can submit a brief description of his invention made and which is not complete. In case of complete, it is mandatory that the inventor provides complete details of his invention. An additional patent is submitted when an inventor has explored further with an invention that is already patented. A divisional application is submitted, where there is more than one invention in a patent. The inventions are necessary to be submitted with the prescribed application forms.

Inventions not Patentable

Subject matter that is frivolous, natural law, intended for commercial exploitation, contrary to public order or morality, serious prejudice to human, animal, plant life or health or the environment, mere discovery, scientific discovery, abstract theory, mere discovery of new form of known substance, mere admixture, mere arrangement or re-arrangement or duplication of known devices, method of agriculture, process for the medicinal, surgical, curative, prophylactic or treatment of human beings/animals, whole plant, whole animals, mathematical methods, business methods, computer program, literary, dramatic, musical, artistic, cinematography, television productions, mere scheme, method of performing mental act, method of playing game, presentation of information, topography of integrated circuits, traditional knowledge, relating to atomic energy are not patentable.

Content of a Patent

A patent document contains Title, Bibliography, Abstract, Prior art, Summary, Description of invention with best mode,

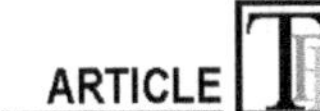
ARTICLE

Tables, Figures, Claims comprising of independent and dependent claims. It is necessary to understand that scientists, academicians involved in research are used to drafting research articles for journal publications and it is necessary to understand that persons skilled in the research activity can draft their own provisional/complete specifications.

Procedure for Filing a Patent Application

A provisional specification is submitted by the inventor where he conducted a superficial research activity and submitting the details. A complete specification may be either submitted after provisional specification or as directly. In other words, a provisional application contains in brief the research conducted by the inventor where as a complete specification gives the complete details of the invention with all the contents of a patent. Necessary forms must be accompanied with the specification. Several industries may apply directly to a country of their interest and later opt through PCT. If biological resources are used for the invention, it is necessary to mention the details of sources and geographical origin and submit permission details from the National Biodiversity Authority (NBA). If the invention relates to a biological material which is not possible to be described in a sufficient manner and which is not available to the public, the application shall be completed by depositing the material to an International Depository Authority (IDA) within a stipulated time so that the reference numbers of deposits made are mentioned in the specification. Indian patent office accepts applications for grant of patents within India and applications for grant of patents through PCT. Where an application has to be filed directly in a foreign country patent office, it is mandatory that the patentee gets prior permission from the controller general of patents.

Types of Patents

A patent can be a process patent, product patent. An in house terminology of platform patents is used in several industries. A process patent mainly describes about the methods of conducting the invention where in the process is exclusively claimed. A product patent mainly claims for new chemical entity, active ingredient, drug moiety. A product patent additionally may describe the method of conducting the invention for the entity/moiety. A product patent may be for a new chemical entity or formulation where in all the drugs available in the market are claimed (platform patent). When an application is submitted through PCT, the application is phased out into national and international phases.

Is there any World patent?

As such there is no provision of protecting an invention as one patent (World patent) for the entire countries in the World. However, Patent Co-operation Treaty provides a provision of single time application to get patents in different countries subject to the condition that countries are members of the treaty; else the inventor has to apply to the specific country of his interest.

Who can apply for a Patent?

The inventor always has the provision of filing of patent applications at the Indian patent office both at the national and international level. In most of the cases it is preferable to file a patent application through patent agents, patent attorneys as they are qualified for prosecutions.

First to invent or first to file

Currently, first to file concept is practiced. Country like USA, earlier practiced first to invent system and changed to first to file system.

What is the expenditure incurred for filing, procedural and maintenance of patent?

The expenditure incurred for filing, procedural and maintenance of a patent is about Rs. 1,00,000/- for a natural person. The total expenditure may increase or decrease based on the official procedures followed by the inventor. If the expenditure is burdensome, an individual may get granted with a patent and later license it out to a party interested. The initial cost may be up to Rs. 15,000/- to file and receive a granted patent.

Family patent

When an invention is patented in the native country, the innovator may also wish to have granted patents in other countries of the World. All the patents of the countries that are reflecting to the invention are considered as family patents. Identifying and sorting family patents may minimize duplicate study of the invention during innovation mining.

Innovation mining

For a new invention, it is necessary that the scientific work fulfills the patentability criteria. It is now a day necessary to completely examine the work already done relating to the scientific work and plan the work so that the outcome is eligible for patentability.

Compulsory License

Compulsory license is a provision wherein an invention is patented and not further worked or put into use, the marketed products of the inventions are not manufactured in India, the marketed products of the invention are commercially of high value and not reachable to common man. If inventions are not further worked after three years, a third party may apply for a compulsory license. If an invention in not manufactured in India, commercially of high value, a third party may approach the patent holder for license and if not fruitful, may approach the Controller of patents for a compulsory license of the invention. If special circumstances such as where a country does not have a manufacturing infrastructure may opt for a compulsory license. In addition to this, the government may grant a compulsory license under the circumstances of national emergency etc. In several cases, it is mandatory that the patent holder has to provide details of working of the patented invention to the authority to ensure that a compulsory license is not granted for an invention or to bring awareness that a third party who is interested for a compulsory license be aware that the invention is being worked and may not be opted for compulsory license.

Infringement And Its Types

When a new party involves in his invention which is in the purview of claims made in a patent, the new party is liable for an act of infringement. Infringement is categorized into direct (literal), doctrine of equivalence, and prosecution history estoppels. If a new party's invention coincides directly with the claims of a patent, the invention is an act of direct infringement. In several circumstances, pharmaceutical inventions fall under the category of doctrine of equivalence wherein the new party's invention have same function, same way and same result with respect to a patent and under such circumstances, the new party's invention may not be granted for a patent. In case of prosecution history estoppels, an inventor might have narrowed the claims of his invention for a grant of a patent. Under such circumstances, if a new party files an application for a patent, his invention is tested for the triple identity test, prosecution history and finally decided whether to grant a patent to the new party or not. Parallel import is a provision by which importing patented products from an authorized license holder being exempted from act of infringement. Several disputes were witnessed in the past relating to transit of pharmaceutical goods from India to destination countries. The goods were considered as an act of infringement while halting at different country before reaching the destination country. Several discussions are in progress relating to this issue at the diplomatic level. Use of patented information for research and development,

for regulatory approvals is not an act of infringement since no commercial activity is made. Stock piling of goods for commercial activity before a patent has expired is considered as an act of infringement. Several generic companies try to file drug approval applications, especially at USFDA for early entry of their product into the market before the patent expiry of the innovator's patent, challenging as an act of non-infringement or invalidating the patent for various reasons.

Procedure Involved at the Patent Office

The procedure involved in application submissions to grant ranges from simple to very complex conditions depending on the various parameters. If very well planned an application filed may be granted with a patent at the earliest possible stipulated

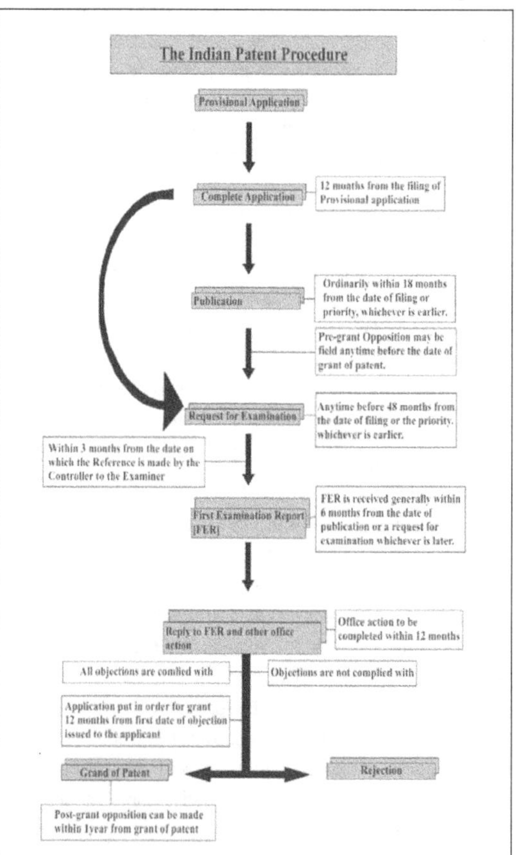

Time line for grant of patent at IPO

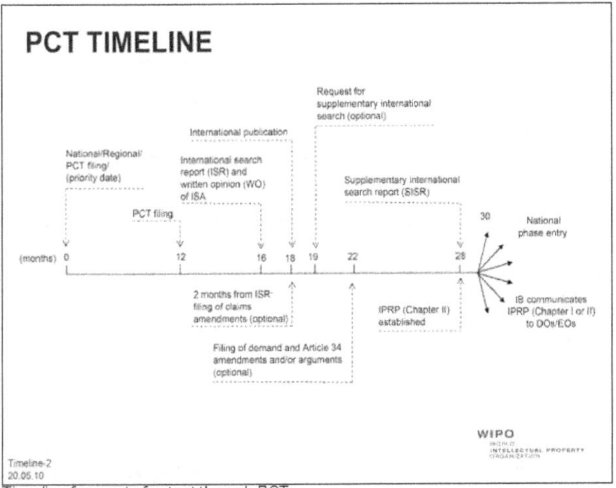

Time line for grant of patent through PCT

time schedules mentioned in The Patents Act, 1970 and The Patent Rules, 2003. When considered in brief, the procedure involves with submission of provisional specification → complete specification → publication in patent journal → pre-grant opposition (if any) → grant of patent → publication of granted patent → post grant opposition (if any).

Evergreen Patent

A word commonly used is ever green for a patent wherein the invention patented is being protected more than the stipulated time especially due to extended inventions of the patented invention. Such research activity hinders entry of the generic versions into the market.

Freedom to Operate

An invention patented in a specific country may not be patented in entire countries of the World. In addition to this, prior to treaties and conventions, countries are independent of patent grants taking into consideration of territorial limits. Currently, several new countries are emerging with legislations to protect intellectual property of its nationals. As there is no uniformity, a product that is developed in a country may be patent protected in another country. Hence, it is necessary to identify whether a drug product or the process has been patent protected in a specific country of interest or not. The act of freedom to operate helps an exporter whether his drug product if exported to a specific country lead to an act of infringement in the said country or not.

Patent Mapping

Patent mapping deals with identifying by hierarchy from innovator to current status of technology available by means of patents for a particular drug product. Patent mapping helps to identify the white space that may lead to patentability of subject matter of current interest with respect to past work. Patent mapping helps is developing process for bulk drugs, identifying drugs going off patent as pipeline drugs for releasing as generics.

Necessity of Identifying The Legal Status of A Patent

In several cases the patent granted may be revoked for different reasons such as lack of patentability criteria, the invention falling under the purview of traditional knowledge, granted patent was not further maintained by prescribed fee by the patentee. In addition to this, several patents are extended in their term over 20 years for justified and accepted reasons like the invention patented being used under the category of orphan, pediatric drug (especially in US).

Whether An Invention Disclosed in Conferences, Public Meetings, Published in Journals Patentable?

Inventions that are disclosed in conferences, public meetings, published in journals can be applied for a patent, but within a stipulated time after disclosure.

Differences In Patent System Among Countries

In United States, patents are granted as plant, utility and design patents. In addition to this patents are also granted for new indication/use. Computer programming is patented in United States. In India, plants and designs are protected by registration. Computer programming is protected by copyright in India. It is necessary to understand that international treaties and conventions suggest the minimum criteria of protection of intellectual property within a country and it is up to the country's policies and local needs the stringency prevails.

Pre-Grant Opposition, Post-Grant Opposition, Revoking, Invoking Of Applications, Grants Relating To Patent

Several applications were rejected after opposition at the pre-grant and post-grant level. A patent granted was later identified to be traditionally practiced and the patent was revoked. Social welfare associations are playing critical role in monitoring the innovations filed for patent grants. Several applications were rejected based on the mere admixture of different components/drugs and not having significant biological/pharmacological activity.

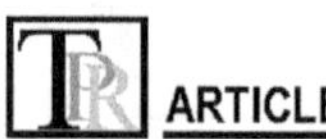 ARTICLE

Current Status of Statistics on Patent Applications/ Grants at Indian Patent Office

Currently, scientific work is either published as research publications in journals (as non-patent literature), or as granted patents. It is not until an invention is published in official journal of Indian patent office, the other innovators are aware of the existing technology as prior art. It is necessary to review all the granted patents, published patent applications as well as the non-patented literature so as to understand whether the current scientific work is a patentable subject matter. There is still a necessity of bringing awareness of statistics of filed application, grants at Indian patent office and an attempt is made. Table 1 provides the details of patent grants relating to chemical, drug and biotechnology.

Indian patent office has granted about 361 Pharma related patents (Apr, 2012 to July, 2013). Among the granted patents 3488 (2005-10) are product patents, 119 [Foreign (26), India (93)] patents are relating to Ayurveda and Herbal based medicines (until 31st March, 2013).

Year	Chemical	Drug	Biotechnology
1997-1998	503	291	---
1998-1999	609	150	---
1999-2000	516	307	---
2000-2001	353	276	---
2001-2002	483	320	---
2002-2003	399	312	---
2003-2004	609	419	---
2004-2005	573	192	71
2005-2006	1140	457	51
2006-2007	1989	798	89
2007-2008	2662	905	341
2008-2009	2376	1207	1157
2009-2010	1420	530	449
2010-2011	1899	596	165
2011-2012	1168	282	309
2012-2013	1289	344	144

Table 1: Statistics of Patents Granted at Indian Patent Office 1997-2013

Source: Indian Patent Office website

Conclusion

During the last five years, Indian patent office has taken necessary steps and made easier the free access of information relating to application status, patents granted. All patented innovations indicate that the subject matter qualified for patentability, but all innovations made need not qualify for patentability criteria. It is necessary that pharmaceutical educational institutions refer to such literature to bring out research thesis that fulfill patentability criteria either being published as research papers in journals or filed for a patent. It is necessary that innovation mining, patent mining being conducted right from the student level so that, new ideas pour in leading to intellectual property protection. It is the time to re-consider that intellectual property rights, especially patents, not only belongs to discipline of law but also to the discipline of technology. Intellectual property rights have become a new generation concept like the scenario of computerization in India during 1990s. There is a need that creators have to be encouraged. A lot of literature is not available in public domain and efforts are in progress to facilitate for persons skilled in art to quest for innovations that are patentable. A drug price control mechanism for patented drugs in India is in process. India's Innovation Index may increase if efforts from educational institutes are extended from research thesis leading to research paper journal publication to patent grants.

Disclaimer

1. All the time limits for filing and submissions, at the Indian patent office and international
    bureau is to be monitored from official sources whenever necessary.

2. Application fee and maintenance fee has to be monitored from official sources whenever necessary.

3. All the information and interpretations are purely of the author.

4. The article is to bring awareness and for knowledge purpose.

References

1. An Overview of Innovation Policy and Innovation Index, The Pharma Review, Mar-Apr, 2014, p: 75-80

2. www.ipindia.nic.in

3. www.wipo.int

ARTICLE 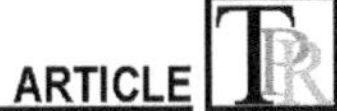

An Overview of Trade Marks in Pharmaceuticals

Dr. Bayya Subba Rao

Abstract: Provenance of Trade Marks dates back to Indian Harappa Civilization. Trade Marks presented on a product or a service represent a company from which originated. Registration of Trade Marks at the Government authority is beneficial, as intellectual property rights are currently non-territorial both at the national and international levels. It has been observed that several national level trademarks being available at international territories and an ambiguity arise whether Indian or foreign national origin. The current article is a brief understanding of the concepts of Trade Marks.

Introduction:

Trade Marks are alphabets, numerical, words, alphanumeric, pictorial (multi-dimensional), sound, olfactory (fragrance), symbols, touch sensible, colour representations, monograms, signatures etc., and that are incorporated on goods registered/ unregistered by a company. Trade Mark on a product indicates the products (or services) have originated from a company representing maintenance of quality standards set forth. Trade Marks representing from service oriented organisations are usually called as Service Marks. Trade Marks that are commonly used by several companies are called as collective marks.

Some of the examples of Trade Marks are A1, TV5, Vicco Turmeric, Anacin, Sare Jahan Se Achhi, Agmark, Indian Standard Institute (ISI) mark, Apollo Pharmacy, India Post specially fragmented envelops, living person pictures, embossed symbols that are touch sensible, a special rhythmic sounds etc.,

In contrast to Trade Marks, Geographical indications are specially considered as separate category where in the geographical name of origin of the product is indicated. Geographical indications of a product indicate its uniqueness in quality featuring the uniqueness in climatic conditions in which the product has been developed, cultivated. Some of the examples of geographical indications are Kondapalli toys, Tirupati Laddu, Agra Halwa, Basmati rice, etc.

Hence, a trade mark represents a company where as a geographic indicator represents the geographical location of origin of the product. The current article is aimed in understanding the concepts.

History of Indian Trade Mark System:

Indian origin Trade Marks were indentified on pottery remains of Harappa Civilization, one of the oldest civilizations. In India, it is only after 1940 official sources of recognition of Trade Marks and their registrations are witnessed. Currently, in India, The Trade Marks Act, 1999 and The Trade Mark Rules, 2002/2012 (amendment) are in force. Table 1, illustrates some of the oldest trademarks registered in India.

S. No	Brand Name	Year (Journal date)	Year (Used since)
1	Anacin	1944	-
2	Disprin	1947	-
3	Vicks	1955	-
4	Amrutanjan	1947	1906
5	Woodwards	1952	1890
6	Vicco	1960	1950
7	Hajmola	1960	1950
8	Dabur Limited	1948	1884
9	ZindaTilismath	1966	-
10	Dabur Iodised Sarsa	1949	-

Table 1: Indicative list of some of the oldest Trade Marks in India relating to Pharmaceuticals

International Agreements Relating to Trademarks

After India signing WTO agreement, India is obliged to fulfill TRIPS agreement. In addition to this India is a member to GATT, WTO, WIPO, Paris Convention etc., International treaties (agreements) such as Paris Convention (for national treatment, priority date), Trademarks Law Treaty (for standardization and streamline of national and regional trademark registration procedures), Singapore Treaty (for harmonization of administrative trademark registration procedures), Madrid agreement/protocol (for international registration of marks), Nice agreement (for

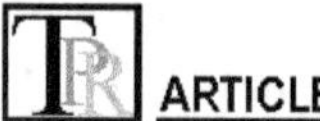

ARTICLE

classification of goods and services), Vienna agreement (for international classification of figurative elements of marks) are to be fulfilled for harmonization in administration, prevent duplication of applications and examinations. Such a harmonization is expected to grant/register marks at the earliest possible. As per Nice classification, goods and services are classified into 34 and 11 categories respectively. Relating to pharmaceuticals, among goods, class 5 is dealt with medical and veterinary preparations and articles. Among the services, relating to pharmaceuticals, class 34 (for business assistance/management/administrative services), class 42 (for science and technology services), class 44 (for human healthcare services) and class 45 (for legal services).

Category of Trade Marks

Trademarks can be categorised into individual, collective, certification, associated, series, in part, concurrent. Individual trademarks are registrations by an individual company. In case of collective, the mark may be used by group of companies registered and maintaining quality standards set, for using the mark. A collective mark is usually seen for Geographical indicators. Certification marks are set for different range of products to different companies maintaining the same quality standards for a product in question. Several independent/autonomous/government organizations set the standards that meet at national and international levels and upon a product meet the quality standards, issues/grants/register the product/company, in using the mark. Certification marks are Agmark, ISI, WHOGMP, ISO etc.

Associated marks are those marks which are identical or similar in marks of same or different goods belonging to either the same or different individuals and such marks are designated to prevent confusion by the consumer of products. For instance, M/s. ABC (India) Limited and M/s. ABC (US) Inc., are associated companies belonging to one.

When an individual has several marks with same name (in-part) but different suffix (or prefix), such marks are designated as series marks. For instance, Alex (for cough lozenges) and Alex-P(for syrup); Betadine, Betadine Gargle, Betadine STD SOLN, Betadine Surgical Scrub, Betadine-AD etc.

Under special circumstances, a concurrent mark is issued to more than one company/proprietor, whether a product is same or similar, upon discretion of the authority. For instance, BITS (Pilani) and BIT (Ranchi) confuses an individual as being owned by one

individual, but are not. However, the names of the organisations are concurrent and are accepted based on the reason that they belong to two different geographical locations, which is distinctive enough and does not confuse and have their national popularity.

Role of Coloured Marks

As long as a mark has been applied for a specific colour (or combination of colours) of interest, upon final decisions, the mark is registered for the exclusive colour/s, else by default, it is claimed for all the colours.

Role of Un-Registered and Living Person Trade Marks

Figure 1, is an illustrative example (modified) of the living person with an un-registered trade mark. Such un-registered trademarks may in future can be registered and if a trade mark contains a non-living person as a picture, such marks may be registered within a limited time upon representation by the legal heirs.

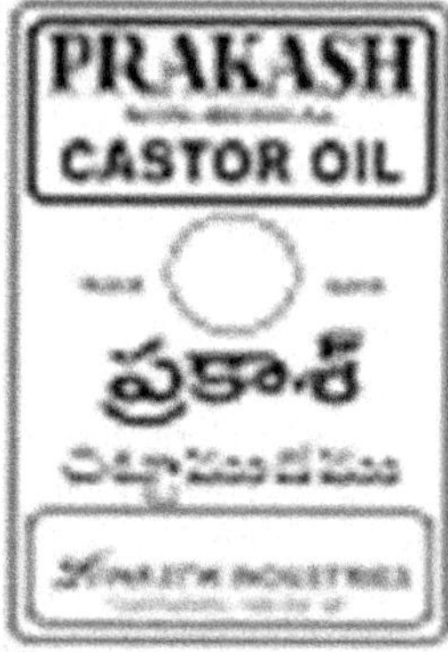

Figure 1

Some of the well-known words that are available officially are DR. Reddy (un-registered well known word/mark), Vicks VapoRub, Balaji, Asoka Chakra, Gandhi etc. For instance, DR. Reddy was not a registered trademark, not until 2001 (after an issue), but the company was established in 1984 and is now considered as well-known mark.

Eligibility Criteria for Registration/Grant of a Trade Mark

For a trade mark to be registered/granted, the mark should be novel, non-obvious, and original. A trade mark must not directly indicate the kind, quality, quantity, intended purpose, values, geographical origin, time of production etc. As a thumb rule, trademarks that deceive or confuse a consumer are not eligible for registration. Section 9, of the Act indicates a "Test of Similarity" where in, a conclusion whether to grant/register a mark in question with respect to other already registered, it is not mandatory to keep aside to each other to make a decision in grant/register. It is also not necessary to monitor any un-registered marks while registering/granting a trade mark in question. A well-known mark or names are usually not encouraged for registration of a product. In several cases, a similar trademark may be granted for a different product as the consumer does not have any confusion in deciding purchase of the product. Especially relating to pharmaceuticals, World Health Organisation has notified 3113 International Non-proprietary Names (INN) that cannot be used as trademarks. In several cases, Trade Mark planned has to be ensured and is free from copyright registrations. Trademarks are mentioned with ® or ™, indicating former for registered whereas the later indicates an application has been filed and in the process of registration. However, in several cases, where un-registered, TM was widely used in the past. Using of ®, without registration is an offence.

Procedure and Time Line of Registration of Trade Mark

A trade mark application can be filed by an individual, company or through an attorney (agent). A trade mark application can be filed in India at various registries in Indian Intellectual Property Offices (Trade Mark Registry) located at Mumbai, Ahmadabad, Kolkata, Chennai and New Delhi. An applicant has to file an application at the right registry based on the jurisdiction and the principal place of business. Registries have a provision to accept applications both at the national and international levels. Figure 2 illustrates the layout of sequence of procedures followed at the Indian Trade mark registry.

Before submission of an application for a trade mark, an initial search whether similar mark is already registered or applied for registration can be checked at the registry. A provision of accelerated search is available at a charge of fivefold when compared to conventional. An application is received at the office and upon fulfilling the formalities; a receipt is generated along with the file number and date. Within three months from date of filing, an examination report is provided to the applicant. Upon fulfilling the deficiencies (within one month) by the applicant, and upon acceptance by the authority, the trade mark, applicant name, domicile etc., are published in Trade Mark journal (which is usually published twice monthly i.e., 1st, 16th of every month). From date of advertisement/publication in journal, a third

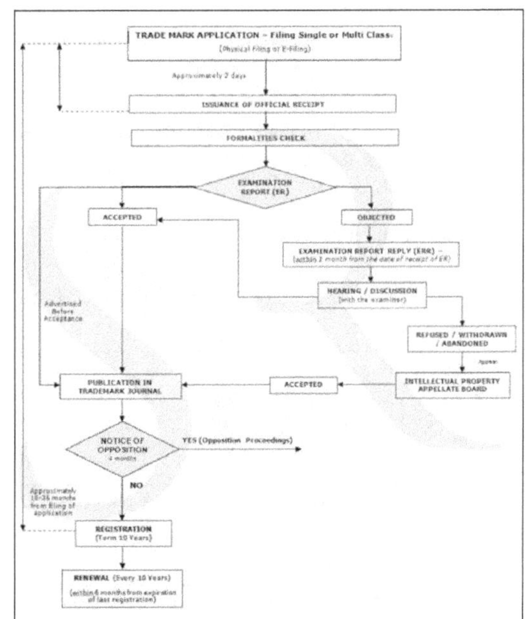

Figure 2: Trade Mark Registration Procedure

party within a period of four months can file an opposition for the application. If no opposition, the trade mark is registered and a certificate is issued that is valid for 10 years and can be renewed periodically. A third party who wish to oppose, a notice of opposition is submitted at the cash section along with the application and fee. The notice of opposition is intimated by the office to the applicant. A process of evidence from opponent and a process of counter statement from applicant are being submitted by the parties. Upon hearing, a final decision for registration or refusal is decided. If the application is refused upon hearing, an appeal at the Intellectual Property Appellate Board (IPAB) may be submitted and upon review, if in favor of registration, published in journal, and at a later stage registered.

Madrid protocol provides, uniformity, single application procedure for a Trade Mark to be registered at various member countries (97). For the international level, the application may be submitted in French, English or Spanish languages. It is necessary that the 'Basic Mark' must either be registered or applied at the parent country office, later through which the application is forwarded to WIPO. As the second stage, the international application is examined and the mark is recorded in the international register and published in WIPO Gazette of International Marks (published

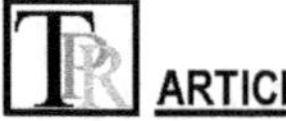

ARTICLE

every week) with issuing a certificate of international registration (within about 3 months). At the national phase (stage 3), the application is examined and at the discretion of the foreign country's law, within a period limit of 12 or 18 months, a decision is intimated through WIPO, which records the decisions in the international register. A statement of grant is issued by the foreign country.

Forms and Fees for Application/Registration of Trade Mark

Table 2, illustrates the basic application forms and the stipulated fee especially in India.

Form Number	Purpose	Fees
TM-1	Application to register a trade mark for a specification of goods or services included in one class	Rs. 3, 500=00
TM-2	Application to register a trade mark for goods or services included in a class from a convention country	Rs. 3, 500=00
TM-51	One single application for registration of a trade mark for different classes of goods or services	Rs. 3, 500=00 for each class
TM-52	One single application for registration of a trade mark for different classes of goods or services from a convention country	Rs. 3, 500=00 for each class
TM-5	Notice of opposition	Rs. 2, 500=00
TM-10	Application of renewal within six months from the expiration of last registration of the trade mark	Rs. 3, 000=00 as surcharge
TM-60	Application for search and issue of certificate	Rs. 5, 000=00
TM-72	Application requesting for an expedited search and issuance of a certificate	Rs. 25, 000=00

Table 2: List of Forms and Fees relating to Trade Mark application (limited and selective list)

Term of Trade Mark Registration

A trade mark for a product is an exclusive right of the applicant forever until the company/company product exists. However, a trade mark registered is valid for 10 years and has to be renewed periodically for every 10 years.

Infringement

Any third party who uses a Trade Mark already registered (or un-registered) and sell products is an act of infringement. For a registered mark, the Act provides a provision for legal proceedings. In case of legal proceeding for a non-registered product, a passing of provision is available wherein general law safeguards from infringements. In the current day scenario, several un-registered Trade Marks are applied for registration, prior registration are being advised for public news paper advertisement so that public can oppose/object registration (within a specified period of time).

Conclusion

Trademarks are the most widely known intellectual property rights both at the literate and the illiterate levels. To achieve branding of a product, it has been observed that developing a trademark has a strong scientific and research approach. In majority of the cases, colour trademark has its impact on the product. India Post initiated an individual's photo as stamps for promoting services. Several counterfeits such as one company using other company product labels/names, tampering products were witnessed and to combat such issues, current Trace and Track technologies implemented in India are expected as a prophylactic.

Disclaimer

1. All the information is to the interpretation of the author.
2. The information is basic and is for awareness purpose.
3. Timelines and fees are indicative and may vary from one country to another.

References

1. www.ipindia.nic.in

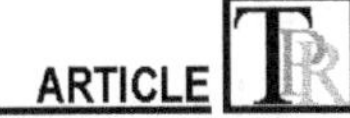

ARTICLE

Influence of Intellectual Property Matters in Pharmaceutical Manufacturing and Exports

'Dr. Bayya Subba Rao, Dr. P. V. Appaji & Ashutosh Gupta

Abstract: Post GATT scenario a silent expected change is seen in the intellectual property system in several countries of the World, including India. The scenario changed from territorial limits of intellectual property to non-territorial limits. Several stake holders are in ambiguity in understanding whether a drug product as API or formulation can be manufactured in India and can be exported into a country of specific interest. The current article is aimed in acquiring basic knowledge.

Introduction

Even though intellectual property system existed since ages in India, influence of British legislation can be witnessed. However, significant indigenous legislation date backs with The Patents Act, 1970; the Post GATT scenario (after India signing WTO agreement) has made a revolutionary change in intellectual property system of India. The Patents Act, 1970 was amended thrice so as to provide a 20 year patent exclusivity term as well as a product patent system (in addition to process patent system). Since 2005, product patents are granted by Indian Patent Office (IPO). Grant of patents for internationals in Indian territory is significantly increasing and even though Indian legislation is preventing grant of patents relating to subject matters that influence on section 3d, 3e, 3f and traditional knowledge especially relating to pharmaceuticals, opposition filings are usually witnessed from social welfare associations, Indian pharmaceutical companies and not from pharmaceutical teaching intellectuals who are also expected as skilled persons for a technology in question. The current article is a lead to understand for initiators who wish to innovate as well as export and is purely for understanding the basic concepts.

Doubts that Arise While Planning Manufacturing of Pharmaceutical Products Keeping in Mind Intellectual Property Rights

1. Whether an API/Formulation Process Can Be Manufactured Without Infringing?

This can be achieved in such a way by compiling all the available processes for an API/formulation (both patented and not patented) and establishing a new process that was not patented (so as to fulfill non-infringement) or not available as prior art. Indian Pharmaceutical Industry has pioneered in developing processes that are economical as well as non-infringing.

Establishing a new economical process for an API may be saturated in several cases and in addition to this usage of certain chemicals is prohibited in several circumstances. Several challenges persist over researchers.

2. Who is An Infringer and How to Identify?

Any patented invention (API or process) that is illegally used by a person (manufacturer, third party business holder) and making business without paying royalty either directly or indirectly to the patent holder is an infringer. Developing the product under non-commercial conditions for launch of the product after patent expiry may not be an act of infringement (Bolar provision), but stock piling the product is an act of infringement. Innovators can file legally for compensation and in several cases, the innovator has technology collaborations with process/generic manufacturers. Innovators have APIs that have product patents with limited process patents. This gives a benefit to the pharmaceutical manufacturers to quest for non-patented process development and launch of the product especially in collaboration with innovator. An innovator has to establish scientific proof in several cases that an API/formulation process developed is infringing and this can be monitored by impurity profiles (for APIs) etc by collecting and analyzing similar products (bulk drugs) available in market. Trace and track technologies can also be expected to minimize infringements. It is the duty of the innovator to identify infringers and not the duty of the Government.

3. Whether a Formulation Containing an API or A Combination Can Be Manufactured?

Currently, India has both product and process patent systems. Such patented inventions are either Indian or foreign origin. A formulation invention can claim for a product (API-innovator's), process or platform patents. Other than conventional technologies, as India has majority of generic manufacturers, it is necessary whether a formulation planning with an API (or a combination) can be first manufactured in India and can be exported. Such doubts are currently persisting since India has several product and process patents in force. Platform formulation patents involve with the development of technology (process claim) and are being claimed for all the APIs available in market (product claim). Hence, product, process, platform, product by process/ process by product etc., patents have to be monitored.

4. Whether a Formulation Can Be Manufactured And Can Be Exported to The Country of Interest?

Every country in the World has a system of protection of intellectual property rights. Global harmonization and WTO agreements (including TRIPS) have brought mutual predictable business, uniformity of administration (with limitations) and protection of intellectual property by foreign nationals (national treatment). Several patent offices have online search system to know whether a patent exists or in the process of grant or lapsed or withdrawn or abandoned. Several countries are in the process of making the information available online and this is currently hindering as a communication gap to know whether a product can be exported to a specific country (especially developing countries). Such a situation is currently sorted out by using services of local patent agents who have direct collaboration with foreign country patent office or agents. A "Freedom to operate" analysis is sorting out such doubts. The analysis is done with respect to a country. In several cases drug products were delayed (or destroyed) to destination country by the authority where the products intermittently halted. So, it is necessary to prior intimate/ take permission from halting authority/patent holder saying that the product is not infringing.

For instance, whether a patent is available to the innovator in a country "xyz" is a subject of doubt due to lack of individual country patent office online patent search database (or in the process of development or in the conversion of hard copies to soft copies). In addition to this, several countries do not furnish information to regional patent offices. Currently, several patent high end

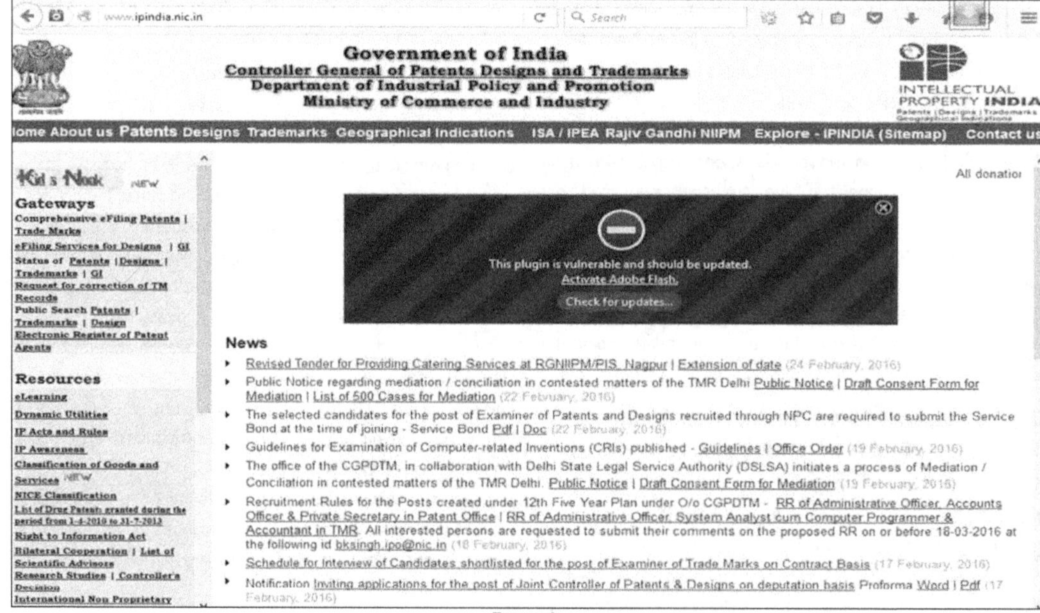

Figure: 1

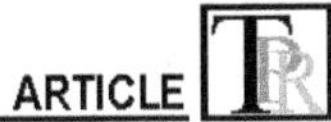

paid databases even do not provide all country legal status of applications/patent grants. Then how can we expect information whether a patent is in force in a country "xyz", until unless by a person who is a native of the country of interest. Currently, this is achieved by local agents in the specific country or research conducted by importer or a global database that is WIPO database, which even does not give the information whether the applicant stated protection (designated state) has a protection in the country of interest or not.

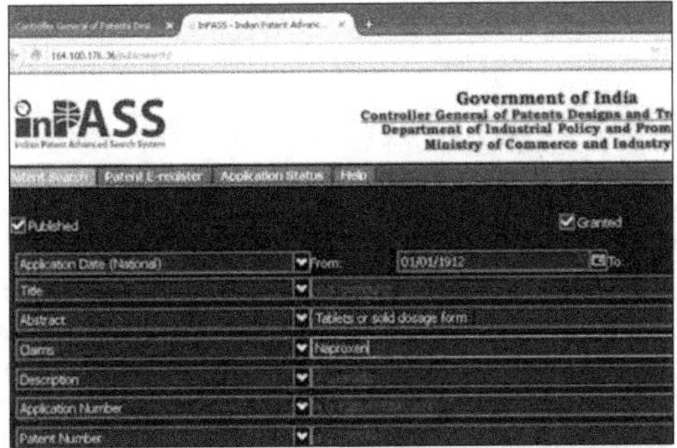

Figure: 2

Figure: 3

As a live example, with the available resources, an attempt is made in how to monitor available patents in India and country of interest for a formulation planned to manufacture in India and export to Sri Lanka.

Industry is aware that Naproxen and Eletriptan are well established drugs and are available in the market. Research indicated that Naproxen is available either as individual or combination with Omeprazole or Sumatriptan etc. Eletriptan is the next generation to Sumatriptan. If a drug combination of Naproxen and Eletriptan in tablet dosage form has to be planned (empirical and has to be scientifically established for compatibility), the first line of doubts whether such combination is acceptable and it is necessary to establish strengths, dosage form, route of administration,

analytical method to quantify individual drugs when available in combination, are there any patents in India, Sri Lanka for such combination, dosage form etc.

To see availability of patents at Indian patent office, Figure 1, indicates Indian Patent Office Web portal (www.ipindia.nic.in). Using InPass patent database, a limited search was conducted

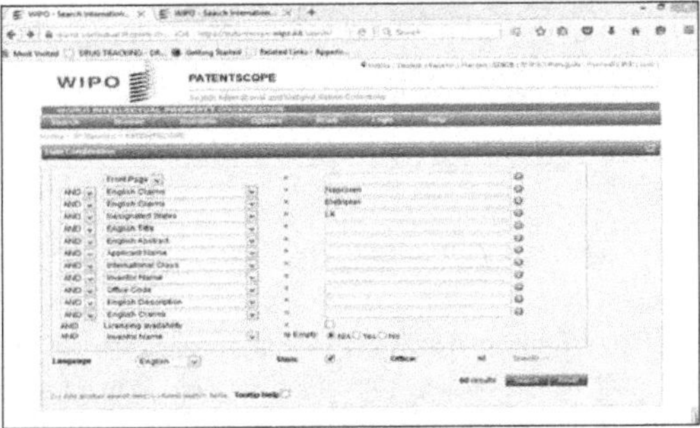

Figure: 4

Figure: 5

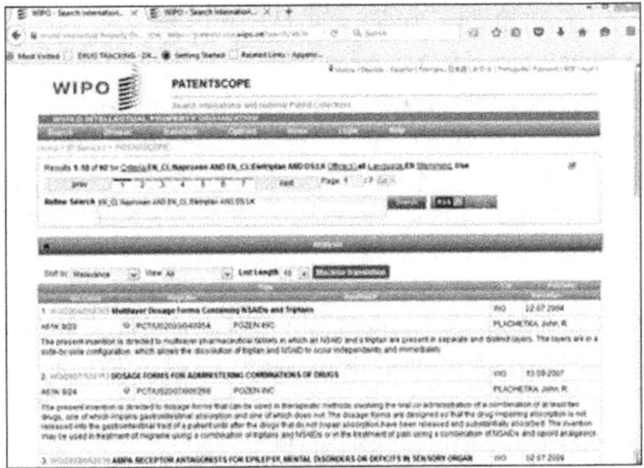

Figure: 6

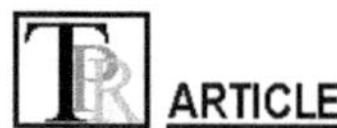ARTICLE

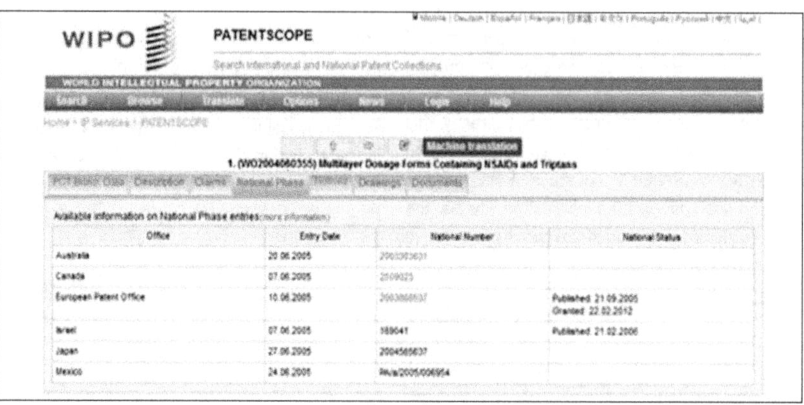

Figure: 7

and Figure 2, Figure 3 indicates available patents/applications. The patents/applications contain a dosage form design, estimation of Naproxen and Omeprazole, liquid oral suspension, sustained release composition etc. The applications/patents have to be clearly checked for our objective of combination drugs by referring to text, claims of the patent/application, process etc.

When a search was made of similar kind to Eletriptan, the end result was nil at a point of time. When a review of the complete specification of a few granted/applications indicate claiming APIs and therapeutic classes currently available which indicates a platform patent.

Figures 4, 5, 6, 7 are a quest of patents granted/applications filed at International Bureau (IB). Research indicates that several patents/applications are available either for Eletriptan or Naproxen or as platform. Figure 7 in specific illustrates a patent granted for European region which later enters into national phase of individual country of EU. Our objective of whether a patent is in force or going to be granted is still a question un-answered and this might be solved by individual country patent office database or at a suitable time being reflected at WIPO when the application entered national phase. It is necessary to understand that country designated provides an opportunity to innovator to decide within a stipulated time whether to get a granted patent in the country.

Several New Chemical Entities (NCEs) possess with a product patent by the innovator. Whether a product patent exists for the NCE in a specific country or not is the subject of question. In several cases, identifying the NCE name with product patent is not easy. The easy source is from USFDA orange book database, Merck Index etc., where the NCE along with the patents are mentioned. Using this first line of information, NCE patented in USA, is usually available in other countries (developed) as a

patent that is being reflected as family patent, that can be referred in Espace.net (EU Regional Patent Office database).

In the current analysis, despite several platform patents exist, a process developed can be non-infringing and may provide an opportunity to export and if a product patent claiming for NCE/s exists, a royalty has to be paid to the innovator with prior permission from innovator.

Conclusion

Harmonization is a process of re-organizing administration protocols at the state, national and international levels. This does not mean that a country does not have systematic protocols. Harmonized, systematic, local country needs are expected to bring out minimum requirements in administration. Every country's drug regulatory or patent database is expected to clarify first line ideas whether a project has to be initiated or not. In the current day scenario, language is not considered but, information non-availability is considered as communication gap. IPR matters have majority of their influence at the researcher level questing for non-infringing exploration. Planning, manufacturing and marketing a product in India itself needs a review of territorial exclusivities and at a later stage has to overcome non-territorial exclusivities so as to fulfill export criteria. Several prior art technologies may provide a room for non-infringing technologies even though platform patents persist.

Disclaimer

1. All the information provided are basics and extensive study has to be conducted in all possible directions.

2. All the information is to the knowledge of the author and is only for propagation of information/knowledge resources.

3. The information is only a lead to initiators and Indian Pharmaceutical fraternity is well versed with such resources.

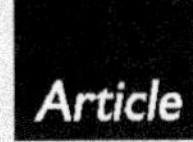

An Analysis of Para IV Certifications of USFDA

A. Nagarani, M. Swathi, Dr. Bayya Subba Rao*
*Professor, Geethanjali College of Pharmacy, Cheeryal, Keesara, Hyderabad, Telangana State, India

Abstract:
Para IV certification filing at USFDA, for approval of generic or tentative needs through back ground of formulation technology knowledge, innovator's patented technologies and its drawbacks. A para IV challenge makes the entry of the generic or tentative drug product into the market before patent expiry. Such filings are usually made by high end generic industries. The current study is an analysis of various Para-IV filings at USFDA.

Introduction

Hatch-Waxman Act, commonly called as Drug Price Control and Patent Term Restoration Act, is a balance mechanism among the innovator, generic and the end user of medicines. The Act provides a provision of early entry of generic (or tentative) by filing a drug product application, claiming for challenging of the innovator's active patents[1]. The difference among ANDA and Tentative are identical and similar drug products respectively.

Filing a para IV certification indicates that the generic manufacturer is challenging his drug product technology with patented technology claiming as non-infringement. Usually, a para IV challenger claims the patented technology is invalid, obvious, mere commercial exploitation, guilty on disclosure of best mode, double patenting, limited use, lack of novelty etc. Unlike in India, the most critical aspect with US patent system is the exclusivity claim for a specific clinical condition use.

Methodology

Compiled and available Para IV certifications of USFDA was reprocessed and correlated with orange book for interpretations.

The most critical part in the analysis is not with relating to which product, which innovator company and which patent, but the applicant who has filed the challenge for the patent. Such information needs a thorough review from US court database, PACER. However, an attempt is made from US court of appeals database which has free access.

Analysis of Paragraph IV Certifications
Over all Certifications

A total of 1082 para IV certifications were submitted since 2001, taking into consideration as such the official data[2]. Among these, after fine tuning the data with respect to drug name, dosage form, innovator and the brand name of drug product, and after removal of 47 certifications due to ANDA withdrawal/exclusivity relinquished a final total of 832 certifications was observed.

Para IV Certifications (Year Wise)

Analysis, Table 1, indicates year wise number of certifications made at USFDA. Among the total 1082, the lowest (1) is observed in the year 2001 and the highest (97) is observed in the year 2008 with respect to the available data. It is necessary to understand that several drug products having different strengths being claimed for para IV certification.

Table 1: Year Wise Submission of Application with Para IV Certification (as on 22nd September, 2016)

Year	No. of Drug Products	Year	No. of Drug Products
2001	1	2011	63
2004	47	2012	60
2005	56	2013	59
2006	55	2014	55
2007	84	2015	62
2008	97	2016	19
2009	96	Prior 2009	3
2010	78	No data	247
		Total	1082

Para IV Certification (Type Wise)

A para IV certification filed by a generic applicant at USFDA is with respect to innovator's NDA or ANDA application. Analysis, Table 2, indicates that majority (1049, 97 %) of the para IV certification filings are with respect to NDA filings of the innovator.

Table 2: No. of Para IV Certifications w.r.t Innovator's Application Type (as 22nd Sep, 2016)

Innovator's Application Type	No. of Para IV filings
ANDA	6
NDA	1049
No Data	27
Total	1082

Time duration to file para IV Certification

In order to find out the duration taken by the generic applicant to file a para IV certification w.r.t innovator's drug product approval date, a compilation of USFDA para IV data and orange book data was made. From the compiled data, among the available dates, a difference of date of submission of para IV certification from date of approval of innovator's drug product was calculated. It has been observed that para IV certification filing ranges from [Minimum (14 days) to Maximum (28 years)], but on an average it has been observed that 5 ± 4.5 years to file a certification.

*E-mail: drbayyasubbarao@yahoo.com

Para IV Certifications (Molecule Wise)

Analysis was made with respect to molecule wise and it has been observed 832 certifications were filed among 565 molecules (includes base, salt or combination form). Molecule wise along with corresponding certifications ranges from lowest (1) to highest (7).

Para IV Certifications (Dosage Form Wise)

With respect to the certifications filed, dosages forms were classified more specific to technology back ground (i.e., tablets are classified as tablets, extended release, orally disintegrating, delayed release, chewable, sublingual, buccal, delayed release orally disintegrating, extended release chewable, extended release orally disintegrating, vaginal) and it has been observed that 832 certifications were filed among the 87 technology based dosage forms.

Table 3: Number of Para IV Certifications at USFDA-Dosage Form Wise-Top 20

S. No	Dosage Form	No. of Para IV Certification Filings	Percentage Contribution
1	Tablets	262	31.5
2	Injection	96	11.5
3	Extended-release Tablets	81	9.7
4	Capsules	73	8.8
5	Extended-release Capsules	38	4.6
6	Ophthalmic Solution	28	3.4
7	Oral Solution	25	3
8	Gel	16	1.9
9	Orally Disintegrating Tablets	16	1.9
10	Nasal Spray	15	1.8
11	Oral Suspension	15	1.8
12	Delayed-release Tablets	14	1.7
13	Chewable Tablets	11	1.3
14	Delayed-release Capsules	11	1.3
15	Transdermal System	11	1.3
16	Cream	7	0.8
17	Inhalation Solution	6	0.7
18	Sublingual Tablets	5	0.6
19	Topical Gel	4	0.5
20	Topical Solution	4	0.5
	Top 20 Sub Total	738	88.6
	Subtotal of remaining 67 dosage forms	94	11.4
	Grand Total	832	100

Table 3, illustrates top 20 dosage form wise and their corresponding para IV certifications. It has been observed that among the 832 certifications, the contribution of top 20 dosage forms and their corresponding para IV certifications is about 90 percent. Among the top 20 dosage forms, tablets have the highest para IV certifications (262, 31.5%) and topical gel as well as topical solution has the lowest para IV certifications (4 each, 0.5% each).

Para IV certifications (Innovator Company Wise)

Innovator companies provide all the information relating to all the active patents (crucial) for the approved product and it is mandatory that it is listed in the orange book. Based upon this, the innovator company was identified and an analysis was made. It has been observed that a total of 196 companies' products were challenged by para IV certifications. Among these three Indian company patents i.e., M/s. Dr. Reddy's, M/s. Lupin, M/s. Ranbaxy were challenged for their NDA filings. Table 4, illustrates the top 20 innovator companies whose products were challenged by para IV certification. It has been observed that amongst the top 20 innovator companies, M/s. Novartis was challenged for its 47 products (highest, 5.6 percent) and M/s. Allergan, M/s. Apil, M/s. Takeda, M/s. Teva and M/s. Wyeth were challenged for their 11 products each (lowest, 1.3 percent each)

Table 4: Innovator Company Name wise Number of Products for Which Para IV certifications filed by Generic applicants (Indicative)

S. No	Innovator Company Name (Indicative)	No. of Products	Percentage
1	M/s. Novartis	47	5.6
2	M/s. Pfizer	28	3.4
3	M/s. Janssen	24	2.9
4	M/s. GlaxoSmithKline	23	2.8
5	M/s. Merck Sharp Dohme	21	2.5
6	M/s. Sanofi Aventis US	19	2.3
7	M/s. Valeant	18	2.2
8	M/s. Abbvie	17	2
9	M/s. Bayer Health Care	17	2
10	M/s. Baxter Health Care	14	1.7
11	M/s. Merck	14	1.7
12	M/s. Boehringer Ingelheim	13	1.6
13	M/s. Bristol Myers Squibb	13	1.6
14	M/s. Ucb Inc	13	1.6
15	M/s. J and J Consumer Inc	12	1.4
16	M/s. Lilly	12	1.4
17	M/s. Purdue Pharma	12	1.4
18	M/s. Roche	12	1.4
19	M/s. Allergan	11	1.3
20	M/s. Apil	11	1.3
21	M/s. Takeda	11	1.3
22	M/s. Teva	11	1.3
23	M/s. Wyeth	11	1.3
	Sub Total of Top 20	384	46
	Sub Total of Remaining 173 companies	448	54
	Grand Total	832	100

Number of patents innovator has respect to orange book and para IV challenges

An analysis of orange book for average number of patents per application was calculated and it was observed that a range of minimum of (1) to maximum of (30) patents per application of a drug product approved. When average number of patents per application was calculated, it was observed that 4 ± 4 (Mean $\pm$ SD) patents per application. A similar kind of analysis (as information available) was conducted for the data of para IV certified innovator products and it was observed that a range of minimum of (1) to maximum of (27) patents per application of a drug product approved. When average number of patents per application with respect to para iv certified innovator products, it was observed that 4.08 ± 3.78 (Mean ± SD) patents per application.

Indicative list of Indian Companies having patent litigations at US Court of Appeals

Indicative list[3] of Indian pharmaceutical companies who are active in para IV certifications are M/s. Dr. Reddy's Laboratories Limited, M/s. Ranbaxy Laboratories Limited, M/s. Aurobindo Pharma Limited, M/s. Natco Pharma Limited, M/s. Sun Pharma, M/s. Zydus Pharmaceutical Limited, M/s. Lupin Pharmaceuticals, M/s. Glenmark Pharmaceuticals Limited, M/s. Caraco Pharmaceutical Laboratories, M/s. Matrix Laboratories Limited.

Conclusion

In general there are about 78 dosage forms and 47 routes of administration in pharmaceuticals. Development of a formulation is witnessed with very strong strategies. Development of a drug product to export to United States not only needs formulation technology but also with drug regulatory and patent legislation back grounds. Especially, similar drug development needs strong understanding of clinical condition, need of new dosage form, new route of administration and new combinations.

References

1. Bayya Subba Rao, Strategies and Lead Resources for Generic Drug Development, The Pharma Review, Nov-Dec, 2012, pp:96-104

2. www.fda.gov

3. http://www.cafc.uscourts.gov

ARTICLE 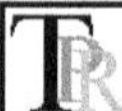

An Overview of Innovation Policy and Innovation Index

Bayya Subba Rao

Abstract: Even though intellectual property persists in every country, the economic growth of a country with respect to innovations is compared with several factors. The article is in brief and a reproduction from reports in bringing awareness.

1.0 Introduction

After the World Wars, it is believed that not Wars, but technology that decides the supremacy of a country. Intellectual status of citizens in a country is found to play a critical role in the economic growth of a country. Ideas generated by the citizens, have to be best protected so that the country's economic growth further increases. Signing WTO, TRIPS agreement, it is mandatory for the members and several countries like India update already existing legislations and vest new legislations for those not existing earlier with respect to intellectual property protection. With respect to trade, legislations were also tuned to trade services. The objective of the article is to analyze two reports made and emphasize the status of different countries in the World in terms of trade, intellectual property, governance etc. One of the reports "Global Innovation Policy Index" is released by The Information Technology and Innovation Foundation (ITIF), and Kauffman Foundation, USA. The second report "Global Innovation Index" released by World Intellectual Property Organisation (WIPO). The former report emphasizes and assesses the status of government policies and implementations whereas the later assess the status of innovations in a country.

2.0 Global Innovation Policy Index-2012

2.1.1 Selection of Countries

As per the report, a country's innovation policy depends on science policy, promotion of high-tech product development, improving productivity across the board in all economic sectors, skills, scientific research, information and communications technologies (ICTs), tax, trade, intellectual property, government procurement, standards, and regulations in an integrated approach designed to drive economic growth through innovation.

Fifty five countries belonging to Organisation for Economic Co-operation and Development (OECD), all European Union (EU) member states, and nineteen of the twenty-one Asia-Pacific Economic Cooperation (APEC) member economies, as well as the large developing nations of Argentina, Brazil, India, and South Africa were considered for comparison. As per World Bank, the countries selected belong to the categories high income, upper middle income, lower middle income, and low income.

2.1.2 Methodology

Comparison of the selected countries was assessed based on seven core policy areas (Table 1.1) with respect to weightage given and finally the countries were grouped under the categories upper tier, upper-mid tier, lower-mid tier and lower tier.

Core Policy Area	Share of Overall Weight
Trade and Foreign Direct Investment	17.5%
Science and R & D	17.5%
Domestic Market Competition	15.0%
Intellectual Property Rights	15.0%
Digital/Information and Communications Technology	17.5%
Government Procurement	10.0%
High-Skill Immigration	7.5%

Table 1.1: Policy Areas and weightage given for comparison

The weightage considered for individual policy area is based on a set of several indicators considered. The report is an analysis of the data submitted by various countries on various indicators to World Bank, World Trade Organisation, ITC, Fraser

Associate Professor, RBVRR Women's College of Pharmacy, Barkatpura, Hyderabad, A.P.

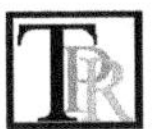 **ARTICLE**

institute, Peterson Institute, The World Economic Forum (WEF), Organisation for Economic Co-operation and Development (OECD).

2.1.3 Assessment on Trade and Foreign Direct Investment

Several indicators and their sub-indicators were assessed based on the data submitted by the countries to various international organisations. Indicators such as open market access (tariffs rates, complexity of tariffs, share of duty-free imports, index of non-tariff measures, non-tariff trade barriers, GATS commitments restrictiveness index, currency manipulation, participation in regional trade agreements), trade facilitation (customs services index, time to import goods, documents to import goods, irregular payments in exports and imports), openness to Foreign Direct Investment (foreign equity restrictions, screening and approval requirements, key personnel restrictions, operational restrictions) were assessed.

Upper-Tier	Upper-Mid Tier	Lower-Mid Tier	Lower-Tier
Australia, Austria, Belgium, Canada, Chile, Czech Republic, Denmark, Estonia, Finland, France, Germany, Greece, Hungary, Ireland, Italy, Latvia, Lithuania, Luxembourg, Netherlands, New Zealand, Norway, Romania, Portugal, Singapore, Slovak Republic, Slovenia, Spain, Sweden, United Kingdom, United States	Bulgaria, Cyprus, Hong Kong, Iceland, Malta, Mexico, Peru, Poland, Switzerland	Chinese Taipei, Israel, Japan, Malaysia, South Africa, South Korea, Turkey, Vietnam	Argentina, Brazil, China, India, Indonesia, Philippines, Russia, Thailand

Table 1.2: Country Ranks for Trade and Foreign Direct Investment

A total of fifteen indicators were considered and Table 1.2 illustrates tier wise the countries based on the assessment made.

2.1.4 Assessment on Science, R & D

Indicators such as R & D tax incentives, government R & D expenditure (non-defense, defense, higher education R & D performance, industry cluster development) were considered for comparison of the countries and Table 1.3 illustrates the ranks of the countries.

Upper-Tier	Upper-Mid Tier	Lower-Mid Tier	Lower-Tier
Australia, Austria, Canada, Chinese Taipei, Denmark, Finland, France, Netherlands, Norway, Singapore, South Korea, Spain, Sweden	Brazil, China, Czech Republic, Estonia, Germany, Hong Kong, Iceland, India, Israel, Italy, Japan, Lithuania, Portugal, Russia, Slovenia, Switzerland, United Kingdom, United States	Argentina, Belgium, Chile, Cyprus, Greece, Hungary, Ireland, Latvia, New Zealand, Poland, Romania, South Africa, Turkey	Bulgaria, Indonesia, Luxembourg, Malaysia, Malta, Mexico, Peru, Philippines, Slovak Republic, Thailand, Vietnam

Table 1.3: Country Ranks on Science and R & D policy

2.1.5 Assessment on Domestic Market Competition and Entrepreneur ship

Indicators such as regulatory environment (starting a business – number of procedures to start a business, time to start a business, cost to start a business), (acquiring property - number of procedures in buying/renting property, time involved in buying/renting property), (enforcing contracts - number of procedures to enforce a contract, time involved in enforcing contracts, cost involved in enforcing contracts), (acquiring talent - rigidity of employment, impact of pay on productivity), (closing a business - recovery rate when closing a business, time needed to close a business, cost involved in closing a business), (operating in a corruption free environment - irregular payment and bribes, regulatory and administrative opacity), competitive environment (intensity of local competition, extent of market dominance, efficiency of legal framework in challenging regulations, barriers to competition), entrepreneurial environment (number of new firms, administrative burdens on startups) were considered for comparison and Table 1.4 illustrates the ranks of the countries.

Upper-Tier	Upper-Mid Tier	Lower-Mid Tier	Lower-Tier
Australia, Canada, Denmark, Hong Kong, Singapore, Switzerland United Kingdom, United States	Austria, Belgium, Chinese Taipei, Cyprus, Czech Republic, Estonia, Finland, Germany, Iceland, Ireland, Japan, Malaysia, Malta, Netherlands, New Zealand, Norway Slovak Republic, Sweden	Bulgaria, Chile, China, France, Hungary, Israel, Latvia, Lithuania, Luxembourg, Poland, Portugal, Slovenia, South Africa, South Korea, Spain, Thailand, Turkey, Vietnam	Argentina, Brazil, Greece, Italy, Indonesia, India, Mexico, Peru, Philippines, Romania, Russia

Table 1.4: Country Ranks on Domestic Market Competition and Entrepreneurship

2.1.6 Assessment on Intellectual Property Rights

Indicators such as IP protection (2005 Park index, IP protection rating), enforcement (legal and political environment, integrity of the legal system), IP theft (software piracy rate, USTR 301 watch list) were considered and Table 1.4 illustrates the ranks of countries.

Upper-Tier	Upper-Mid Tier	Lower-Mid Tier	Lower-Tier
Australia, Austria, Belgium, Canada, Denmark, France, Finland, Germany, Japan, Ireland, Luxembourg, Netherlands, New Zealand, Norway, Singapore, Sweden, Switzerland, United Kingdom, United States	Chile, Chinese Taipei, Cyprus, Czech Republic, Estonia, Hong Kong, Hungary, Iceland, Israel, Italy, Latvia, Malta, Poland, Portugal, Slovak Republic, Slovenia, Spain, South Africa, South Korea	Bulgaria, China, Greece, India, Lithuania, Malaysia, Mexico, Romania, Turkey	Argentina, Brazil, Indonesia, Peru, Philippines, Russia, Thailand, Vietnam

Table 1.5: Country Ranks for Intellectual Property Protection

2.1.7 Assessment on Digital and Information and Communications Technology

Several digital policy indicators such as competitiveness of ICT infrastructure and policy (infrastructure access – broadband penetration, mobile network coverage rate, internet access in schools; infrastructure affordability – price basket for residential fixed line, price basket for mobile call, price basket for internet; ICT policy governance – national broadband plan, separate regulatory body, government prioritization of ICT, importance of ICT to government vision of the future), international openness to ICT and market competition (international openness to ICT-Tariffs on ICT products, WTO/ITA, foreign participation/ownership in telecom sector, long distance termination charges, open interconnection agreement, unregulated VoIP; ICT market competition level – international long distance market competition, mobile telephone market competition, fixed line telephone market competition), legal (legal environment – IP, transparency, privacy and cyber-crime; laws relating to ICT; spam legislation), usage (public sector usage – government success in ICT promotion, ICT use and government efficiency, online service index, e-participation index, public service sector expenditure; business usage-extent of business internet use, ICT impact on new services and products, ICT impact on new organizational models, business sector expenditure; individual usage – internet use, mobile cellular use, use of virtual social networks) were considered and Table 1.6 illustrates tier under which each country falls.

Upper-Tier	Upper-Mid Tier	Lower-Mid Tier	Lower-Tier
Canada, Chinese Taipei, Denmark, Finland, Germany, Hong Kong, Iceland, Luxembourg, Netherlands, New Zealand, Norway, Singapore, South Korea, Sweden, Switzerland, United Kingdom, United States	Australia, Austria, Belgium, Cyprus, Czech Republic, Estonia, France, Hungary, Ireland, Israel, Japan, Lithuania, Malaysia, Malta, Portugal, Spain	Brazil, Bulgaria, Chile, China, Greece, India, Italy, Latvia, Poland, Romania, Slovak Republic, Slovenia, Thailand, Turkey	Argentina, Indonesia, Mexico, Peru, Philippines, Russia, South Africa, Vietnam

Table 1.6: Country Ranks on Digital Policy

2.1.8 Assessment on Government Procurement

Indicators such as participation in WTO government procurement agreement, government enterprise and investment indicator,

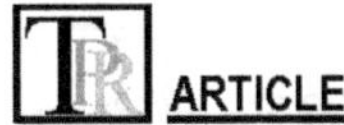

ARTICLE

corruption perception index, government procurement of advanced technology products were assessed and Table 1.7 illustrates ranking of the countries tier wise.

Upper-Tier	Upper-Mid Tier	Lower-Mid Tier	Lower-Tier
Austria, Belgium, Canada, Chinese Taipei, Cyprus, Denmark, Estonia, Finland, France, Germany, Hong Kong, Iceland, Japan, Luxembourg, Netherlands, Norway, Portugal, Slovenia, Singapore, Sweden, Switzerland, United Kingdom, United States	Australia, Bulgaria, Chile, Czech Republic, Greece, Hungary, Ireland, Israel, Italy, Lithuania, Malta, New Zealand, Poland, Slovak Republic, Spain, South Korea	Latvia, Romania, Turkey	Argentina, Brazil, China, India, Indonesia, Malaysia, Mexico, Peru, Philippines, Russia South Africa, Thailand, Vietnam

Table 1.7: Country Ranks on Government Procurement

2.1.9 Assessment of high skill immigration

Indicators such as selection rate for high skill immigrants, ratio of selection rate of high skill immigrants to low skill immigrants, high skill immigrants as a share of total population were assessed and Table 1.8 illustrates ranking of the countries tier wise.

Upper-Tier	Upper-Mid Tier	Lower-Mid Tier	Lower-Tier
Canada, Chinese Taipei, Hong Kong, Israel, Singapore	Australia, Japan, Latvia, Malaysia, New Zealand, Philippines, South Africa, United States	Argentina, Austria, Belgium, Brazil, Chile, China, Cyprus, Denmark, Estonia, France, Germany, Hungary, Iceland, Ireland, India, Indonesia Luxembourg, Netherlands, Norway, Peru, Poland, Russia, South Korea, Sweden, Switzerland, Thailand, United Kingdom, Vietnam	Bulgaria, Czech Republic, Finland, Greece, Italy, Lithuania, Malta, Mexico, Portugal, Romania, Slovak Republic, Slovenia Spain, Turkey

Table 1.8: Country ranks on high skill immigration

3.0 The Global Innovation Index-2013

The Global Innovation Index is a collaborative work among Cornell University, INSEAD, and the World Intellectual Property Organization (WIPO), Johnson Cornell University, Booz & Company, the Confederation of Indian Industry, du, and Huawei.

3.1 Methodology

Global Innovation Index is an outcome of average of two sub-indices i.e., innovation input sub-index and innovation output sub-index. The input sub-index is obtained by considering five input pillars that have a key role in economic growth of the country with respect to innovations i.e., institutions, human capital and research, infrastructure, market sophistication and business sophistication. The output sub-index is obtained by considering the result activity relating to innovations i.e., knowledge and technology output, creative outputs.

Each pillar is divided into three sub-pillars and each sub-pillar is composed of individual indicators for a total of 84 indicators.

Innovation efficiency ratio is the ratio of output sub-index over the input sub-index. The parameter helps in assessing a country with respect to the innovation output with corresponding inputs of the country.

For the year 2013, a total of 142 economies were compared and ranked.

3.2 Innovation Input Sub-Index-In Detail

The input sub-index concentrates on five pillars with an objective of availability of environment for innovations.

3.2.1 Institutional pillar

The institutional pillar mainly discusses and assesses on political environment (political stability, government effectiveness, press freedom), regulatory environment (regulatory quality, rule of law, cost of redundancy dismissal, salary weeks), business environment (ease of starting a business, ease of resolving insolvency, ease of paying taxes).

3.2.2 Human Capital and Research pillar

The human capital and research pillar discusses and assesses on education (current expenditure on education-% GNI, public expenditure/pupil-% GDP/cap, school life expectancy-years, PISA scale-reading/maths/science, pupil-teacher ratio-secondary), tertiary education (tertiary enrolment-% gross, graduates in science & engineering-%, tertiary inbound mobility-%, gross tertiary outbound enrolment-%), research & development (researchers-headcounts/mn pop, gross expenditure on R&D-%GDP, QS University ranking, average score top).

3.2.3 Infrastructure pillar

The infrastructure pillar discusses and assesses on information & communication technologies (ICT access, ICT use, government's online service, e-participation), general infrastructure (Electricity output-kWh/cap, Electricity consumption-kWh/cap, logistics performance, gross capital formation-% GDP), Ecological sustainability (GDP/unit of energy use-2000 PPP$/kg oil eq, environmental performance, ISO 14001 environ. certificates/bn PPP$ GDP).

3.2.4 Market sophistication pillar

The market sophistication pillar discusses and assesses on credit (ease of getting credit, domestic credit to private sector-% GDP, microfinance gross loans-% GDP), investment (ease of protecting investors, market capitalization-% GDP, total value of stocks traded-% GDP, venture capital deals/tr PPP$ GDP), trade and competition (applied tariff rate, weighted mean-%, non-agriculture market access weighted tariff-%, intensity of local competition).

3.2.5 Business sophistication pillar

The business sophistication pillar discusses and assesses on knowledge workers (knowledge intensive employment-%, firms offering formal training-% firms, R&D performed by business-% GDP, R & D financed by business-%, GMAT mean score, GMAT test takers/mn pop), innovation linkages (university/industry research collaboration, state of cluster development, R&D financed by abroad-%, JV-strategic alliance deals/tr PPP$ GDP, patent families filed in 3+ offices/bn PPP$ GDP), knowledge absorption (royalty and license fees payments-% service imports, high-tech imports less re-imports-%, communication, computer and information services imports-%, FDI net inflows, % GDP).

3.3 Innovation Output Sub-Index-In Detail

3.3.1 *Knowledge and technology outputs pillar*

The knowledge and technology output pillar discusses and assesses on knowledge creation (domestic resident patent ap/bn PPP$ GDP, PCT resident patent ap/bn PPP$ GDP, domestic resident utility model ap/bn PPP$ GDP, scientific & technical articles/bn PPP$ GDP, citable documents H index), knowledge impact (growth rate of PPP$ GDP/worker-%, new business/th pop, computer software spending-% GDP, ISO 9001 quality certificates/bn PPP$ GDP, high & medium-high tech

manufacturers-%), knowledge diffusion (royalty and license fees receipts-% service exports, high tech exports less re-exports-%, communication, computer and information services exports-%, FDI net outflows-% GDP).

3.3.2 *Creative output pillar*

The creative output pillar discusses and assesses on intangible assets (domestic resident trademark registration/bn PPP$ GDP, Madrid trademark registrations/bn PPP$ GDP, ICT & business model creation, ICT & organizational model creation), creative goods & services (audio-visual & related services exports-%, national feature films/mn pop, paid for dailies, circulation-% pop, creative goods exports-%, printing & publishing manufacturers-%), online creativity (generic top-level domains (TLDs)/th pop, country code TLDs/th pop, Wikipedia monthly edits/mn pop, video loads on YouTube/pop).

3.4 Discussion

3.4.1 *Global Innovation Policy Index-2012*

India is one among the countries which is listed under the category of currency manipulation. Our immediate competitor China is also found to be included under the category. In several issues, India stands in lower tier, lower mid-tier except in R & D policy (upper mid-tier). There is a possibility that India's status of lower mid-tier in intellectual property protection moving to upper-tier. India is one among the countries listed under USTR 301 watch list. Over all, the report indicates that India is under the category of lower-tier with respect to innovation policy capacity.

Upper-Tier	Upper-Mid Tier	Lower-Mid Tier	Lower-Tier
Australia, Austria, Canada, Chinese Taipei, Denmark, Finland, France, Germany, Hong Kong, Japan, Netherlands, New Zealand, Norway, Singapore, Sweden, Switzerland United Kingdom, United States	Belgium, Cyprus, Czech Republic, Estonia, Hungary, Iceland, Ireland, Israel, Lithuania, Luxembourg, Malta, Portugal, Slovenia, South Korea, Spain	Brazil, Bulgaria, Chile, China, Greece, Italy, Latvia, Malaysia, Poland, Romania, Slovak Republic, South Africa, Turkey	Argentina, India, Indonesia, Mexico, Peru, Philippines, Russia, Thailand, Vietnam

Table 1.9: Rank of Countries on Innovation Policy Capacity

3.4.2 *Global Innovation Index-2013*

Among the countries compared, table 1.10 illustrates the top 10 countries in ranking with respect to Global Innovation Index. It

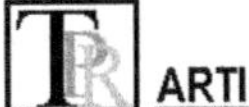 **ARTICLE**

is observed that Switzer Land stands first and United States of America stands tenth among the top ten countries.

Rank	Country Name
1	Switzer Land
2	Sweden
3	United Kingdom
4	Netherlands
5	United States of America
6	Finland
7	Hong Kong (China)
8	Singapore
9	Denmark
10	Ireland

Table 1.10: Global Innovation Index-Top 10/Country wise

Among the 142 countries assessed and compared, the final scoring was found to be at a range of [Yemen-lowest (19.32)-Switzerland-highest (66.59)] with respect to standard score ranging 0-100. India stands 66th rank with a score of 36.17. Our immediate competitor China stands 35th rank with a score of 44.66. Yemen stands with 142nd rank.

With respect to innovation input sub-index ranking, the final scoring was found to be at a range of [Pakistan-lowest (23.68)-Singapore-highest (72.27)] with respect to standard score ranging 0-100. India stands 87th rank with a score of 35.77. Our immediate competitor China stands 46th rank with a score of 45.19.

With respect to innovation output sub-index ranking, the final scoring was found to be at a range of [Sudan-lowest (13.11)-Switzerland-highest (66.65)] with respect to standard score ranging 0-100. India stands 42nd rank with a score of 36.56. Our immediate competitor China stands 25th rank with a score of 44.12.

With respect to innovation efficiency ratio, which indicates more out come with less input, the final ratio was found to be at a range of [Syrian Arab Republic-lowest (0.45)-Mali-highest (1.13)]. India stands 11th rank with a ratio of 1.02. Our immediate competitor China stands 14th rank with a ratio of 0.98.

Among the countries with emerging economies, eighteen were found to increase their status relating to innovation index with respect to previous years and they are, Armenia, China, Costa Rica, Georgia, Hungary, India, Jordan, Kenya, Latvia, Malaysia, Mali, the Republic of Moldova, Mongolia, Montenegro, Senegal, Tajikistan, Uganda, and Viet Nam.

3.5 Conclusion

Several data cited in YouTube, Wikipedia are gaining their importance as a factor in determining the innovation index of a country. Several researches especially made at the academic level are not available to public as it is not published in journals. If such information is made available online, is considered under the purview of public domain and may not be protected as intellectual property by others.

3.6 Disclaimer

1. The article is a reproduction of original work transformed into brief and for quick understanding.
2. The article is only for awareness/knowledge purpose and the author do not have any commercial benefits.
3. It is advised to refer to the original reports where ever necessary in detail for making final conclusions.

3.7 References

1. The Global Innovation Policy Index-2012
2. The Global Innovation Index-2013

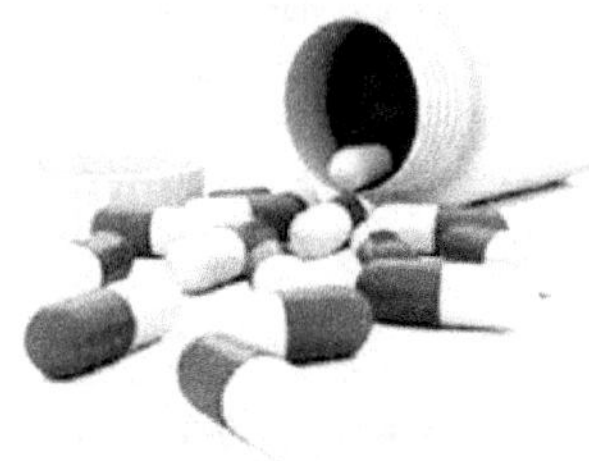

Article

Challenges Ahead for New Government in Pharmaceuticals in Intellectual Property Matters

Bayya Subba Rao*

Associate Professor, RBVRR Women's College of Pharmacy, Barkatpura.

Twenty five years ago computers were new to India and as time passed, computerization and internet has made communication system faster. Later, at one stage we were far away behind in technology of computers and networking, when compared to western countries. The concept has changed the living system in every sector of India. Likewise, liberalization is playing a key role in intellectual property system in India. Earlier Indian legislations were updated to the expected at that time's needs. Policy makers even might not predict such advancements would happen due to lack of updated international knowledge, legislations. Currently, it is believed that our intellectual property system is strong to local needs, but it happens not to be so to the western countries. United States of America through United States Trade Representative monitors WTO member countries and voluntarily interferes with foreign country legislations whether fulfilling international agreements with an objective of safeguarding its national's intellectual property in India. The current article discusses about the concern of the United States and several WTO member countries in safe guarding it's nationals in India relating to intellectual property system and emphasis is made only relating to Indian status in pharmaceuticals relating to patent system.

1.0 Introduction

Post GATT scenario has brought a challenging competitive environment in almost every sector. Trade exchange, intellectual property protection is expected to increase the economic growth especially of developing countries. Trade Related Aspects of Intellectual Property Rights (TRIPS) has indicated minimum guidelines and it is up to individual country's discretion in bringing out stringency of the legislations. Office of United States Trade Representative (USTR), Executive Office of The President of the United States since 25 years is releasing an annual report indicating care taking of its national's intellectual property protection in WTO member countries and simultaneously monitoring, helping, initiating negotiations in strengthening intellectual property regime in countries where needed. In USTR 301, 2014 annual report, India is one of the countries listed in the Priority Watch List. Since 1995, India has brought necessary new legislations and upgraded already existing legislations relating to intellectual property rights. With respect to patents, The Patents Act 1970 was amended thrice to bring out 20 years exclusivity term, compulsory licensing (removing license of right), burden of proof, facility to deposit micro-organisms as per Budapest Treaty, product patent system in addition to process, Bolar provision etc.

The current article is related to issues that The United States is raising to fulfill the WTO/TRIPS agreement.

2.0 TRIPS agreement:

TRIPS agreement is a mandatory guideline once a country becomes a member of World Trade Organization. TRIPS guidelines are minimum guidelines in harmonizing application, scrutiny, granting processes with a single application system of different intellectual property rights. The guideline indicates national treatment, fulfilling international and regional conventions by the member countries. TRIPS agreement provides guidelines on copyrights, trademarks, geographical indications, industrial designs, patents, protection of undisclosed information, and control of anti-competitive practices in contractual licences. The agreement indicates the countries in bringing out administrative bodies for enforcement with respect to legal system, border measures emphasizing on criminal procedure, infringements. A provision of establishing an international council as TRIPS council is proposed to monitor the status of intellectual property regime and enforcement in a member country during the transitional arrangement. United States earlier had made its representation

to the Dispute Settlement Body of WTO relating to India whether fulfilling TRIPS obligation has been done and India by the year 2005 implemented the product patent in addition to process patent regime.

3.0 Current issues raised by the office of the United States trade representative

2014 Special 301 report, released by the Office of United States Trade Representative (USTR) indicates countries under two categories i.e., Priority Watch List (China, India, Russia, Algeria, Argentina, Chile, Indonesia, Pakistan, Thailand, Venezuela) and Watch List (Barbados, Bolivia, Brazil, Bulgaria, Canada, Colombia, Costa Rica, Dominican Republic, Ecuador, Egypt, Finland, Greece, Guatemala, Jamaica, Kuwait, Lebanon, Mexico, Paraguay, Peru, Romania, Tajikistan, Trinidad and Tobago, Turkey, Turkmenistan, Uzbekistan, Vietnam).

Even though, India has made several efforts in strengthening intellectual property regime, post GATT, the report indicates India made a limited progress in 2013.

3.1 Status of patent application filings and grants at Indian patent office

Table 1 illustrates the statistics of applications received and granted relating to chemical, drug and biotechnology over the years at the Indian patent office:

Indian Controller General of Patents has indicated that the office is

Table 1: Statistics of Patents Granted at Indian Patent Office 1997-2013

Year	Grants			Applications (other than PCT national phase)		
	Chemical	Drug	Biotechnology	Chemical	Drug	Biotechnology
1997-1998	503	291	--	2221	1481	--
1998-1999	609	150	--	2023	1555	3
1999-2000	516	307	--	840	1000	9
2000-2001	353	276	--	707	003	4
2001-2002	483	320	--	778	879	2

2002-2003	399	312	---	776	966	46
2003-2004	609	419	---	2952	2525	23
2004-2005	573	192	71	3916	2316	1214
2005-2006	1140	457	51	5810	2211	1525
2006-2007	1989	798	89	6354	3239	2774
2007-2008	2662	905	341	6375	4267	1950
2008-2009	2376	1207	1157	5884	3672	1844
2009-2010	1420	530	449	6014	3070	1303
2010-2011	1899	596	165	6911	3526	1497
2011-2012	1168	282	309	6698	2762	788
2012-2013	1289	344	144	6812	2954	832

Source: Indian Patent Office website

about to appoint 500 patent examiners in the next five years so that the examination and grant process increases.

3.2 Court settlements

Strengthening of civil IPR enforcement is being suggested so as to increase judicial efficiency, reducing court backlogs through electronic case management, fast-track procedures, specialized judges and similar reform measures. With respect to criminal issues, the report indicates launch of raids at counterfeit markets, combat the manufacture, sale and distribution of counterfeit medicines.

3.3 Section 3d of The Patents Act, 1970

Section 3d of The Patents Act, 1970 (Indian) indicates inventions not patentable. The subject matter in an invention if fulfills all the patentability criteria of novelty, non-obviousness, useful (industrial application) and enabling, a patent may be granted.

Section 3d of The Patents Act, 1970 indicates "The mere discovery of a new form of a known substance which does not result in the enhancement of the known efficacy of that substance or the mere discovery of any new property or new use for a known substance or of the mere use of a known process, machine or apparatus unless such known process results in a new product or employs at least one new reactant. Explanation: For the purposes of this clause salts, esters, ethers, polymorphs, metabolites, pure form, particle size, isomers, mixtures of isomers, complexes, combinations and other derivatives of known substance shall be considered to be the same, unless they differ significantly in properties with regard to efficacy". The subsection indicates that, in India, especially pharmaceutical related inventions that are new form of an already existing substance may or may not be granted with a patent. This implies that, based on case by case the examiner decides and makes a decision whether to grant a patent or not. In other words, all the new forms of an existing substance are considered as one substance (existing substance) in India and usually patents are not granted for every new form or in combination. However, if the new form of the existing substance has a statistically significant clinical effect, under such circumstances Indian patent office has granted patents. At the same time, Indian patent office rejected patent applications for inventions in which new forms did not exhibit statistically significant clinical effect with respect to the known (existing) form.

Currently, 2014 USTR 301 report indicates that the current section 3d may have the effect of limiting the patentability of potentially beneficial innovations which would include drugs with fewer side effects, decreased toxicity, improved delivery system, or temperature or storage stability. This may be interpreted that Indian patent system is stringent enough for local needs, but unable to balance the intellectual property right protection mechanism at the global scenario. A time has approached for the policy makers, to discuss if necessary in fine tuning section 3d. This indicates that section 3d to be made bit flexible providing a provision for new forms of known forms to be granted for a patent if they fulfill not only statistically clinical significant effect but also for new forms that exhibit fewer side effects, decreased toxicity, improved delivery system, or temperature or storage stability.

3.4 Trade secrets

It is believed that India is practicing a contract based approach in exchange of business information. Such information may lead to a theft if a contract has been breached. As there is no law relating to trade secrets, claim for the damages is difficult to obtain as courts does not have legal procedures to handle such cases. It is also believed, if a case is taken up by the courts relating to breach of trade secrets, the chances of trade secret information passing to public is more. Currently, European Union has a proposal of bringing out a legislation relating to trade secret and introduced a proposal for the Directive of the European parliament and of the Council on the Protection of Undisclosed Know-How and Business Information (Trade Secrets) against their unlawful acquisition, use and disclosure. The directive is expected to harmonize civil trade secret law throughout the European Union. The directive may act as a lead to Indian policy makers in framing legislations in India as Trade Secrets.

In pharmaceuticals, biopharmaceutical data is first generated by the innovator for a new drug. Such data is submitted to regulatory authority for approval of their products to release into the Indian market. Currently, as there is no data exclusivity term in India, the entry of generics into Indian market is early. Data protection for pharmaceuticals seems to remain under consideration by Ministry of Health and Family Welfare. Currently, the Pesticide Management Bill, before parliament, includes provision for data protection of agriculture chemicals for five years, although that time period begins with the product's first marketing approval anywhere in the World.

3.5 Compulsory licensing

Compulsory licensing is a mechanism where a third party is authorized to use a patented invention. A compulsory licence is granted in India under the grounds of a patented invention not worked in India, commercially exploited in India, unable to fulfill market demands, national emergency conditions, for life threatening disease treatments, where a country do not have pharmaceutical manufacturing facility etc. A third party may approach the Indian patent office after 3 years from grant of patent seeking for a compulsory license provided a patent licensing mechanism between the third party and patent holder failed.

USTR 301 report indicates that Indian inter-ministerial process is considering over a dozen patented medicines as candidates for government initiated compulsory licenses and is urging India to get the inputs from the patent right holders to bring out a balance mechanism.

Moreover, USTR points out that grant of compulsory license merely on 'not working' in India seems to be controversial. In several cases, innovators argued that working requirement could be met solely by importation due to economic factors and hence not manufactured in India. The report indicates that several Indian companies are manufacturing products without the authorization of the patent holder and this is mainly due to communication gap between the state and central government officials, especially regarding the exclusivity status of drug product in India.

3.6 Pre-grant and post-grant opposition

Opposition mechanism in grant of patent helps in careful monitoring of the patentability criteria for an invention. In India, pre-grant and post-grant opposition are in force. A pre-grant opposition can be filed at any time before grant of a patent at the patent office, but after publication in journal of patent. A post-grant opposition can be filed only after grant of patent and its publication in journal of patent, but within one year after publication.

The report indicates that the grounds for either pre-grant or post-grant opposition are identified to be eleven in number and are found to be common. The conditions of opposition are on the grounds of invention in the patent lack inventive step, mere commercial exploitation, patent invalid, traditional knowledge, obvious ness, unable to meet market demands, not worked in India, non-disclosure of best mode, lack of novelty, infringement etc. Such common agenda of pre-grant and post-grant opposition by the same person or others is found to delay the life of patent exclusivity term and the report suggest for a suitable modification of the agenda so that, the applicant enjoy better patent exclusivity term.

4.0 Conclusion

India was several times reported as one among the countries found and prone for intellectual property leak. The reasons may be due to intellectual property rights being a new generation concept, lack of knowledge, lack of trade secret legislation, state and central government communication gap. United States and European Union are now insisting and putting forward a challenge to the Indian new coming government in making changes in the intellectual property legislations where ever necessary for better enforcement of infringement action, early patent grants, minimizing patent prosecutions time, better enjoyment of patent exclusivity rights by the inventor, a genuine rationale of grant of compulsory licence discussing with patent holder. Currently, India has proposals of a drug price control mechanism for patented drug products. Such mechanism may bring out a balance mechanism among the innovator, generic manufacturer and the end user of medicines. Wait and see mechanism may not be fruitful always and forecasting strategies are not strong enough where countries like US and European Union are identifying pitfalls in our legislations only meeting local needs and not withstanding global needs. Several Indian legislations are being updated to current trend and it is time for the policy makers to not only think and determined for local benefits but also for global benefits since Indians are also treated as national in foreign member countries.

Disclaimer

1. All the information in the article is to author's interpretations.
2. The updated information may be obtained from the appropriate authority.
3. It is advised to refer to official resources where ever necessary in taking final decisions.

References

1. www.ustr.gov
2. www.ipindia.nic.in

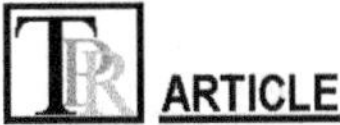 ARTICLE

Strategies and Lead Resources for Generic Drug Development

Bayya Subba Rao

Abstract: *Generic drug approval process is a balance mechanism among innovator, generic manufacturer and the end user of the drug. The provision was made through Hatch-Waxmann Act at United States. The current article brings awareness with emphasis on drug approvals at USFDA with an objective to establish forecast strategies. A forecast strategy is necessary in terms of when a patent period, market exclusivity period is getting expired and how early we should develop a generic drug, complete bioequivalence studies, complete even filing protocols aiming to release possibly as a first generic soon after the innovator's patent, data/market exclusivity period expires. Such forecast strategies may also helps the industry simultaneously plan for approval in other countries in the World.*

Introduction

United States Food and Drug Administration is the whole and sole organization for approval of drugs into the market of United States. At USFDA, drugs are approved as New Drug Application, Abbreviated New Drug Applications (generics), first generics, tentative approvals, New Molecule Entities, Orphan drugs and pediatric drugs. It is necessary to understand drug discovery, drug approval processes with corresponding intellectual property right protection as patents, market exclusivity (data exclusivity) etc. The objective of this article is to bring an awareness so as to be well in hand in the development of products especially by generic manufacturer to release into the US market. It is necessary to understand development and release of a product depends on volume of consumption, quantity already manufactured globally, possible demand to overcome shortage, client's requirements, patent expiry, data/market exclusivity expiry etc., either as bulk drug, different type of formulation, combination products. The current article mainly reflects to USFDA data as countries like India which is a leading manufacturer of pharmaceutical products, and companies can simultaneously get approved upon fulfilling local other country requirements in addition to United States.

Understanding Drug Discovery Process, Intellectual Property Protection as Patents, Data/Market Exclusivity

A drug discovery process involves a lead identification, developing analogues to overcome setbacks inherent with lead molecule, which after preclinical studies finally leading to clinical investigations. Such molecule that is promising has transformed from the stage of New Chemical Entity to Investigational New Drug Application to New Drug Application. Once the drug fulfills the criteria of clinical trials, the drug is approved to release into the market. However, post market surveillance persists.

WTO-TRIPS agreement brought a minimum criterion to fulfill the protection of intellectual property rights in a country. It is upto the country's needs, local legislations are vested that in turn reflects the stringency. It is very clear that protection of intellectual property rights is not uniform throughout the world. The patent law system of United States provides a provision of patenting inventions that have a new use. Data that is generated during the invention/approval process is protected as data protection in United States.

In terms of market exclusivity, at United States the innovator products are approved for 5 years for market exclusivity and later on generics are launched. The first generic launched will have the 180 day exclusivity. Several leading generic manufacturers are at the race of the launching their drug products as first generics since the number of products from companies is less at this level which in turn not only makes the innovator's product available at a fallen price, the first generic company enjoys better margins. As the number of generics later on increases, competition prevails and leads to narrow margins of profit when compared to earlier.

Tentative approvals is a provision similar to the kind of innovator's efforts where in a new indication or dosage form or route of administration etc are developed for the first time and such products requires detailed pharmacodynamic and pharmacokinetic studies.

Monitoring Drug Approvals, Patent Expires, Data/ Market Exclusivity in United States

In United States, drugs are approved as New Drug Application, Abbreviated New Drug Application, First Generics, Tentative Approvals, Pediatric drugs, Orphan drugs.

It is necessary to compile all the drugs approved at United States in terms of drug combinations, strengths, dosage form, route of administration, number of companies with generics approved etc. Simultaneously there is a necessity to monitor whether there is a patent in force for a drug/drug product and simultaneously the possible date of patent, data/market exclusivity expiry. Monitoring such information will provide a lead especially to the generic manufacturer in developing, filing the drug products well in hand under the Bolar provision wherein, research activities as long as they are not made commercial, exempted from the act of infringement.

Filing Certifications for Generic Approvals at USFDA

With the regulations, the FDA publishes all the necessary NDA patent information in the Orange Book. The ANDA applicant for the generic has to submit the reference-listed drugs (RLD) i.e., the NDA related patents for the approval. The FDA cannot approve the ANDA application until the NDA listed patents are expired.

In order to get approved for a generic, the ANDA applicant has to make certifications as per the provisions of the Hatch Waxman Act [21 USC §355 (j)(2)(A)(vii)(I)-(IV)] and regulations [21 CFR 314.94(A)(12)(i)]. The ANDA applicant has to choose the 4 certifications in addressing each patent. The four certifications are commonly referred as paragraph I, II, III and IV.

Paragraph I Certification: An ANDA applicant chooses Paragraph I certification when there is no patent listed in the Orange Book. Even though the NDA holder possess a patent and decided not to list as an RLD, the FDA approves immediately an ANDA provided the holder meets the approval requirements.

Paragraph II Certification: An ANDA applicant chooses Paragraph II certification when there is a patent listed in the Orange Book, but expired. If the applicant meets the approval criteria, the FDA approves immediately for a generic.

Paragraph III Certification: An ANDA applicant chooses Paragraph III certification when there is a patent listed as RLD but not expired and plans to market the product prior patent expiration. In such cases the law inhibits the FDA from approval until the patent expires.

Paragraph IV Certification: An ANDA applicant chooses Paragraph IV certification when he wishes to challenge one or more patents listed and intends to market the generic product before the patent expires. The ANDA holder would challenge by saying that the patent is invalid, unenforceable, or will not be infringed by the manufacture, use or sale of the generic product. Soon after receiving the certification IV and on accepting for a review, the FDA sends acknowledgement for review. Soon after the ANDA applicant receives the notice from the FDA, he has to bring to the notice of the patent holder with the ANDA application number, description of the proposed drug product and the patent numbers with expiration dates that are being challenged. In addition to these, the ANDA applicant must describe the facts that the patent is not infringed, is invalid or unenforceable. If within 45 days of receipt of the notice from the ANDA holder, the NDA holder files a lawsuit at the federal district court, the FDA is inhibited in approving the ANDA for a period of 30 months. During this 30 months stay, both the NDA and ANDA applicants can litigate.

Statistics Relating To Drug Approvals At USFDA

IPR & Regulatory Centre at Pharmexcil is extending its research activities not only in terms of increasing intellectual property awareness for protection of inventions but also in providing awareness with lead resources that help new industries who need to develop strategies for IPR protection, approval of drug products at least as generics into the market. The objective of these statistics is to understand that competition induces price control mechanism but such competition also deteriorate the pharmaceutical industry if the number of competitors is large leading to deterioration of the ecosystem of manufacturing sector etc. The statistics are provided to bring awareness that such analysis is necessary, possible and must be part as a dry laboratory research activity in every pharmaceutical industry. All the statistical data provided is cleaned to our interpretations and there is necessity to periodically update for the current status.

USFDA Approved Products-Ingredient Wise

Our research in terms of drug, drug combination and the

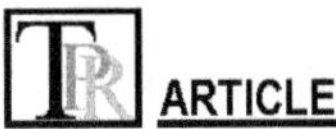 ARTICLE

corresponding number of products approved at USFDA, Table 1 reveals listing of some of the products. It has been observed that there are 195 products approved relating to Ibuprofen as single ingredient at USFDA.

USFDA Approved Products-Ingredient/Dosage form/route of Administration

Our research in terms of ingredient against dosage form and route of administration, Table 2 reveals that Abacavir Sulphate was approved in solution, tablet dosage forms for oral route of administration.

USFDA Approved Products-Dosage form and Route of Administration

Our research in terms of dosage form and route of administration, Table 3 indicates alphabetical listing where in amongst, 59 are approved as Aerosol, metered; inhalation irrespective of ingredient.

S. No	Ingredient Name	No. of Approvals
1	IBUPROFEN	195
2	RISPERIDONE	183
3	PROPRANOLOL HYDROCHLORIDE	172
4	HEPARIN SODIUM	161
5	HYDROCORTISONE	161
6	THEOPHYLLINE	156
7	AMITRIPTYLINE HYDROCHLORIDE	153
8	ACETAMINOPHEN; HYDROCODONE BITARTRATE	152
9	LEVETIRACETAM	141
10	DILTIAZEM HYDROCHLORIDE	140

Table 1: USFDA Approved Products-Ingredient wise

S. No	Ingredient Name	SOLUTION; ORAL	TABLET; ORAL	Grand Total
1	ABACAVIR SULFATE	1	1	2

Table 2: USFDA Approved Products-Ingredient/dosage form/route of administration

S. No	Dosage Form; Route of Administration	No. of Approvals Ingredient wise
1	AEROSOL, FOAM; TOPICAL	12
2	AEROSOL, METERED; INHALATION	59
3	AEROSOL, METERED; INTRAPLEURAL	1
4	AEROSOL, METERED; NASAL	4
5	AEROSOL, METERED; RECTAL	1
6	AEROSOL, METERED; SUBLINGUAL	1
7	AEROSOL, METERED; TOPICAL	3
8	AEROSOL; NASAL	1
9	AEROSOL; ORAL	1
10	AEROSOL; SUBLINGUAL	1

Table 3: USFDA Approved Products-Dosage form; Route of Administration wise

S. No	Applicant Full Name	ANDAs	NDAs	Total
1	WATSON LABORATORIES INC	1316	74	1390
2	SANDOZ INC	932	38	970
3	TEVA PHARMACEUTICALS USA INC	877	17	894
4	MYLAN PHARMACEUTICALS INC	808	12	820
5	HOSPIRA INC	416	325	741
6	IVAX PHARMACEUTICALS INC SUB TEVA PHARMACEUTICALS USA	421	15	436
7	ROXANE LABORATORIES INC	352	28	380
8	GLAXOSMITHKLINE	69	300	369
9	NOVARTIS PHARMACEUTICALS CORP	19	328	347
10	MUTUAL PHARMACEUTICAL CO INC	324	7	331

Table 4: USFDA Approved Products as ANDAs, NDAs-Company wise

USFDA Approved Products as ANDAs, NDAs-Company Wise

Our research reveals that approved products at USFDA when observed company wise (irrespective of parent, subsidiary, sister company), Table 4 provides company wise the number of ANDAs, NDAs that are approved and as per the mentioned statistics, it is observed that Watson Laboratories Inc has a total approvals of 1390 with 1316, 74 as ANDAs, NDAs respectively.

USFDA Approved Products-Ingredient, Strength Wise

Our research in terms of a specific drug, available approved strengths irrespective of dosage form, Table 5 reveals that USFDA has approved Abacavir sulphate at strengths of 20, 300 mg with respect to base.

Ingredient/Strength	ABACAVIR SULFATE
EQ 20MG BASE/ML	1
EQ 300MG BASE	1

Table 5: USFDA Approved Products-Strength

USFDA Approved Products-Ingredient Specific, Company Wise

Our research in terms of ingredient wise, the number of companies that have approved products, Table 6 reveals that Abacavir sulphate as single ingredient was approved for VIIV Healthcare Co irrespective of dosage form, route of administration.

USFDA Approved Products as First Generics-Year Wise/Drug Product/Dosage form

As discussed earlier, releasing a drug product as a first generic implies well established forecast strategies being used by the generic companies. Table 7 indicates that Acarbose tablets were approved as first generics in the year 2008. It is necessary to understand that the generic drug may be developed well in advance before patent, data/market exclusivity expiry. The generic companies have utilized the time before the patent, data/market exclusivity period expiry in developing the formulation, undertaking especially bioequivalence studies and being as the first applicant to file for a generic drug approval.

S. No	Ingredient Name/ Applicant Full Name	VIIV HEALTHCARE CO	Grand Total
1	ABACAVIR SULFATE	2	2

Table 6: USFDA Approved Products-Ingredient/Company wise

USFDA Approved Products As First Generics-Indian Company/Year Wise

Our research Table 8 reveals that Indian origin drug manufacturers Ranbaxy Laboratories Limited, Dr. Reddy's Laboratories Limited were the first companies to file for first generics with 3, 2 products respectively in the year 2002.

USFDA Approved Products as First Generics-Ingredient/Strength/Dosage form/Manufacturer/Brand Name

Our research as per Table 9, reveals that Lamivudine Tablets of strengths 150, 300 mg were approved for Aurobindo Pharma USA, Inc in the year 2011. Such information has to be compiled as a whole so that strength wise, dosage form wise, ingredient wise etc may act as a lead to develop as first generics or generics. It is necessary to understand that first generics are

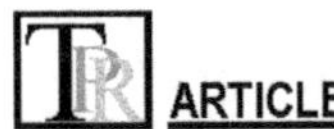 **ARTICLE**

S. No	Generic Drug Name (First Generic)	2001	2003	2008	2010	Grand Total
1	ACARBOSE TABLETS			2		2
2	ACETAMINOPHEN AND CODEINE PHOSPHATE TABLETS USP		2			2
3	ACETAMINOPHEN ASPIRIN AND CAFFEINE TABLETS RESPECTIVELY (OTC) USP	1				1
4	ACETAZOLAMIDE EXTENDED RELEASE CAPSULE			1		1
5	ADAPALENE CREAM				1	1

Table 7: USFDA Approved Products as First Generics-Ingredient/Dosage form/Year of approval

S. No	Generic Manufacturer Name	2001	2002	2003	2004	2005	2006	2007	2008	2009	2010	2011	Grand Total
1	RANBAXY LABORATORIES LIMITED		3	9	9	5	2	6	1	3	1	1	36
2	DR. REDDY'S LABORATORIES LIMITED		2			2	4	2	1	4	6	6	30
3	SUN PHARMA							3	2	5	2	2	14
4	AUROBINDO PHARMA LIMITED					2	1	1	3	3		1	12
5	GLENMARK GENERICS LIMITED						1	2		1	5	3	12
6	LUPIN LIMITED						3	2	1		2	2	12
7	ZYDUS PHARMACEUTICALS USA, INC.					2	1	2	2	2	1		10
8	ORCHID HEALTHCARE							1		2	1		4
9	TORRENT PHARMACEUTICALS									1	1	2	4
10	WOCKHARDT LIMITED					1		1		1		1	4
11	MATRIX LABORATORIES LIMITED								1	1	1		3
12	CLARIS LIFESCIENCES LIMITED								2				2
13	UNICHEM LABORATORIES LIMITED								1	1			2
14	ALEMBIC LIMITED										1		1
15	AUROBINDO PHARMA USA, INC.											1	1
16	CIPLA LIMITED									1			1
17	HETERO DRUGS LIMITED								1				1
18	MICRO LABS LIMITED										1		1
19	NATCO PHARMA LIMITED										1		1
20	SUN PHARMA GLOBAL FZE											1	1
21	SUN PHARMACEUTICAL INDUSTRIES, LTD.											1	1
	Grand Total		5	9	9	12	12	20	15	25	23	21	153

Table 8: USFDA Approved Products as First Generics-Indian Company/Year wise

similar to innovator's products where in bioequivalence studies are mandatory.

USFDA Tentative Approvals for Drug Products-Ingredient, Dosage form, Strength, Year of approval

A tentative approval at USFDA is for a drug product that has been developed for a new indication, new strength, new route of administration, new combination etc wherein, investment is necessary similar to innovator for pharmacodynamic, pharmacokinectics and have to be established separately unlike generics. Tentative approvals made by USFDA are finally approved at the right time to be released into the market. Our research Table 10, indicates tentative approvals for Abacavir sulphate was made in the year 2008, 2010, 2011, where as a tentative approval for Abacavir sulphate oral solution of strength 20 mg/ml was made in the year 2006.

USFDA Tentative Approvals for Drug Products-

S. No	Generic Drug Name	Dosage 1	Dosage 2	Dosage 3	Dosage 4	Generic Manufacturer	Brand Name	Approval Date
1	LAMIVUDINE TABLETS	150 MG	300 MG			AUROBINDO PHARMA USA, INC.	EPIVIR TABLETS	11/17/2011
2	PHENYLBUTYRATE TABLETS	500 MG				AMPLOGEN PHARMACEUTICALS, LLC	BUPHENYL TABLETS	11/18/2011
3	CARBOPLATIN INJECTION PACKAGED IN PHARMACY BULK PACKAGES	10 MG/ML	1000 MG/100 ML			ONCO THERAPIES LIMITED	PARAPLATIN INJECTION	11/23/2011
4	GUAIFENESIN EXTENDED-RELEASE TABLETS (OTC)	600 MG				PERRIGO R&D COMPANY	MUCINEX EXTENDED-RELEASE TABLETS	11/23/2011
5	ENOXAPARIN SODIUM INJECTION USP 100 MG/ML; PACKAGED IN MULTIPLE-DOSE VIALS (WITH PRESERVATIVE)	300 MG/3 ML				SANDOZ INC.	LOVENOX INJECTION	11/28/2011
6	ATORVASTATIN CALCIUM TABLETS	10 MG (BASE)	20 MG (BASE)	40 MG (BASE)	80 MG (BASE)	RANBAXY LABORATORIES LIMITED	LIPITOR TABLETS	11/30/2011
7	METHYLPHENIDATE HYDROCHLORIDE EXTENDED-RELEASE CAPSULES (LA)	20 MG	30 MG	40 MG		ACTAVIS SOUTH ATLANTIC LLC	RITALIN LA CAPSULES	12/1/2011
8	FELBAMATE ORAL SUSPENSION	600 MG/5 ML				AMNEAL PHARMACEUTICALS	FELBATOL ORAL SUSPENSION	12/16/2011
9	FENOFIBRATE TABLETS	48 MG	145 MG			LUPIN LIMITED	TRICOR TABLETS	12/23/2011
10	TRAMADOL HYDROCHLORIDE EXTENDED-RELEASE TABLETS(ONCE DAILY)	100 MG	200 MG	300 MG		SUN PHARMA GLOBAL FZE	RYZOLT TABLETS	12/30/2011

Table 9: USFDA Approved Products as First Generics-Ingredient, Strengths, Dosage form, Manufacturer, Brand Name, Approval Date

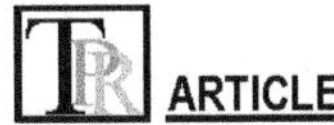

ARTICLE

Ingredient, Company Name

Our research Table 11 reveals, that six tentative approvals made for Abacavir Sulphate are for Aurobindo Pharma Limited, Cipla Limited, Invagen Pharmaceuticals Inc, Matrix Labs Ltd, Mylan Pharmaceuticals Inc. This justifies our claim made earlier.

USFDA Approved Products-Patent Use Codes

Innovator products approved through New Drug Application usually reflect to a patent that is active. Such patents reflect the invention of either API or formulation. Patents may indicate for several uses of the invention but, during market approval of a product it may be indicated for a specific use. Such product may be developed as generics/tentative for approvals.

USFDA Approved Products-Patent Expiry Dates

Especially innovator drug products approved are listed in orange book. Some of the data relating to patent details, patent expiry of such products are to be published in the orange book. The patents published have to be thoroughly observed whether they are for a product patent, process patent, new use etc. Orange book provides an indication of patents that are getting expired in United States especially for products approved by USFDA. Table 13 clearly indicates some of the patents with corresponding expiry dates for Cyclosporine approved products. It is necessary to understand that the status of patent expiry date to be monitored

S. No	Generic Drug Name	2003	2006	2007	2008	2009	2010	2011	Grand Total
1	ABACAVIR SULFATE				1		2	3	6
2	ABACAVIR SULFATE ORAL SOLUTION, 20 MG/ML		1						1
3	ABACAVIR SULFATE TABLETS, 300 MG (BASE)		2						2
4	ABACAVIR SULFATE; LAMIVUDINE				2	1	1	1	5
5	ADENOSINE			1	1		1		3
6	ADENOSINE INJECTION USP, 3 MG/ML; 20 ML AND 30 ML VIALS		1						1
7	ADENOSINE INJECTION, USP 3 MG/ML PACKAGED IN 6 MG/2 ML AND 12 MG/4 ML SINGLE-DOSE VIALS	2							2
8	ADENOSINE INJECTION, USP 3 MG/ML PACKAGED IN 6 MG/2 ML SINGLE-DOSE SYRINGES	1							1
9	ADENOSINE INJECTION, USP 3 MG/ML PACKAGED IN 6 MG/2 ML SINGLE-DOSE VIALS	1							1
10	ALBUTEROL SULFATE INHALATION SOLUTION, USP 0.042% (BASE) PACKAGED IN 1.5 MG (BASE)/3 ML UNIT-DOSE VIALS	1							1

Table 10: USFDA Tentative Approvals for Drug Products-Ingredient, dosage form, strength, year of approval

S. No	Generic Drug Name/Applicant Name	AUROBINDO PHARMA LIMITED	CIPLA LIMITED	INVAGEN PHARMACEUTICALS, INC.	MATRIX LABS LTD	MYLAN PHARMACEUTICALS, INC.	Grand Total
1	ABACAVIR SULFATE	1	2	1	1	1	6

Table 11: USFDA Tentative Approvals for Drug Products-Ingredient, Company Name

periodically.

USFDA Approved Products-Market Start, End Dates

Drug products approved by USFDA, Table 14 reveals that Ranitidine syrup was approved to market from 2011 to 2020, but at USFDA data/market exclusivity period is usually for 5 years, which means the product is also patent protected which is hindering others into the market as generic. In case of Insulin lispro, subcutaneous injection, it is a innovator's product approved as a NDA with a market start date from 1999 to 2013 indicating patent protection, data/market exclusivity.

USFDA Approved Orphan Drug Products

In United States of America, drugs approved for orphan diseases are given special benefits in terms of patent term extension, an extended market exclusivity period than usual. This is because of occurrence of the disease in a fewer population (less than 2,00,000 in United States). Such drugs products are developed by very few manufacturers. Table 15 indicates the orphan drugs approved by USFDA since 1983 and development of such products also have to be monitored for their patent, data/market exclusivity, ingredients, strengths, route of administration in similar grounds discussed earlier. There are about 399 drugs approved under the category of Orphan drugs.

USFDA Approved Products-Market Exclusivity

At USFDA, drug products are approved under different categories of market exclusivity. Table 16 reveals some of the products approved as NDAs for various categories of market exclusivity. Such market exclusivity can be compared with corresponding method of use in patents so as to establish new generic/tentative approvals.

Conclusion

Several Indian large companies are competing for release as first generics at United States market. A present day approval

U	PATENT USE CODE (SEE INDIVIDUAL REFERENCES)
U-1	PREVENTION OF PREGNANCY
U-2	TREATMENT OR PROPHYLAXIS OF ANGINA PECTORIS AND ARRHYTHMIA
U-3	TREATMENT OF HYPERTENSION
U-4	PROVIDING PREVENTION AND TREATMENT OF EMESIS AND NAUSEA IN MAMMALS
U-5	METHOD OF PRODUCING BRONCHODILATION
U-6	METHOD OF PRODUCING SYMPATHOMIMETIC EFFECTS
U-7	INCREASING CARDIAC CONTRACTILITY
U-8	ACUTE MYOCARDIAL INFARCTION
U-9	CONTROL OF EMESIS ASSOCIATED WITH ANY CANCER CHEMOTHERAPY AGENT
U-10	DIAGNOSTIC METHOD FOR DISTINGUISHING BETWEEN HYPOTHALMIC MALFUNCTIONS OR LESIONS IN HUMANS

Table 12: USFDA Patent Use Codes

S. No	Ingredient	Dosage Form/Route of Administration	Strength	Applicant	Patent Number	Patent Expiry Date
1	Cyclosporine	Solution; Oral	100Mg/ML	Novartis Pharmaceuticals Corp	5342625	30-Aug-11
2	Cyclosporine	Solution; Oral	100Mg/ML	Novartis Pharmaceuticals Corp	5741512	30-Aug-11

Table 13: USFDA Approved Products-Patent Expiry Date

S. No	COMPANY NAME	DRUG NAME	DOSAGE FORM	ROUTE OF ADMINISTRATION	MARKET START DATE	MARKET END DATE	DRUG APPLICATION TYPE
1	Sandoz Inc.	Ranitidine	SYRUP	TOPICAL	20111025	20201025	ANDA
2	Eli Lilly and Company	Insulin lispro	INJECTION, SOLUTION	SUBCUTANEOUS	19990201	20130921	NDA

Table 14: USFDA Approved Products-Market Start, End Dates

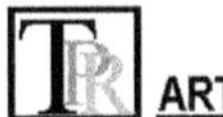 **ARTICLE**

Country Name	Approved
CANADA	5
FINLAND	1
FRANCE	2
GERMANY	3
JAPAN	1
NETHERLANDS	1
SWEDEN	1
SWITZERLAND	2
UNITED STATES	383
Grand Total	399

Table 15: Orphan Drugs Approved at USFDA for Different Countries since 1983

for a first generic reflects to well established forecast strategies co-relating the intellectual property rights, regulatory approvals, market exclusivities, demand of the product in terms of combinations, strengths, routes of administration. It is necessary to understand that companies monitor with USFDA whether any filings are made for specific combination, strengths, route of administration, dosage form so that products are developed well in hand. It is also necessary to understand that several products are filed and are in the approval process and such products are developed well in advance and are not known to public as long as the FDA approves the product. Several countries approve drug products as similars wherein generic versions have to comply to pharmacopoeial standards wavering from bioequivalence studies.

Reference

1. www.fda.gov

S. No	Ingredient	DF; Route	Trade Name	Applicant	Exclusivity	Exclusivity Date
1	TAPENTADOL HYDROCHLORIDE	TABLET, EXTENDED RELEASE; ORAL	NUCYNTA ER	JANSSEN PHARMS	NEW CHEMICAL ENTITY	20-Nov-13
2	VARDENAFIL HYDROCHLORIDE	TABLET, ORALLY DISINTEGRATING; ORAL	STAXYN	BAYER HLTHCARE	NEW DOSAGE FORM	17-Jun-13
3	AMLODIPINE BESYLATE; HYDROCHLOROTHIAZIDE; OLMESARTAN MEDOXOMIL	TABLET; ORAL	TRIBENZOR	DAIICHI SANKYO	NEW COMBINATION	23-Jul-13
4	PRAMIPEXOLE DIHYDROCHLORIDE	TABLET, EXTENDED RELEASE; ORAL	MIRAPEX ER	BOEHRINGER INGELHEIM	TREATMENT OF SIGNS AND SYMPTOMS OF ADVANCED IDIOPATHIC PARKINSON'S DISEASE	19-Mar-13
5	PALIPERIDONE PALMITATE	SUSPENSION, EXTENDED RELEASE; INTRAMUSCULAR	INVEGA SUSTENNA	JANSSEN PHARMS	PEDIATRIC EXCLUSIVITY	31-Jan-13
6	LAPATINIB DITOSYLATE	TABLET; ORAL	TYKERB	SMITHKLINE BEECHAM	FOR USE IN COMBINATION WITH LETROZOLE FOR THE TREATMENT OF POSTMENOPAUSAL WOMEN WITH HORMONE RECEPTOR POSITIVE METASTATIC BREAST CANCER THAT OVEREXPRESSES THE HER2 RECEPTOR FOR WHOM HORMONAL THERAPY IS INDICATED	29-Jan-13

Table 16: USFDA Approved Products-Market Exclusivity

ANNEXURE 23

LIST OF GLOBAL COUNTRIES AND THEIR MEMBERSHIP WITH INTERNATIONAL CONVENTIONS/TREATIES/AGREEMENTS

List of Global Countries and their Membership with International Conventions/Treaties/Agreements-as on 3rd March, 2018

S. No	Contracting Party	PCT (In Force)	S. No	Contracting Party	Paris Convention (In force)	S. No	Contracting Party	WIPO Convention (In Force)	S. No	Name of Country	WTO (In Force)	S. No	Country Name	GATT Members Up to 1994
1	Albania	October 4, 1995	1	Afghanistan	May 14, 2017	1	Afghanistan	December 13, 2005	1	Afghanistan	29 July 2016	1	Angola	April 8, 1994
2	Algeria	March 8, 2000	2	Albania	October 4, 1995	2	Albania	June 30, 1992	2	Albania	8 September 2000	2	Antigua and Barbuda	March 30, 1987
3	Angola	December 27, 2007	3	Algeria	March 1, 1966	3	Algeria	April 16, 1975	3	Angola	23 November 1996	3	Argentina	October 11, 1967
4	Antigua and Barbuda	March 17, 2000	4	Andorra	June 2, 2004	4	Andorra	October 28, 1994	4	Antigua and Barbuda	1 January 1995	4	Australia	January 1, 1948
5	Argentina		5	Angola	December 27, 2007	5	Angola	April 15, 1985	5	Argentina	1 January 1995	5	Austria	October 19, 1951
6	Armenia	December 25, 1991	6	Antigua and Barbuda	March 17, 2000	6	Antigua and Barbuda	March 17, 2000	6	Armenia	5 February 2003	6	Bahrain	December 13, 1993
7	Australia	March 31, 1980	7	Argentina	February 10, 1967	7	Argentina	October 8, 1980	7	Australia	1 January 1995	7	Bangladesh	December 16, 1972
8	Austria	April 23, 1979	8	Armenia	December 25, 1991	8	Armenia	April 22, 1993	8	Austria	1 January 1995	8	Barbados	February 15, 1967
9	Azerbaijan	December 25, 1995	9	Australia	October 10, 1925	9	Australia	August 10, 1972	9	Bahrain, Kingdom of	1 January 1995	9	Belgium	January 1, 1948
10	Bahrain	March 18, 2007	10	Austria	January 1, 1909	10	Austria	August 11, 1973	10	Bangladesh	1 January 1995	10	Belize	October 7, 1983
11	Barbados	March 12, 1985	11	Azerbaijan	December 25, 1995	11	Azerbaijan	December 25, 1995	11	Barbados	1 January 1995	11	Benin	September 12, 1963
12	Belarus	December 25, 1991	12	Bahamas	July 10, 1973	12	Bahamas	January 4, 1977	12	Belgium	1 January 1995	12	Bolivia	September 8, 1990
13	Belgium	December 14, 1981	13	Bahrain	October 29, 1997	13	Bahrain	June 22, 1995	13	Belize	1 January 1995	13	Botswana	August 28, 1987
14	Belize	June 17, 2000	14	Bangladesh	March 3, 1991	14	Bangladesh	May 11, 1985	14	Benin	22 February 1996	14	Brazil	July 30, 1948
15	Benin	February 26, 1987	15	Barbados	March 12, 1985	15	Barbados	October 5, 1979	15	Bolivia, Plurinational State of	12 September 1995	15	Brunei Darussalam	December 9, 1993
16	Bosnia and Herzegovina	September 7, 1996	16	Belarus	December 25, 1991	16	Belarus	April 26, 1970	16	Botswana	31 May 1995	16	Burkina Faso	May 3, 1963
17	Botswana	October 30, 2003	17	Belgium	July 7, 1884	17	Belgium	January 31, 1975	17	Brazil	1 January 1995	17	Burundi	March 13, 1965
18	Brazil	April 9, 1978	18	Belize	June 17, 2000	18	Belize	June 17, 2000	18	Brunei Darussalam	1 January 1995	18	Cameroon	May 3, 1963
19	Brunei Darussalam	July 24, 2012	19	Benin	January 10, 1967	19	Benin	March 9, 1975	19	Bulgaria	1 December 1996	19	Canada	January 1, 1948
20	Bulgaria	May 21, 1984	20	Bhutan	August 4, 2000	20	Bhutan	March 16, 1994	20	Burkina Faso	3 June 1995	20	Central African Republic	May 3, 1963
21	Burkina Faso	March 21, 1989	21	Bolivia (Plurinational State of)	November 4, 1993	21	Bolivia (Plurinational State of)	July 6, 1993	21	Burundi	23 July 1995	21	Chad	July 12, 1963

Table *Contd…*

22	Cambodia	December 8, 2016	22	Bosnia and Herzegovina	March 1, 1992	22	Bosnia and Herzegovina	March 1, 1992	22	Cabo Verde	23 July 2008	22	Chile	March 16, 1949
23	Cameroon	January 24, 1978	23	Botswana	April 15, 1998	23	Botswana	April 15, 1998	23	Cambodia	13 October 2004	23	Colombia	October 3, 1981
24	Canada	January 2, 1990	24	Brazil	July 7, 1884	24	Brazil	March 20, 1975	24	Cameroon	13 December 1995	24	Congo, Republic of	May 3, 1963
25	Central African Republic	January 24, 1978	25	Brunei Darussalam	February 17, 2012	25	Brunei Darussalam	April 21, 1994	25	Canada	1 January 1995	25	Costa Rica	November 24, 1990
26	Chad	January 24, 1978	26	Bulgaria	June 13, 1921	26	Bulgaria	May 19, 1970	26	Central African Republic	31 May 1995	26	Côte d'Ivoire	December 31, 1963
27	Chile	June 2, 2009	27	Burkina Faso	November 19, 1963	27	Burkina Faso	August 23, 1975	27	Chad	19 October 1996	27	Cuba	January 1, 1948
28	China	January 1, 1994	28	Burundi	September 3, 1977	28	Burundi	March 30, 1977	28	Chile	1 January 1995	28	Cyprus	July 15, 1963
29	Colombia	February 28, 2001	29	Cambodia	September 22, 1998	29	Cabo Verde	July 7, 1997	29	China	11 December 2001	29	Czech Republic	April 15, 1993
30	Comoros	April 3, 2005	30	Cameroon	May 10, 1964	30	Cambodia	July 25, 1995	30	Colombia	30 April 1995	30	Denmark	May 28, 1950
31	Congo	January 24, 1978	31	Canada	September 1, 1923	31	Cameroon	November 3, 1973	31	Congo	27 March 1997	31	Djibouti	December 16, 1994
32	Costa Rica	August 3, 1999	32	Central African Republic	November 19, 1963	32	Canada	June 26, 1970	32	Costa Rica	1 January 1995	32	Dominica	April 20, 1993
33	Croatia	July 1, 1998	33	Chad	November 19, 1963	33	Central African Republic	August 23, 1978	33	Côte d'Ivoire	1 January 1995	33	Dominican Republic	May 19, 1950
34	Cuba	July 16, 1996	34	Chile	June 14, 1991	34	Chad	September 26, 1970	34	Croatia	30 November 2000	34	Egypt	May 9, 1970
35	Cyprus	April 1, 1998	35	China	March 19, 1985	35	Chile	June 25, 1975	35	Cuba	20 April 1995	35	El Salvador	May 22, 1991
36	Czech Republic	January 1, 1993	36	Colombia	September 3, 1996	36	China	June 3, 1980	36	Cyprus	30 July 1995	36	Fiji	November 16, 1993
37	Côte d'Ivoire	April 30, 1991	37	Comoros	April 3, 2005	37	Colombia	May 4, 1980	37	Czech Republic	1 January 1995	37	Finland	May 25, 1950
38	Democratic People's Republic of Korea	July 8, 1980	38	Congo	September 2, 1963	38	Comoros	April 3, 2005	38	Democratic Republic of the Congo	1 January 1997	38	France	January 1, 1948
39	Denmark	December 1, 1978	39	Costa Rica	October 31, 1995	39	Congo	December 2, 1975	39	Denmark	1 January 1995	39	Gabon	May 3, 1963
40	Djibouti	September 23, 2016	40	Croatia	October 8, 1991	40	Cook Islands	October 27, 2016	40	Djibouti	31 May 1995	40	The Gambia	February 22, 1965
41	Dominica	August 7, 1999	41	Cuba	November 17, 1904	41	Costa Rica	June 10, 1981	41	Dominica	1 January 1995	41	Germany	October 1, 1951
42	Dominican Republic	May 28, 2007	42	Cyprus	January 17, 1966	42	Croatia	October 8, 1991	42	Dominican Republic	9 March 1995	42	Ghana	October 17, 1957

Table *Contd...*

43	Ecuador	May 7, 2001	43	Czech Republic	January 1, 1993	43	Cuba	March 27, 1975	43	Ecuador	21 January 1996	43	Greece	March 1, 1950
44	Egypt	September 6, 2003	44	Côte d'Ivoire	October 23, 1963	44	Cyprus	October 26, 1984	44	Egypt	30 June 1995	44	Grenada	February 9, 1994
45	El Salvador	August 17, 2006	45	Democratic People's Republic of Korea	June 10, 1980	45	Czech Republic	January 1, 1993	45	El Salvador	7 May 1995	45	Guatemala	October 10, 1991
46	Equatorial Guinea	July 17, 2001	46	Democratic Republic of the Congo	January 31, 1975	46	Côte d'Ivoire	May 1, 1974	46	Estonia	13 November 1999	46	Guinea	December 8, 1994
47	Estonia	August 24, 1994	47	Denmark	October 1, 1894	47	Democratic People's Republic of Korea	August 17, 1974	47	European Union (formerly EC)	1 January 1995	47	Guinea Bissau	March 17, 1994
48	Finland	October 1, 1980	48	Djibouti	May 13, 2002	48	Democratic Republic of the Congo	January 28, 1975	48	Fiji	14 January 1996	48	Guyana	July 5, 1966
49	France	February 25, 1978	49	Dominica	August 7, 1999	49	Denmark	April 26, 1970	49	Finland	1 January 1995	49	Haiti	January 1, 1950
50	Gabon	January 24, 1978	50	Dominican Republic	July 11, 1890	50	Djibouti	May 13, 2002	50	France	1 January 1995	50	Honduras	April 10, 1994
51	Gambia	December 9, 1997	51	Ecuador	June 22, 1999	51	Dominica	September 26, 1998	51	Gabon	1 January 1995	51	Hong Kong	April 23, 1986
52	Georgia	December 25, 1991	52	Egypt	July 1, 1951	52	Dominican Republic	June 27, 2000	52	Gambia	23 October 1996	52	Hungary	September 9, 1973
53	Germany	January 24, 1978	53	El Salvador	February 19, 1994	53	Ecuador	May 22, 1988	53	Georgia	14 June 2000	53	Iceland	April 21, 1968
54	Ghana	February 26, 1997	54	Equatorial Guinea	June 26, 1997	54	Egypt	April 21, 1975	54	Germany	1 January 1995	54	India	July 8, 1948
55	Greece	October 9, 1990	55	Estonia	August 24, 1994	55	El Salvador	September 18, 1979	55	Ghana	1 January 1995	55	Indonesia	February 24, 1950
56	Grenada	September 22, 1998	56	Finland	September 20, 1921	56	Equatorial Guinea	June 26, 1997	56	Greece	1 January 1995	56	Ireland	December 22, 1967
57	Guatemala	October 14, 2006	57	France	July 7, 1884	57	Eritrea	February 20, 1997	57	Grenada	22 February 1996	57	Israel	July 5, 1962
58	Guinea	May 27, 1991	58	Gabon	February 29, 1964	58	Estonia	February 5, 1994	58	Guatemala	21 July 1995	58	Italy	May 30, 1950
59	Guinea-Bissau	December 12, 1997	59	Gambia	January 21, 1992	59	Ethiopia	February 19, 1998	59	Guinea	25 October 1995	59	Jamaica	December 31, 1963
60	Holy See		60	Georgia	December 25, 1991	60	Fiji	March 11, 1972	60	Guinea-Bissau	31 May 1995	60	Japan	September 10, 1955
61	Honduras	June 20, 2006	61	Germany	May 1, 1903	61	Finland	September 8, 1970	61	Guyana	1 January 1995	61	Kenya	February 5, 1964
62	Hungary	June 27, 1980	62	Ghana	September 28, 1976	62	France	October 18, 1974	62	Haiti	30 January 1996	62	Korea, Republic of	April 14, 1967
63	Iceland	March 23, 1995	63	Greece	October 2, 1924	63	Gabon	June 6, 1975	63	Honduras	1 January 1995	63	Kuwait	May 3, 1963

Table Contd...

#	Country	Date	#	Country	Date	#	Country	Date	#	Country	Date	#	Country	Date
64	India	December 7, 1998	64	Grenada	September 22, 1998	64	Gambia	December 10, 1980	64	Hong Kong, China	1 January 1995	64	Lesotho	January 8, 1988
65	Indonesia	September 5, 1997	65	Guatemala	August 18, 1998	65	Georgia	December 25, 1991	65	Hungary	1 January 1995	65	Liechtenstein	March 29, 1994
66	Iran (Islamic Republic of)	October 4, 2013	66	Guinea	February 5, 1982	66	Germany	September 19, 1970	66	Iceland	1 January 1995	66	Luxembourg	January 1, 1948
67	Ireland	August 1, 1992	67	Guinea-Bissau	June 28, 1988	67	Ghana	June 12, 1976	67	India	1 January 1995	67	Macao	January 11, 1991
68	Israel	June 1, 1996	68	Guyana	October 25, 1994	68	Greece	March 4, 1976	68	Indonesia	1 January 1995	68	Madagascar	September 30, 1963
69	Italy	March 28, 1985	69	Haiti	July 1, 1958	69	Grenada	September 22, 1998	69	Ireland	1 January 1995	69	Malawi	August 28, 1964
70	Japan	October 1, 1978	70	Holy See	September 29, 1960	70	Guatemala	April 30, 1983	70	Israel	21 April 1995	70	Malaysia	October 24, 1957
71	Jordan	June 9, 2017	71	Honduras	February 4, 1994	71	Guinea	November 13, 1980	71	Italy	1 January 1995	71	Maldives	April 19, 1983
72	Kazakhstan	December 25, 1991	72	Hungary	January 1, 1909	72	Guinea-Bissau	June 28, 1988	72	Jamaica	9 March 1995	72	Mali	January 11, 1993
73	Kenya	June 8, 1994	73	Iceland	May 5, 1962	73	Guyana	October 25, 1994	73	Japan	1 January 1995	73	Malta	November 17, 1964
74	Kuwait	September 9, 2016	74	India	December 7, 1998	74	Haiti	November 2, 1983	74	Jordan	11 April 2000	74	Mauritania	September 30, 1963
75	Kyrgyzstan	December 25, 1991	75	Indonesia	December 24, 1950	75	Holy See	April 20, 1975	75	Kazakhstan	30 November 2015	75	Mauritius	September 2, 1970
76	Lao People's Democratic Republic	June 14, 2006	76	Iran (Islamic Republic of)	December 16, 1959	76	Honduras	November 15, 1983	76	Kenya	1 January 1995	76	Mexico	August 24, 1986
77	Latvia	September 7, 1993	77	Iraq	January 24, 1976	77	Hungary	April 26, 1970	77	Korea, Republic of	1 January 1995	77	Morocco	June 17, 1987
78	Lesotho	October 21, 1995	78	Ireland	December 4, 1925	78	Iceland	September 13, 1986	78	Kuwait, the State of	1 January 1995	78	Mozambique	July 27, 1992
79	Liberia	August 27, 1994	79	Israel	March 24, 1950	79	India	May 1, 1975	79	Kyrgyz Republic	20 December 1998	79	Myanmar, Union of	July 29, 1948
80	Libya	September 15, 2005	80	Italy	July 7, 1884	80	Indonesia	December 18, 1979	80	Lao People's Democratic Republic	2 February 2013	80	Namibia	September 15, 1992
81	Liechtenstein	March 19, 1980	81	Jamaica	December 24, 1999	81	Iran (Islamic Republic of)	March 14, 2002	81	Latvia	10 February 1999	81	Netherlands	January 1, 1948
82	Lithuania	July 5, 1994	82	Japan	July 15, 1899	82	Iraq	January 21, 1976	82	Lesotho	31 May 1995	82	New Zealand	July 30, 1948
83	Luxembourg	April 30, 1978	83	Jordan	July 17, 1972	83	Ireland	April 26, 1970	83	Liberia	14 July 2016	83	Nicaragua	May 28, 1950
84	Madagascar	January 24, 1978	84	Kazakhstan	December 25, 1991	84	Israel	April 26, 1970	84	Liechtenstein	1 September 1995	84	Niger	December 31, 1963
85	Malawi	January 24, 1978	85	Kenya	June 14, 1965	85	Italy	April 20, 1977	85	Lithuania	31 May 2001	85	Nigeria	November 18, 1960
86	Malaysia	August 16, 2006	86	Kuwait	December 2, 2014	86	Jamaica	December 25, 1978	86	Luxembourg	1 January 1995	86	Norway	July 10, 1948
87	Mali	October 19, 1984	87	Kyrgyzstan	December 25, 1991	87	Japan	April 20, 1975	87	Macao, China	1 January 1995	87	Pakistan	July 30, 1948

Table *Contd…*

88	Malta	March 1, 2007	88	Lao People's Democratic Republic	October 8, 1998	88	Jordan	July 12, 1972	88	Madagascar	17 November 1995	88	Papua New Guinea	December 16, 1994
89	Mauritania	April 13, 1983	89	Latvia	September 7, 1993	89	Kazakhstan	December 25, 1991	89	Malawi	31 May 1995	89	Paraguay	January 6, 1994
90	Mexico	January 1, 1995	90	Lebanon	September 1, 1924	90	Kenya	October 5, 1971	90	Malaysia	1 January 1995	90	Peru	October 7, 1951
91	Monaco	June 22, 1979	91	Lesotho	September 28, 1989	91	Kiribati	July 19, 2013	91	Maldives	31 May 1995	91	Philippines	December 27, 1979
92	Mongolia	May 27, 1991	92	Liberia	August 27, 1994	92	Kuwait	July 14, 1998	92	Mali	31 May 1995	92	Poland	October 18, 1967
93	Montenegro	June 3, 2006	93	Libya	September 28, 1976	93	Kyrgyzstan	December 25, 1991	93	Malta	1 January 1995	93	Portugal	May 6, 1962
94	Morocco	October 8, 1999	94	Liechtenstein	July 14, 1933	94	Lao People's Democratic Republic	January 17, 1995	94	Mauritania	31 May 1995	94	Qatar	April 7, 1994
95	Mozambique	May 18, 2000	95	Lithuania	May 22, 1994	95	Latvia	January 21, 1993	95	Mauritius	1 January 1995	95	Romania	November 14, 1971
96	Namibia	January 1, 2004	96	Luxembourg	June 30, 1922	96	Lebanon	December 30, 1986	96	Mexico	1 January 1995	96	Rwanda	January 1, 1966
97	Netherlands	July 10, 1979	97	Madagascar	December 21, 1963	97	Lesotho	November 18, 1986	97	Moldova, Republic of	26 July 2001	97	Senegal	September 27, 1963
98	New Zealand	December 1, 1992	98	Malawi	July 6, 1964	98	Liberia	March 8, 1989	98	Mongolia	29 January 1997	98	Sierra Leone	May 19, 1961
99	Nicaragua	March 6, 2003	99	Malaysia	January 1, 1989	99	Libya	September 28, 1976	99	Montenegro	29 April 2012	99	Singapore	August 20, 1973
100	Niger	March 21, 1993	100	Mali	March 1, 1983	100	Liechtenstein	May 21, 1972	100	Morocco	1 January 1995	100	Slovak Republic	April 15, 1993
101	Nigeria	May 8, 2005	101	Malta	October 20, 1967	101	Lithuania	April 30, 1992	101	Mozambique	26 August 1995	101	Slovenia	October 30, 1994
102	Norway	January 1, 1980	102	Mauritania	April 11, 1965	102	Luxembourg	March 19, 1975	102	Myanmar	1 January 1995	102	Solomon Islands	December 28, 1994
103	Oman	October 26, 2001	103	Mauritius	September 24, 1976	103	Madagascar	December 22, 1989	103	Namibia	1 January 1995	103	South Africa	June 13, 1948
104	Panama	September 7, 2012	104	Mexico	September 7, 1903	104	Malawi	June 11, 1970	104	Nepal	23 April 2004	104	Spain	August 29, 1963
105	Papua New Guinea	June 14, 2003	105	Monaco	April 29, 1956	105	Malaysia	January 1, 1989	105	Netherlands	1 January 1995	105	Sri Lanka	July 29, 1948
106	Peru	June 6, 2009	106	Mongolia	April 21, 1985	106	Maldives	May 12, 2004	106	New Zealand	1 January 1995	106	Saint Kitts and Nevis	March 24, 1994
107	Philippines	August 17, 2001	107	Montenegro	June 3, 2006	107	Mali	August 14, 1982	107	Nicaragua	3 September 1995	107	Saint Lucia	April 13, 1993
108	Poland	December 25, 1990	108	Morocco	July 30, 1917	108	Malta	December 7, 1977	108	Niger	13 December 1996	108	Saint Vincent and the Grenadines	May 18, 1993
109	Portugal	November 24, 1992	109	Mozambique	July 9, 1998	109	Marshall Islands	December 11, 2017	109	Nigeria	1 January 1995	109	Suriname	March 22, 1978
110	Qatar	August 3, 2011	110	Namibia	January 1, 2004	110	Mauritania	September 17, 1976	110	Norway	1 January 1995	110	Swaziland, Kingdom of	February 8, 1993

Table Contd...

No.	Country	Date	No.	Country	Date	No.	Country	Date	No.	Country	Date	No.	Country	Date
111	Republic of Korea	August 10, 1984	111	Nepal	June 22, 2001	111	Mauritius	September 21, 1976	111	Oman	9 November 2000	111	Sweden	April 30, 1950
112	Republic of Moldova	December 25, 1991	112	Netherlands	July 7, 1884	112	Mexico	June 14, 1975	112	Pakistan	1 January 1995	112	Switzerland	August 1, 1966
113	Romania	July 23, 1979	113	New Zealand	July 29, 1931	113	Monaco	March 3, 1975	113	Panama	6 September 1997	113	Tanzania	December 9, 1961
114	Russian Federation	March 29, 1978	114	Nicaragua	July 3, 1996	114	Mongolia	February 28, 1979	114	Papua New Guinea	9 June 1996	114	Thailand	November 20, 1982
115	Rwanda	August 31, 2011	115	Niger	July 5, 1964	115	Montenegro	June 3, 2006	115	Paraguay	1 January 1995	115	Togo	March 20, 1964
116	Saint Kitts and Nevis	October 27, 2005	116	Nigeria	September 2, 1963	116	Morocco	July 27, 1971	116	Peru	1 January 1995	116	Trinidad and Tobago	October 23, 1962
117	Saint Lucia	August 30, 1996	117	Norway	July 1, 1885	117	Mozambique	December 23, 1996	117	Philippines	1 January 1995	117	Tunisia	August 29, 1990
118	Saint Vincent and the Grenadines	August 6, 2002	118	Oman	July 14, 1999	118	Myanmar	May 15, 2001	118	Poland	1 July 1995	118	Turkey	October 17, 1951
119	San Marino	December 14, 2004	119	Pakistan	July 22, 2004	119	Namibia	December 23, 1991	119	Portugal	1 January 1995	119	Uganda	October 23, 1962
120	Sao Tome and Principe	July 3, 2008	120	Panama	October 19, 1996	120	Nepal	February 4, 1997	120	Qatar	13 January 1996	120	United Arab Emirates	March 8, 1994
121	Saudi Arabia	August 3, 2013	121	Papua New Guinea	June 15, 1999	121	Netherlands	January 9, 1975	121	Romania	1 January 1995	121	United Kingdom	January 1, 1948
122	Senegal	January 24, 1978	122	Paraguay	May 28, 1994	122	New Zealand	June 20, 1984	122	Russian Federation	22 August 2012	122	United States of America	January 1, 1948
123	Serbia	February 1, 1997	123	Peru	April 11, 1995	123	Nicaragua	May 5, 1985	123	Rwanda	22 May 1996	123	Uruguay	December 6, 1953
124	Seychelles	November 7, 2002	124	Philippines	September 27, 1965	124	Niger	May 18, 1975	124	Saint Kitts and Nevis	21 February 1996	124	Venezuela	August 31, 1990
125	Sierra Leone	June 17, 1997	125	Poland	November 10, 1919	125	Nigeria	April 9, 1995	125	Saint Lucia	1 January 1995	125	Yugoslavia	August 25, 1966
126	Singapore	February 23, 1995	126	Portugal	July 7, 1884	126	Niue	January 8, 2015	126	Saint Vincent and the Grenadines	1 January 1995	126	Zaire	September 11, 1971
127	Slovakia	January 1, 1993	127	Qatar	July 5, 2000	127	Norway	June 8, 1974	127	Samoa	10 May 2012	127	Zambia	February 10, 1982
128	Slovenia	March 1, 1994	128	Republic of Korea	May 4, 1980	128	Oman	February 19, 1997	128	Saudi Arabia, Kingdom of	11 December 2005	128	Zimbabwe	July 11, 1948
129	South Africa	March 16, 1999	129	Republic of Moldova	December 25, 1991	129	Pakistan	January 6, 1977	129	Senegal	1 January 1995			
130	Spain	November 16, 1989	130	Romania	October 6, 1920	130	Panama	September 17, 1983	130	Seychelles	26 April 2015			
131	Sri Lanka	February 26, 1982	131	Russian Federation	July 1, 1965	131	Papua New Guinea	July 10, 1997	131	Sierra Leone	23 July 1995			
132	Sudan	April 16, 1984	132	Rwanda	March 1, 1984	132	Paraguay	June 20, 1987	132	Singapore	1 January 1995			

Table Contd...

No.	Country	Date	No.	Country	Date	No.	Country	Date	No.	Country	Date
133	Swaziland	September 20, 1994	133	Saint Kitts and Nevis	April 9, 1995	133	Peru	September 4, 1980	133	Slovak Republic	1 January 1995
134	Sweden	May 17, 1978	134	Saint Lucia	June 9, 1995	134	Philippines	July 14, 1980	134	Slovenia	30 July 1995
135	Switzerland	January 24, 1978	135	Saint Vincent and the Grenadines	August 29, 1995	135	Poland	March 23, 1975	135	Solomon Islands	26 July 1996
136	Syrian Arab Republic	June 26, 2003	136	Samoa	September 21, 2013	136	Portugal	April 27, 1975	136	South Africa	1 January 1995
137	Tajikistan	December 25, 1991	137	San Marino	March 4, 1960	137	Qatar	September 3, 1976	137	Spain	1 January 1995
138	Thailand	December 24, 2009	138	Sao Tome and Principe	May 12, 1998	138	Republic of Korea	March 1, 1979	138	Sri Lanka	1 January 1995
139	Togo	January 24, 1978	139	Saudi Arabia	March 11, 2004	139	Republic of Moldova	December 25, 1991	139	Suriname	1 January 1995
140	Trinidad and Tobago	March 10, 1994	140	Senegal	December 21, 1963	140	Romania	April 26, 1970	140	Swaziland	1 January 1995
141	Tunisia	December 10, 2001	141	Serbia	April 27, 1992	141	Russian Federation	April 26, 1970	141	Sweden	1 January 1995
142	Turkey	January 1, 1996	142	Seychelles	November 7, 2002	142	Rwanda	February 3, 1984	142	Switzerland	1 July 1995
143	Turkmenistan	December 25, 1991	143	Sierra Leone	June 17, 1997	143	Saint Kitts and Nevis	November 16, 1995	143	Chinese Taipei	1 January 2002
144	Uganda	February 9, 1995	144	Singapore	February 23, 1995	144	Saint Lucia	August 21, 1993	144	Tajikistan	2 March 2013
145	Ukraine	December 25, 1991	145	Slovakia	January 1, 1993	145	Saint Vincent and the Grenadines	August 29, 1995	145	Tanzania	1 January 1995
146	United Arab Emirates	March 10, 1999	146	Slovenia	June 25, 1991	146	Samoa	October 11, 1997	146	Thailand	1 January 1995
147	United Kingdom	January 24, 1978	147	South Africa	December 1, 1947	147	San Marino	June 26, 1991	147	The former Yugoslav Republic of Macedonia	4 April 2003
148	United Republic of Tanzania	September 14, 1999	148	Spain	July 7, 1884	148	Sao Tome and Principe	May 12, 1998	148	Togo	31 May 1995
149	United States of America	January 24, 1978	149	Sri Lanka	December 29, 1952	149	Saudi Arabia	May 22, 1982	149	Tonga	27 July 2007
150	Uzbekistan	December 25, 1991	150	Sudan	April 16, 1984	150	Senegal	April 26, 1970	150	Trinidad and Tobago	1 March 1995
151	Viet Nam	March 10, 1993	151	Suriname	November 25, 1975	151	Serbia	April 27, 1992	151	Tunisia	29 March 1995

Table Contd…

152	Zambia	November 15, 2001	152	Swaziland	May 12, 1991	152	Seychelles	March 16, 2000	152	Turkey	26 March 1995
153	Zimbabwe	June 11, 1997	153	Sweden	July 1, 1885	153	Sierra Leone	May 18, 1986	153	Uganda	1 January 1995
154	the former Yugoslav Republic of Macedonia	August 10, 1995	154	Switzerland	July 7, 1884	154	Singapore	December 10, 1990	154	Ukraine	16 May 2008
			155	Syrian Arab Republic	September 1, 1924	155	Slovakia	January 1, 1993	155	United Arab Emirates	10 April 1996
			156	Tajikistan	December 25, 1991	156	Slovenia	June 25, 1991	156	United Kingdom	1 January 1995
			157	Thailand	August 2, 2008	157	Somalia	November 18, 1982	157	United States	1 January 1995
			158	Togo	September 10, 1967	158	South Africa	March 23, 1975	158	Uruguay	1 January 1995
			159	Tonga	June 14, 2001	159	Spain	April 26, 1970	159	Vanuatu	24 August 2012
			160	Trinidad and Tobago	August 1, 1964	160	Sri Lanka	September 20, 1978	160	Venezuela, Bolivarian Republic of	1 January 1995
			161	Tunisia	July 7, 1884	161	Sudan	February 15, 1974	161	Viet Nam	11 January 2007
			162	Turkey	October 10, 1925	162	Suriname	November 25, 1975	162	Yemen	26 June 2014
			163	Turkmenistan	December 25, 1991	163	Swaziland	August 18, 1988	163	Zambia	1 January 1995
			164	Uganda	June 14, 1965	164	Sweden	April 26, 1970	164	Zimbabwe	5 March 1995
			165	Ukraine	December 25, 1991	165	Switzerland	April 26, 1970			
			166	United Arab Emirates	September 19, 1996	166	Syrian Arab Republic	November 18, 2004			
			167	United Kingdom	July 7, 1884	167	Tajikistan	December 25, 1991			
			168	United Republic of Tanzania	June 16, 1963	168	Thailand	December 25, 1989			
			169	United States of America	May 30, 1887	169	Timor-Leste	December 12, 2017			
			170	Uruguay	March 18, 1967	170	Togo	April 28, 1975			
			171	Uzbekistan	December 25, 1991	171	Tonga	June 14, 2001			
			172	Venezuela (Bolivarian Republic of)	September 12, 1995	172	Trinidad and Tobago	August 16, 1988			

Table *Contd...*

492

173	Viet Nam	March 8, 1949	173	Tunisia	November 28, 1975
174	Yemen	February 15, 2007	174	Turkey	May 12, 1976
175	Zambia	April 6, 1965	175	Turkmenistan	December 25, 1991
176	Zimbabwe	April 18, 1980	176	Tuvalu	June 4, 2014
177	the former Yugoslav Republic of Macedonia	September 8, 1991	177	Uganda	October 18, 1973
			178	Ukraine	April 26, 1970
			179	United Arab Emirates	September 24, 1974
			180	United Kingdom	April 26, 1970
			181	United Republic of Tanzania	December 30, 1983
			182	United States of America	August 25, 1970
			183	Uruguay	December 21, 1979
			184	Uzbekistan	December 25, 1991
			185	Vanuatu	March 2, 2012
			186	Venezuela (Bolivarian Republic of)	November 23, 1984
			187	Viet Nam	July 2, 1976
			188	Yemen	March 29, 1979
			189	Zambia	May 14, 1977
			190	Zimbabwe	December 29, 1981
			191	the former Yugoslav Republic of Macedonia	September 8, 1991

ANNEXURE 24

LIST OF INDIAN ORGANISATIONS ACTIVE IN PATENTING PHARMACEUTICAL TECHNOLOGIES (INDICATIVE)

S. No	Name of Company/Institute
1	Advanced Enzymes Technologies Limited
2	Ajanta Pharma Limited
3	Alembic Limited
4	Alkem Laboratories Limited
5	Amoli Organics Private Limited
6	Apex Laboratories Private Limited
7	Arjuna Natural Extracts
8	Astron Research Limited
9	Aurobindo Pharma Limited
10	Bharat Biotech International Limited
11	Bharat Serums and Vaccines Limited
12	Biocon India Limited
13	Bombay Drugs and Pharmaceuticals Limited
14	Cadila Pharmaceuticals Ltd
15	Cipla Limited
16	Council of Scientific and Industrial Research
17	Dabur India Limited
18	Dabur Pharma Limited
19	Dabur Research Foundation
20	Department of Biotechnology, Government of India
21	Department of Science and Technology, Government of India
22	Divi's Laboratories Limited
23	DR. Reddy's Research Foundation
24	Emcure Pharmaceuticals Limited
25	FDC Limited
26	Fermenta Biotech Limited
27	Genesen Labs Limited
28	Glenmark Generics Ltd
29	Glenmark Pharmaceuticals Limited
30	Green Chem
31	Hetero Drugs Limited
32	Hetero Research Foundation
33	Himalaya Global Holding Limited
34	Ideal Cures Private Limited
35	Ind Swift Laboratories Limited

S. No	Name of Company/Institute
36	Indian Institute of Science
37	Indian Institute of Technology
38	Indoco Remedies Limited
39	IPCA Laboratories Limited
40	Jagat Pharma
41	JB Chemicals and Pharmaceuticals Limited
42	Jubilant Organosys Limited
43	Laila Impex
44	Laila Nutraceuticals
45	Lupin Limited
46	Macleods Pharmaceuticals Limited
47	Matrix Laboratories Limited
48	Megafine Pharma Private Limited
49	Mercury Laboratories Limited
50	Morepen Laboratories Limited
51	MSN Laboratories Limited
52	Mylan Laboratories Limited
53	Name of Company/Institute
54	Natco Pharma Limited
55	National Institute of Pharmaceutical Education (NIPER)
56	Nicholas Piramal India Limited
57	Nisarga Biotech Private Limited
58	Omniactive Health Technologies Limited
59	Orchid Chemicals and Pharmaceuticals Limited
60	Padmavati Pharmaceuticals
61	Panacea Biotech Limited
62	Piramal Enterprises Limited
63	Piramal Healthcare Limited
64	Piramal Life Sciences Limited
65	Poly Medicure Limited
66	Ranbaxy Laboratories Limited
67	Reliance Industries Limited
68	Reliance Life Sciences Private Limited
69	Rubicon Research Private Limited
70	Sami Labs Limited

Annexure 24 Contd...

S. No	Name of Company/Institute
71	Sentiss Pharma Private Limited
72	Shasun Pharmaceuticals Limited
73	Shilpa Medicare Limited
74	Sun Pharma Advanced Research Company Limited
75	Sun Pharmaceutical Industries Ltd
76	Suven Life Sciences Limited
77	Symed Labs Limited
78	Torrent Pharmaceuticals Ltd
79	Unichem Laboratories Limited
80	USV Limited
81	Venus Remedies Limited
82	Wockhardt Limited
83	Zydus Cadila Healthcare Limited

ANNEXURE 25

CGPDTM ORGANISATION STRUCTURE

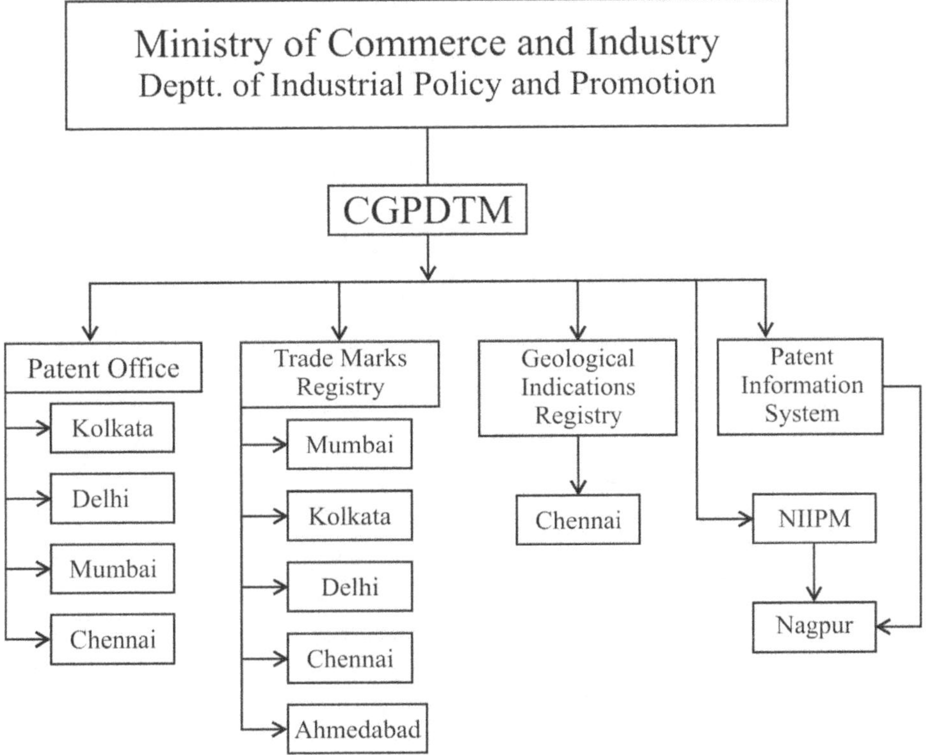

Ministry of Commerce and Industry
Deptt. of Industrial Policy and Promotion
CGPDTM
Patent Office
Kolkata
Delhi
Mumbai
Chennai
Trade Marks Registry
Mumbai
Kolkata
Delhi
Chennai
Ahmedabad
Geological Indications Registry
Chennai
Patent Information System
NIIPM
Nagpur